MATERNAL-INFANT
CARE PLANNING

Third Edition

Kathryn A. Melson, RN, MSN
Marie S. Jaffe, RN, MS (deceased)
Carole Kenner, RN,C, DNS, FAAN
Stephanie Amlung, RN, PhD

Springhouse Corporation
Springhouse, Pennsylvania

Staff

Vice President
Matthew Cahill

Clinical Director
Judith Schilling McCann, RN, MSN

Art Director
John Hubbard

Managing Editor
David Moreau

Clinical Consultant
Patricia Kardish Fischer, RN, BSN

Editors
Karen Diamond, Margaret MacKay Eckman

Copy Editors
Cynthia C. Breuninger (manager), Barbara Hodgson,
Brenna H. Mayer, Pamela Wingrod

Designers
Arlene Putterman (associate art director), Mary
Ludwicki

Manufacturing
Deborah Meiris (director), Patricia K. Dorshaw (manager), Otto Mezei (book production manager)

Editorial Assistants
Beverly Lane, Marcia Mills, Liz Schaeffer

Indexer
Judith Schaeffer Young

The clinical procedures described and recommended in this publication are based on research and consultation with nursing, medical, and legal authorities. To the best of our knowledge, these procedures reflect currently accepted practice; nevertheless, they cannot be considered absolute and universal recommendations. For individual application, all recommendations must be considered in light of the patient's clinical condition and, before administration of new or infrequently used drugs, in light of the latest package-insert information. The author and the publisher disclaim responsibility for any adverse effects resulting directly or indirectly from the suggested procedures, from any undetected errors, or from the reader's misunderstanding of the text.

Printed in the United States of America.

MICP3-011198

A member of the Reed Elsevier plc group

Library of Congress Cataloging-in-Publication Data

Maternal-infant care planning/Kathryn A. Melson... [et al.]. — 3rd ed.
      p. cm.
  Includes bibliographical references and index.
  1. Maternity nursing. 2. Infants (newborn)—Diseases—Nursing. 3. Nursing care plans. I. Melson, Kathryn A. II. Melson, Kathryn A.
  [DNLM: 1. Maternal-Child Nursing. 2. Patient Care Planning.
WY157.3M4255 1999]
RG951.J341999
6100.73'678—dc21

DNLM/DLC   98-36726
ISBN 0-87434-951-6 (alk. paper)   CIP

Contents

Appendices, references, and index

Clinical consultants

Cynthia Chatham,
RN,C, DSN
Associate Professor
University of Southern Mississippi
Long Beach

Lynne H. Conrad,
RN,C, MSN, MHA
Patient Progressions Coordinator
Albert Einstein Healthcare Network
Philadelphia

Nancy Donoho,
RN,C, MSN
Maternal-Infant Clinical Nurse Specialist
Covenant Health
Knoxville, Tenn.

Sheila H. Stewart,
RN, MSN, CRNP
Nursing Instructor
Alvernia College
Family Nurse Practitioner
Amanda Stout Family Health Center
Reading, Pa.

Acknowledgments

The authors wish to thank the following individuals whose contributions to the preparation of this book have been invaluable:

Leslie Altimier, RN,C, MSN
Manager of Neonatal Services, Tri-Health, Good Samaritan Hospital, Cincinnati

Sister Sharon Becker, RN, MSN, CNM
Director, Healthy Beginnings–New Avenues, Apple Valley, Calif.

Libby Bragg, RN, PhDc
Perinatal Clinical Nurse Specialist, Health Alliance, Cincinnati

Susan Johnson, RN,C, PhD
Assistant Professor, Mount St. Joseph College, Cincinnati

Denise Lucas, RN,C, MSN
Perinatal Clinical Nurse Specialist, TriHealth, Bethesda North Hospital, Cincinnati

Kathleen Murray, RNC, MSN,
Minot (N.D.) Air Force Base

Carolyn H. Routledge Simmons, RN, MSN, CNM
Director, Nurse-Midwifery Program, Texas Tech University Health Science Center at El Paso

Margaret T. Steinbach, RN, RN,C, MSN
Mountain Regional Neonatal Practitioner Leader, Pediatrix, Medical Group, El Paso, Tex.

Tina Weitkamp, RN,C, MSN
Associate Professor of Clinical Nursing, University of Cincinnati

Preface

These plans of care are designed to serve as a tool to guide nurses in providing safe and effective perinatal and infant care.

The maternal section of this book covers antepartum, intrapartum, and postpartum care; the infant section covers preterm and full-term conditions, with care provided in the newborn nursery or neonatal intensive care nursery. These sections address normal and common abnormal conditions.

Each plan uses these organizational headings:
- definition of the condition and the focus of the plan
- etiology and precipitating factors — causes or predisposing or contributing factors — that place the mother or infant at risk
- physical findings organized by body system; in the maternal plans, the findings begin in the signs and symptoms; in the infant plans, the findings include maternal history, infant status at birth, and signs and symptoms
- diagnostic studies that assist in formulating nursing diagnoses
- nursing diagnoses and collaborative problems that focus primarily on nursing functions but include independent and interdependent actions; the former are exclusive to nursing, whereas the latter are nursing and medically oriented
- expected outcomes — measurable statements of expectations for the patient based on the nursing diagnoses
- interventions and rationales that give specific patient or nurse activities with appropriate physiologic or descriptive explanations for their use
- additional individualized interventions to provide for specific patient interventions related to aspects of care not included in the plan
- associated plans and appendices that cross-reference to other plans and to the appendices and related resources
- additional nursing diagnoses to identify other problems that may need to be addressed and integrated into the care
- documentation checklists, new to this edition, to encourage appropriate charting for quality assurance and improvement of care in health care settings; any family teaching should be culturally sensitive, and the nurse should note on the chart that such teaching has included this aspect of care.

In most health care settings, the quality improvement program includes the use of clinical pathways (sometimes called care maps). These pathways provide managed care groups with milestones for progress toward discharge or termination of treatment. They reflect a multidisciplinary team approach to care, with progress based on expected outcomes. Selected pathways currently being used in the United States have been included in this text. Because they were created for use in a specific institution, they may vary somewhat from the general guidelines found in the care plans. The pathways are meant only to serve as samples; they can be adapted to meet the specific needs of a given institution.

Nursing diagnoses are derived from the North American Nursing Diagnosis Association (NANDA) system of classification. (See appendix A for NANDA-approved diagnoses.) Collaborative problems are included and may or may not reflect the approved NANDA statements.

Although the guidelines for nursing interventions are specific, they serve only as guidelines for care and do not override or replace safe alternatives based on patient condition or profile, doctor's order, drug information inserts, agency policy or protocol, position papers, or official standards of care. All plans must be adapted to the population being served and must be culturally sensitive to and considerate of the specialized needs of the disadvantaged population.

In this book, the term *parents* is used to signify two parents, a single parent, or a guardian.

Part 1

Antepartum

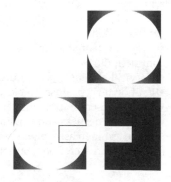

Normal antepartum

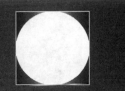

Definition
The antepartum or prenatal period of pregnancy begins with the fertilization of the ovum and ends before the onset of labor. Pregnancy imposes marked anatomic, physiologic, and biochemical changes on the woman. The nurse must recognize these normal adaptations and differentiate them from any deviations. This plan of care focuses on identifying the pregnant patient, promoting health measures to ensure good maternal and fetal outcomes, and preventing and recognizing the discomforts associated with pregnancy.

Etiology and precipitating factors
Conjoining of an ovum and sperm results in fertilization; ovulatory function is one of the requisites and, without contraception, an 85% pregnancy rate will occur within 1 year.

Physical findings
Cardiovascular
• Arterial blood pressure essentially unchanged from baseline values; slight decrease in diastolic pressure during second trimester
• Resting pulse increased by 10 to 20 beats/minute
• Shift of apex and apical pulse (point of maximal intensity) upward and ⅜″ to ⅝″ (1 to 1.5 cm) left, depending on degree of uterine displacement; usually heard in fourth rather than fifth intercostal space; electrocardiogram (ECG) shows displacement along with increased size of cardiac silhouette
• S_1 — exaggerated splitting and loudness
• Physiologic S_3
• Systolic murmurs that intensify with respiratory activity (common); soft, diastolic, or continuous murmurs (less common)
• Fatigue
Genitourinary
• Amenorrhea
• Progressive uterine enlargement, with an ultimate 500- to 1,000-fold increase in capacity and eventual dextroversion
• Irregular, painless uterine contractions (Braxton Hicks contractions)
• Cervical softening with bluish discoloration
• Leukorrhea (profuse, thick, white vaginal discharge)
• Vaginal discoloration and lengthening
• Breast tenderness and tingling; enlargement and nodularity; increased pigmentation of nipple and areola; colostrum secretion near term

• Presence of fetal heart tones (FHT), uterine souffle, and funic or umbilical souffle
• Quickening
Integumentary
• Chloasma (mask of pregnancy)
• Linea nigra from top of fundus to symphysis pubis
• Striae gravidarum (stretch marks)
• Vascular spiders (nevi)
• Palmar erythema
• Epulis; bleeding gums
Musculoskeletal
• Progressive lordosis
• Waddle gait
• Integrity of teeth unchanged
• Backache
• Quickening
Renal
• Glycosuria
• Increase in glomerular filtration rate of 30% to 50%
• Increase in renal plasma flow of 30%
• Urinary frequency in first and third trimesters
Gastrointestinal
• Morning sickness
• Decreased hydrochloric acid
• Decreased peristalsis
• Delayed gastric emptying
• Increased appetite
Respiratory
• Respiratory rate essentially unchanged; depth increased
• Shortness of breath near term
• Thoracic breathing pattern as pregnancy progresses
• Flaring of rib cage and elevated diaphragm as pregnancy progresses
• Nasal congestion, occasional epistaxis

Diagnostic studies
• Accurate and complete history and physical examination may render a diagnosis of presumptive, probable, or positive pregnancy.
• Radioimmunoassay reveals human chorionic gonadotropin in maternal plasma or urine.

NURSING DIAGNOSIS

Anxiety related to anatomic and physiologic changes associated with pregnancy

Expected outcomes

The patient will express minimal anxiety as evidenced by verbalization of well-being, coping, and a positive attitude.

Interventions

1. Introduce yourself to the patient. Refer to her as Ms. if marital status is unknown.

2. Be nonjudgmental. If pregnancy is likely, do not assume it is welcome.

3. Assess progression through psychological tasks of pregnancy.

4. Assess teaching receptivity. Note presence of partner, family, and friends and allow them to stay with the patient before and after examination, according to the patient's wishes.

5. Note and document signs and symptoms that suggest past or present sexual or physical abuse:
• bruising anywhere on body
• frequent unexplained or implausible accidents, falls, burns, or fractures; scarring from past incidents
• course of past pregnancies; incidence of spontaneous abortion
• marked resistance to disrobing or undergoing physical examinations and invasive procedures
• ambivalence toward authority figures
• aversion to either all male or all female caregivers
• controlling behaviors regarding all aspects of care
• inability to sleep; nightmares.

6. Additional individualized interventions: _____

Rationales

1. Establishment of good rapport is essential to a trusting relationship. By assuming the patient is married, the nurse implies a personal value that may be destructive to the nurse-patient relationship.

2. Reactions to pregnancy vary among prospective mothers and depend on age, parity, marital status, health, financial status, education, culture, ethnic background, and desire for children. Emotional responses to pregnancy may include disbelief, joy, fear, ambivalence, a sense of being intruded on, egocentrism, introversion, emotional lability, change in decision-making patterns, change in self-image, and altered sexual desires.

3. Tasks include accepting the pregnancy; working through past experiences, expectations, and conflicts related to pregnancy and parenting; working through age-related developmental tasks; and preparing for the practical aspects of parenthood. Progression through tasks may indicate acceptance of pregnancy and readiness for motherhood.

4. Health awareness and teaching help prevent or minimize deviations from normal and increase patient compliance. Health teaching increases maternal and fetal well-being. Partner, family, and friends may reinforce health care information presented.

5. Evidence of current abuse warrants referral to appropriate social and psychological services for crisis intervention. Police action might be indicated. Pregnancy may trigger suppressed memories of sexual abuse. Confusion about trust, control, authority, self-image, boundary setting, and sexuality is typical. Caregivers must recognize the patient's needs, include her in the decision-making process, and allow her to control and direct as much of her care as possible.

6. Rationales: _____

Evidence of pregnancy

The following chart highlights presumptive, probable, and positive signs of pregnancy. Indications can also be categorized as subjective or objective.

Presumptive	Probable	Positive
• Amenorrhea • Increased breast size; nodularity; tenderness and tingling; colostrum secretion; increased pigmentation of nipple and areola • Chadwick's sign: blue-purple discoloration of cervix and vaginal mucosa (at 6 weeks) • Increased skin pigmentation; abdominal striae • Subjective accounts of fatigue and morning sickness; increased appetite; urinary frequency; quickening	• Progressive increase in uterine size and abdomen by 20 weeks • Progressive uterine shape change from pear to globular to ovoid • Hegar's signs: softening of uterine isthmus (at 6 to 8 weeks) • Goodell's sign: softening of cervix (at 6 to 8 weeks) • Braxton Hicks contractions in second and third trimesters • Ballottement: fetal rebound after release of uterine pressure (at midpregnancy) • Positive pregnancy test (human chorionic gonadotropin present in maternal plasma or urine)	• Fetal heart tones distinct from mother's (at 12 weeks with Doppler device; at 20 weeks with fetoscope) • Fetal activity (at 20 weeks) • Sonographic identification (at 5 to 8 weeks) or radiographic identification (after 16 weeks) • Fetal movement palpated by examiner • Externally visible fetal movement

COLLABORATIVE PROBLEM

Altered anatomy, physiology, and metabolism related to pregnancy (two expected outcomes)

Expected outcome 1

The patient will express understanding of the changes associated with her pregnancy and the date of her pregnancy.

Interventions

1. Obtain a complete history, including obstetric and gynecologic histories.

2. Note regularity of menses, date of last menstrual period (LMP), and use of contraceptives. (See *Evidence of pregnancy.*) Perform physical examination and correlate data.

3. Estimate the menstrual or gestational age, and determine the estimated date of confinement (EDC) using Nägele's rule: Add 7 days to the date of the 1st day of the LMP; count back 3 months.

4. Additional individualized interventions: _____

Rationales

1. A complete history and physical examination assist in diagnosis. Amenorrhea and the presumptive and probable signs of pregnancy may suggest various gynecologic or endocrine disorders. Diagnosis is most difficult in early pregnancy, when the uterus is still located in the pelvic cavity. Subsequent examination usually proves more definitive.

2. Estimation of time of ovulation helps determine the time of fertilization and allows dating of the pregnancy.

3. Duration of pregnancy is about 280 days, 10 lunar months, or 40 weeks. Note that the EDC is just that — an estimate; labor may begin 7 to 14 days before or after this date.

4. Rationales: _____

Expected outcome 2

Once the patient understands the changes of pregnancy, she will express feelings of maternal well-being.

Interventions

1. Codify the obstetric history to show the number of total pregnancies, abortions, and living children, using the four-digit system separated by dashes:
digit 1 — number of term infants
digit 2 — number of preterm infants
digit 3 — number of abortions
digit 4 — number of living children
For example, 1-1-0-2 would indicate 1 term, 1 preterm, 0 abortions, and 2 living children.

2. Coach the patient on deep breathing for relaxation during the vaginal examination. Have the patient void before the procedure. Assist with the vaginal examination, Papanicolaou smear, and cultures, as indicated. Refer to the laboratory for serologic testing.

3. After the 12th week of gestation, assess fundal height. Measure from the superior aspect of the symphysis pubis to the top of the fundus.

4. Assess vital signs. Take resting pulse and blood pressure. Allow time for a second reading if the patient seems apprehensive or values are outside established norms. Note variations with each visit.

5. Aid in laboratory tests as follows:

• Perform fingerstick for hemoglobin (Hb) measurement.

• Obtain a clean-catch urine specimen for dipstick analysis. Test for glucose, protein, and nitrites.

Rationales

1. Various systems may be used, each summarizing the patient's obstetric history for quick integration into a complete clinical profile. Most systems determine basic gravidity and parity before listing the number of previous term and preterm deliveries and miscarriages.

2. Vaginal examination and testing monitor tissue integrity and discharge and detect the presence of lesions; they also allow monitoring of progressive vaginal and cervical changes associated with pregnancy. In the latter part of pregnancy, another vaginal examination may be performed to estimate pelvic size, capacity, and adequacy.

3. Increasing fundal height indicates advancing pregnancy and fetal growth. Greater than normal height may be attributed to full rectum or bladder (bladder should be emptied before examination), multiple pregnancy, obesity, hydramnios, or myomata; less than normal height may be attributed to lack of certainty about LMP or to intrauterine growth retardation.

4. Higher values may be attributed to sympathetic reflex action. An accurate resting value is critical in establishing a baseline and evaluating adaptations associated with pregnancy or maladaption associated with pregnancy-induced hypertension (PIH) or chronic hypertension.

5. Laboratory results help establish baseline values and allow for monitoring.
• Hb values of 12 to 16 g/dl are consistent with adequate circulatory volume and iron stores. Anemia is defined as an Hb value below 11 g/dl during the first or third trimester and an Hb value below 10.5 g/dl during the second trimester. Anemia in pregnancy is associated most commonly with iron deficiency and acute blood loss.
• Mild glycosuria is usually benign and typically occurs at some point during most pregnancies. A patient with an elevated glucose level or a familial history of diabetes may require further testing because pregnancy can trigger diabetes. Screening should take place at 28 weeks or, if indicated, earlier. Proteinuria of +1 or greater is associated with PIH and needs to be investigated. Sudden weight gain of more than 2 lb (0.9 kg) per week and a significant elevation in blood pressure usually precede proteinuria in the classic triad of symptoms. Nitrites may indicate infection.

6. Note weight: actual, ideal, and changes. Monitor for edema, and differentiate among benign, dependent, and pathologic types. Chart prepregnancy weight and height.

6. A progressive weight gain of 25 lb (11.3 kg) or more is expected and indicates maternal adaptation and well-being. Failure to gain weight is associated with poor fetal outcome; sudden gain, with PIH. Careful assessment is essential in distinguishing true weight gain from fluid retention.

7. Schedule subsequent visits as follows:
• each month for the first 7 months
• every 2 weeks for month 8
• every week thereafter until delivery.
Continue to note vital signs, weight, and fundal height. Modify the schedule according to patient condition. (See *Managing discomforts of pregnancy.*)

7. Systematic appraisal of anticipated changes of pregnancy is necessary to monitor adaptation.

8. Additional individualized interventions: _____

8. Rationales: _____

NURSING DIAGNOSIS

Risk for fetal injury related to dependence on maternal well-being and genetic and environmental factors

Expected outcome

The fetus will experience minimal, if any, injury as evidenced by positive fetal heart rate patterns, fetal movement, and no signs of distress.

Interventions

1. Include a high-risk profile in maternal history, noting:
• maternal weight of less than 100 lb (45 kg) or 20% above appropriate weight for patient's height; pregnant weight gain of less than 15 lb (6.8 kg) or more than 35 lb (15.8 kg)
• medical history of hypertension, diabetes, cardiovascular disorders, infectious and childhood diseases, and Rh and ABO incompatibilities with partner
• family history of genetic disorders
• obstetric history of anemia, bleeding, protracted or precipitous labors, preterm deliveries, delivery of macrosomic infant, deliveries by cesarean section or extraction, and compromised fetal outcome
• unhealthy lifestyle patterns, including multiple sexual partners and use of caffeine, nicotine, alcohol, and over-the-counter, prescribed, or illicit drugs (see *Maternal implications of chemical substance use during pregnancy,* page 8, and appendix C, Substance use and fetal and neonatal abnormalities)
• family history of dysfunctional or abusive relationships or financial instability.

Rationales

1. A high-risk profile allows early recognition of problems that can be prevented or reversed to improve maternal condition and fetal outcome.

Managing discomforts of pregnancy

Problem	Management
Nausea and vomiting (morning sickness)	• Avoid foods that specifically aggravate problem. • Keep dry crackers or other dry carbohydrates at bedside and eat several before arising. • Consume six small meals a day; alternate meal without liquid with one that is only liquid. • Drink liquids 30 minutes after eating solids. • Avoid greasy, fried, highly spiced, and gas-producing foods. • Avoid eating or preparing highly aromatic foods.
Heartburn	• Take sips of milk over a 15-minute period. • Eat smaller meals more frequently. • Avoid greasy, gas-producing foods or those that specifically aggravate symptom. • Avoid lying down after eating; change position if symptom occurs. • Chew gum. • Take low-sodium antacids as a last resort and only if prescribed; do not take any sodium bicarbonate or over-the-counter medicines. • Chew on cracked ice.
Breast tenderness	• Wear support bra day and night.
Backache	• Avoid excessive or undue lifting, bending, or walking. • Use good body mechanics, and perform pelvic tilt exercises regularly. • Avoid exaggerated curving of the lumbar region. • Maintain good posture.
Leg cramps (muscle spasm)	• Have doctor perform evaluation to rule out phlebitis and thrombosis. • Consume adequate dietary calcium or take a calcium supplement. • Wear adequate clothing to prevent chilling extremities. • Apply heat to affected muscle. • Exercise regularly, especially with knee flexion and foot dorsiflexion, to stretch affected muscle. • Avoid standing on cold surfaces.
Varicosities	• Avoid prolonged standing, sitting, and crossing legs at knee. • Avoid constrictive clothing (such as garters). • Take periodic rests with legs elevated. • Wear elastic stockings.
Foot and ankle edema	• Have regular evaluations to rule out edema of hands, face, and body. • Avoid prolonged standing and sitting and constrictive clothing. • Rest in side-lying position. • Elevate legs above level of heart for 10-minute intervals.
Shortness of breath	• For symptoms of malignant cardiovascular or pulmonary disorders, contact doctor. • Recognize that shortness of breath is normal during pregnancy. • Maintain good posture. • Use extra pillows in bed. • Avoid eating large meals.
Vertigo (dizziness)	• Avoid prolonged standing and walking and undue fatigue. • Change position slowly and deliberately. • Eat regular, well-balanced meals.
Constipation	• Ensure adequate hydration and dietary fiber intake. • Exercise moderately. • Defecate when urge presents itself. • Schedule to allow for daily bowel movements. • Do not use laxatives, cathartics, or enemas.
Hemorrhoids	• Take steps to prevent constipation. • Take warm soaks or sitz or tub baths. • Use local anesthetizing agents. • Manually reinsert protruding hemorrhoids into rectum.

Maternal implications of chemical substance use during pregnancy

The pregnant patient who uses chemical substances is at risk for a wide range of problems. Drug diluents and impurities may compound the negative effects of chemical substance use.

Habitual use of chemical substances may be hard to assess; the patient may deny the practice and give an inaccurate or a distorted history. Attempts to dissuade a patient from using chemical substances may prove futile and even cause her to reject prenatal care.

This chart describes the possible consequences of chemical substance use during pregnancy. Although it addresses only single-substance use, the nurse should keep in mind that multiple-substance use is common. (For fetal and neonatal problems linked with maternal substance use, see appendix C, Substance use and fetal and neonatal abnormalities.)

Substance	Possible maternal outcome
Alcohol	Spontaneous abortion, liver damage, GI disorders
Cocaine	Spontaneous abortion, abruptio placentae, preterm or precipitous delivery, stillbirth, sudden death, arrhythmias, myocardial infarction, aortic rupture, cerebrovascular accident, seizures, bowel ischemia, hyperthermia
Opioids	Bacteremia, endocarditis, phlebitis, cellulitis, pneumonia, tetanus, hepatitis, human immunodeficiency virus infection (with I.V. injection)
Tobacco	Spontaneous abortion, abruptio placentae, placenta previa, premature or prolonged rupture of membranes, amnionitis (dose-related)

2. Note the patient's age:
• under age 18

• over age 35.

2. Age can affect fetal outcome.
• The increase in the number of adolescent pregnancies crosses social, economic, and racial lines. Obstetric risks during early adolescence (ages 11 to 15) result from physiologic immaturity. Obstetric risks during late adolescence (ages 16 to 18) are associated with social factors and lifestyle choices, such as poor nutrition, smoking, alcohol and drug abuse, and sexually transmitted diseases. Teenage gravidas are at high risk for anemia, preeclampsia, and term or preterm low-birth-weight infants. Their offspring have an increased incidence of infections, accidents, cognitive defects, and behavioral problems. Failure of the patient to progress through the psychosocial developmental tasks of adolescence commonly perpetuates the cycle — and consequences — of early pregnancy and childbirth.
• Changing women's roles, technological progress, more effective contraception methods, and economic imperatives have resulted in delayed childbearing for many women. The older pregnant patient is at increased risk for chronic hypertension, gestational or type 2 (non-insulin-dependent) diabetes mellitus, placental disorders (such as placentia previa or abruptio placentae), preeclampsia, and various medical and surgical conditions. These chronic, age-related conditions antedate the pregnancy and may affect it profoundly. Other risks for such a patient include ectopic pregnancy, spontaneous abortion, preterm labor, prolonged labor (especially in the nullipara), and preterm delivery. Implications for offspring include chromosomal anomalies, congenital malformations, low birth weight, and macrosomia. Also, perinatal mortality is increased.

3. Review the patient's immunization record, including vaccinations for rubella, measles, mumps, cholera, influenza, plague, typhoid, diphtheria, and tetanus.

3. Rubella vaccine is contraindicated during pregnancy because of its teratogenicity; lack of immunization necessitates immunization in the immediate postpartum period. Immunization for measles or mumps is also contraindicated. Diphtheria and tetanus toxoids may be given if no primary series was given or no booster was given within 10 years. Immunization for cholera, influenza, plague, and typhoid is given to the patient at risk.

4. Continue assessment of fundal height.

4. Increasing fundal height indicates uterine and fetal growth and implies fetal well-being.

5. Assess fetal heart tones (FHTs).

5. FHTs can be detected at 20 weeks' gestation with a fetoscope and as early as 12 weeks' gestation with a Doppler ultrasound device.

6. Assess fetal movement; query the patient about frequency and intensity of fetal activity.

6. Fetal activity is perceivable by the patient at 20 weeks. Movements are sporadic and increase with maternal activity; they become significant when a marked change in frequency occurs. A gradual decrease in fetal activity over a 24-hour period is an ominous sign. No fetal movement usually portends disappearance of FHT within 24 hours.

7. Review family pedigree, including ethnic, racial, and geographic factors. Correlate with maternal age. Assess the need for maternal serum alpha-fetoprotein (MSAFP) screening. If the patient requires MSAFP screening, obtain an accurate maternal weight and gestational age.

7. MSAFP determination is the most common prenatal screening test for inherited disorders. Ideally, it should be performed between weeks 15 and 18 of pregnancy. Elevated MSAFP levels are associated with neural tube defects, other anomalies typified by fetal edema or skin defects, underestimated gestational age, multiple gestation, decreased maternal weight, and fetal death. Low MSAFP levels are associated with chromosomal trisomies, increased maternal weight, overestimated gestational age, gestational trophoblastic disease, and fetal death.

8. Additional individualized interventions: _____

8. Rationales: _____

NURSING DIAGNOSIS

Altered nutrition: less than body requirements secondary to increased needs of pregnancy (two expected outcomes)

Expected outcome 1

The patient will experience no alteration in nutrition; nutritional needs of pregnancy will be met as evidenced by positive weight gain, shiny hair, bright eyes, and nonbrittle nails.

Interventions

1. Assess the patient's height, weight, and frame, and compare these measurements with standardized charts for normal weight ranges. Note changes.

Rationales

1. Assessment establishes baseline information and deviation from norm. A woman whose weight is appropriate for height and frame should have a progressive gain of 25 to 35 lb (11.5 to 16 kg) to support maternal changes and fetal growth. An underweight woman may gain up to 40 lb (18 kg); a heavier or an obese woman should limit weight gain to 15 to 25 lb (7 to 11.5 kg). Appropriate maternal weight gain is necessary for optimal fetal growth and development.

2. Perform a gross physical examination, including assessment of hair, nails, skin, eyes, and neuromuscular system.

3. Take a 24-hour diet recall, noting portion size, method of food preparation, ethnic preferences, food availability, food cravings, and unusual food habits (such as pica, which is a craving for dirt, starch, or other nonnutritive substances).

4. Additional individualized interventions: _____
_____

2. The well-nourished person exhibits shiny hair that is not easily plucked; firm, nonbrittle nails; smooth skin without lesions, rashes, or edema; bright, clear, shiny eyes with pink, moist membranes; and intact muscle innervation, tactile senses, and ability to perform activities of daily living without difficulty.

3. A diet recall identifies nutritional strengths and weaknesses. Teaching the patient about necessary changes and including her suggestions in menu changes increase compliance. Food cravings are usually benign and may be indulged if they do not interfere with or replace a well-balanced diet. Pica represents an aberration and requires treatment.

4. Rationales: _____
_____

Expected outcome 2

The patient will maintain a well-balanced diet as evidenced by adherence to suggested food group and calorie intake guidelines.

Interventions

1. Provide oral and written information on daily dietary requirements, using the food pyramid as a guide to food choices:
• bread, cereal, rice, and pasta group: 6 to 11 servings
• vegetable group: 3 to 5 servings
• fruit group: 2 to 4 servings
• milk, yogurt, and cheese group: 2 to 3 servings
• meat, poultry, fish, dry beans, egg, and nut group: 2 to 3 servings
• added sugars and naturally occurring and added fats and oils: use sparingly.

2. Advise against weight-reduction diets.

3. Advise the patient to supplement her diet with simple iron salts.

Rationales

1. Within the ranges shown, the patient's intake should be increased to meet the additional dietary requirements of pregnancy. (See appendix B, Selected daily dietary allowances — maternal.) Increases should be based on caloric requirements. Generally, pregnant women require an additional 250 to 500 calories/day. Many of these calories should come from protein (preferably from animal sources). Increased servings from the milk, yogurt, and cheese group provide additional required amounts of vitamin D, calcium, and phosphorous as well as calories. Pregnant women should be encouraged to consume fresh fruits, vegetables, and other high-fiber foods.

2. Failure to gain 15 lb (7 kg) or more is associated with catabolism of maternal tissue to provide for fetal growth and maternal accessory tissue. Weight gain is accounted for as follows:
• fetus: 7½ lb (3.4 kg)
• placenta: 1½ lb (0.7 kg)
• amniotic fluid: 1 lb (0.45 kg)
• uterine growth: 2½ lb (1.13 kg)
• increased blood volume: 3½ lb (1.6 kg)
• increased breast tissue: 2 lb (0.9 kg).

3. Even with a well-balanced diet, insufficient iron stores and the limited iron content of the typical diet necessitate supplementation to meet the increased needs of pregnancy. A pregnant woman should take 30 to 60 mg of iron salts daily — preferably after the 4th month, when needs increase and the GI discomforts of early pregnancy have subsided.

4. Advise the patient to take vitamin and mineral supplements as indicated.

5. Advise the patient to take folic acid supplements as indicated, and suggest that she eat foods rich in folic acid, such as green, leafy vegetables and orange juice.

6. Assess the patient's alcohol intake. Discourage alcohol consumption.

7. Additional individualized interventions: _____
_____

4. Adolescents, vegetarians, women with multiple-gestation pregnancies, heavy smokers, and chemical substance abusers may have inadequate nutritional intake and may benefit from vitamin and mineral supplements.

5. Folic acid supplementation before conception is associated with a reduced incidence of neural tube defects. Such supplementation is recommended for women who have had offspring with spina bifida, anencephaly, or encephalocele. The Centers for Disease Control and Prevention (CDC) recommends that pregnant women with this history take 4 mg of folic acid daily, starting 1 month before conception and continuing for the first 3 months of pregnancy. The CDC recommends 0.4 mg of folic acid daily for all fertile women.

6. Alcohol provides "empty" calories. No level of drinking during pregnancy is known to be safe; adverse fetal effects of maternal alcohol consumption may be profound.

7. Rationales: _____
_____

Nursing diagnosis

Activity intolerance, possibly related to increasing hormone levels and demands of pregnancy

Expected outcome

The patient will experience minimal activity intolerance and will receive adequate rest as evidenced by no complaints of excessive fatigue, exercise intolerance to minimal activities, or inability to walk without shortness of breath.

Interventions

1. Assess sleep and rest patterns, home responsibilities, and employment status. Review Hb level and hematocrit.

2. Offer advice about the need for adequate sleep and rest, including the need for:
• 8 hours of uninterrupted sleep per day plus one nap
• scheduled rest period at place of employment during each break
• napping at home while preschoolers are sleeping.

3. Explain that no restrictions on activity or travel are necessary.

4. Encourage exercise, including pelvic lifting or rocking, modified sit-ups, tailor-fashion sitting, and Kegel exercises.

Rationales

1. Assessment provides baseline data and identifies factors that may affect promotion of rest.

2. Although fatigue cannot be prevented, it can be minimized.

3. Only activities of daily living that cause undue fatigue or possible risk to the fetus need to be altered.

4. These exercises help improve muscle tone in preparation for delivery and promote a more rapid return to the patient's prepregnancy physical state.

5. As pregnancy progresses, advise changing position slowly and deliberately and resting and sleeping in a side-lying position.

6. Additional individualized interventions: _____
_____

5. Changing position slowly minimizes vertigo and the risk of falls. A side-lying position (especially left) reduces aortic compression and increases uteroplacental flow.

6. Rationales: _____
_____

NURSING DIAGNOSIS

Risk for maternal urinary tract infection (UTI), possibly related to urinary stasis and silent bacteriuria

Expected outcome

The patient will have no signs of infection as evidenced by no burning on urination, no pelvic or bladder pain, and no hematuria.

Interventions

1. Assess for urinary frequency and urgency, dysuria, and hematuria. Perform urine examination by dipstick.

2. Offer the following advice about hygienic and prophylactic practices and about elimination:
• Maintain adequate hydration.

• Void when the urge presents itself and before going to bed.
• Stress the importance of promptly reporting signs of UTI.
• Wipe from front to back after elimination.

• Wash hands after elimination.

3. Additional individualized interventions: _____
_____

Rationales

1. Urinary frequency in the first and third trimesters is associated with the weight of the gravid uterus on the urinary bladder. The other symptoms strongly suggest infection and should be referred to the doctor.

2. These measures assist in prophylaxis:

• Adequate hydration keeps urine dilute and bacterial colony counts low.
• Frequent voiding minimizes stasis and possible colonization.
• UTIs during pregnancy have been linked to preterm labor.
• Wiping from front to back minimizes contamination by *Escherichia coli*.
• Hand washing minimizes the spread of contaminants

3. Rationales: _____
_____

NURSING DIAGNOSIS

Altered sexuality patterns related to fatigue, genital changes, or fear of fetal injury

Expected outcome

The patient will experience minimal altered sexuality patterns related to pregnancy as evidenced by no complaints of inability to continue sexual relations during most of the pregnancy.

Interventions

1. Advise the patient about the effects of pregnancy on sexual activity:
• Fatigue and breast tenderness in the first trimester and abdominal bulk and fatigue in the third trimester may diminish sexual responsiveness.
• Intercourse need not be restricted unless membranes have ruptured or abortion, preterm labor, or bleeding threatens. (*Note:* Some practitioners advise against coitus during the last month of pregnancy.)
• Sexual responsiveness is usually highest during the second trimester, when the discomforts of pregnancy are lowest.
• Changes in coital position may be necessary to accommodate the enlarged abdomen.
• If effects of the pregnancy preclude intercourse, sexual activity can take place without it.

2. Assess for leukorrhea. Advise washing with mild soap and water after toileting. Explain that douching is prohibited.

3. Additional individualized interventions: _____

Rationales

1. A physiologic response to and perceptions concerning pregnancy may alter responsiveness and spontaneity. These feelings are normal and usually self-limiting; sexual activity is not associated with fetal injury.

2. Copious vaginal secretions are common and benign during pregnancy; their presence may inhibit sexual interest. Douching is associated with air embolism and ascending genital tract infection.

3. Rationales: _____

Nursing diagnosis

Knowledge deficit related to normal pregnancy

Expected outcome

The patient will receive information on normal changes related to pregnancy to minimize knowledge deficit.

Interventions

1. Assess the patient's knowledge of normal pregnancy, noting the patient's age, previous experience, parity, marital status, and cultural expectations.

2. Present information on normal pregnancy sequentially with each visit. Provide pictures of fetal growth. Reinforce earlier teaching on health maintenance and allow time for questions.

3. Advise the patient of danger signs that should be reported immediately, including vaginal bleeding, abdominal pain, swelling of hands or fingers, persistent or severe headache, visual disturbances, persistent vomiting, chills, fever, painful urination, shortness of breath, and significant change in fetal activity.

4. Demonstrate breast preparation for the patient who plans to breast-feed.

Rationales

1. This information provides a baseline for nursing action and teaching.

2. Sequential presentation allows the patient time to internalize and synthesize information.

3. Any one of these signs and symptoms can signal a serious complication.

4. Teaching the patient these techniques facilitates breast-feeding without discomfort or anxiety.

5. Advise the patient about birthing and anesthesia options.

6. Refer the patient to childbirth preparation classes.

7. Teach the patient the signs of impending labor and criteria for going to the hospital:
• rupture of membranes
• regular contractions felt in the abdomen and back that are 5 to 10 minutes apart and increase in intensity and duration.

8. Provide written information at an appropriate reading level, including culturally sensitive information.

9. Additional individualized interventions: _____

5. Understanding her options makes the patient part of the health care team, allows time for informed decision making, and gives the patient a sense of control.

6. These classes involve the parents in the birthing and parenting processes (see appendix J, Parent teaching guides).

7. This information allows the patient to recognize the signs of labor and make an informed decision before taking action.

8. Written information reinforces teaching and allows the patient to review material as needed.

9. Rationales: _____

Documentation checklist
During prenatal visits, document:
❏ family history, including genetic risk factors, history of previous pregnancies and their outcomes, and assessment findings
❏ patient status at each visit
❏ any changes in patient status since the last visit
❏ fundal height, the patient's weight, and FHT
❏ pertinent laboratory and diagnostic findings
❏ nutritional intake
❏ reaction of the patient and her partner to pregnancy
❏ patient and family teaching guidelines.

Associated appendices
❏ Selected daily dietary allowances — maternal (appendix B)
❏ Substance use and fetal and neonatal abnormalities (appendix C)
❏ Aspects of psychological care — maternal (appendix D)

Additional nursing diagnoses
❏ Altered role performance related to anticipation of new family member
❏ Constipation related to decreased peristalsis and increased water and electrolyte absorption
❏ Risk for fetal poisoning or trauma related to maternal use of nicotine or intoxicants
❏ Sleep pattern disturbance related to change in body size and contour

Abortion

Definition
Abortion is the spontaneous or induced loss of the products of conception before the occurrence of fetal viability, measured as a gestational age of less than 20 weeks or a fetal weight of 500 g or less. Abortions that occur before the 12th week of gestation are termed early or first-trimester abortions; those occur between the 12th and 20th week are termed late or second-trimester abortions. This distinction is necessary because anatomic and physiologic changes in the latter weeks of gestation make treatment more difficult. Spontaneous abortions are classified as threatened, inevitable, missed, incomplete, complete, habitual, and septic. Septic abortion is most commonly associated with self-induced instrumentation. Complications include hemorrhage, septic or endotoxic shock, acute renal failure, and death.

Etiology and precipitating factors
• First-trimester abortions are associated with embryonic, fetal, or placental abnormalities caused by congenital or genetic defects and by alterations in the intrauterine environment due to endocrine imbalance or exposure to teratogens.
• Second-trimester abortions are primarily associated with maternal problems, such as infection, endocrine dysfunction, severe malnutrition, drug ingestion (including alcohol or tobacco), manipulation or abnormalities of the reproductive viscera and, possibly, Rh isoimmunization and blood group incompatibility between the parents. The role of physical and emotional trauma is suspect.

Physical findings
Cardiovascular
• Tachycardia
• Tachypnea
• Hypotension
• Restlessness
• Fever
Genitourinary
Threatened
• Protracted vaginal spotting or slight bleeding for days or weeks
• Mild, menstrual-like cramps or low backache
• Closed cervix
• No passage of tissue
• Uterine size congruent with length of pregnancy
Inevitable
• Moderate vaginal bleeding; passage of clots
• Uterine contractions, pain

• Dilated cervix
• Ruptured membranes
• Uterine size congruent with length of pregnancy
Incomplete
• Profuse, bright red vaginal bleeding
• Severe uterine cramping
• Dilated cervix
• Partial or full placental retention in utero; passage of some placental tissue
• Uterine size smaller than warranted by length of pregnancy
Complete
• Possibly scant vaginal bleeding
• Possibly mild menstrual-like cramps
• Passage of fetus, membranes, and placenta
• Closed cervix after passage
• Uterine size smaller than warranted by length of pregnancy
Septic
• Possibly vaginal or cervical lacerations or puncture wounds; gross trauma
• Possibly bleeding; foul-smelling, purulent vaginal discharge
• Possibly uterine cramping or tenderness
• Cervical pain on palpation
• Possibly dilated cervix
• Uterine size smaller than warranted by length of pregnancy; possibly larger in cases of pronounced infectious process
• Fever

Diagnostic studies
• Accurate and complete history and physical examination, including pelvic examination, may furnish enough data for a definitive diagnosis.
• Sonography identifies poorly formed or absent gestational sac in impending abortion, uterine abnormalities, and placental location and abnormalities; it also confirms presence or absence of fetal viability.
• Urine pregnancy test may be negative or weakly positive.
• Hemoglobin (Hb) level and hematocrit (HCT) generally decrease.
• White blood cell (WBC) count increases, most often in complete and septic abortions.
• Blood and urine cultures may be positive anaerobic or aerobic in septic abortion.
• Tissue cytology may confirm fetal or placental tissue.
• Serial beta human chorionic gonadotropin levels drop or fail to increase appropriately.

NURSING DIAGNOSIS

Risk for injury related to pregnancy termination caused by maternal or fetal abnormality (three expected outcomes)

Expected outcome 1

The patient will experience minimal risk for injury related to pregnancy termination as evidenced by minimal vaginal bleeding and pain.

Interventions

1. Monitor for signs of threatened abortion. Begin by determining date of last menstrual period (LMP), estimation of gestational age, and pregnancy test results. Then assess for the following:
• vaginal bleeding or spotting
• menstrual-like cramping or low backache, notably after onset of bleeding
• loss of pregnancy symptoms (such as nausea and breast tenderness).

2. Prepare patient for ultrasonography, as ordered. Tell the patient not to void or drink fluids before examination.

3. Additional individualized interventions: _____
_____

Rationales

1. Identifying LMP assists in confirming and dating pregnancy. A positive pregnancy test may help confirm the diagnosis. Painless vaginal spotting or bleeding early in pregnancy is common. Fewer than one-half of the patients with such bleeding abort. If pain accompanies the bleeding, the prognosis is poorer. Loss of pregnancy symptoms can signify pregnancy loss.

2. Ultrasonography assists in determining placental site and integrity, stage of abortion and, possibly, fetal viability. The distended bladder pushes the uterus out of the pelvis and facilitates imaging. Although drinking fluids helps produce urine, food and fluids are usually withheld from the patient in anticipation of possible surgery.

3. Rationales: _____
_____

Expected outcome 2

The patient will receive treatment as soon as early signs of threatened abortion occur.

Interventions

1. Assess for risk factors for cervical incompetence, including:
• history of cervical trauma
• dilation of the cervical os in the second or possibly early in the third trimester during previous pregnancies
• absence of pain
• in utero exposure to diethylstilbestrol
• repeated, unexplained late-term abortions or preterm deliveries.

2. Additional individualized interventions: _____

Rationales

1. If cervical incompetence is identified, cerclage can be performed if dilation is less than 4 cm.

2. Rationales: _____

Expected outcome 3

The patient will maintain a viable pregnancy.

Interventions

1. Assess for current use of intrauterine device (IUD); if one is present, assist the doctor in its removal.

2. Instruct the patient about the at-home medical regimen, including:
• bed rest
• no sexual activity, especially intercourse, orgasm, and nipple stimulation; no douching or use of cathartics
• need to report persistent or increased bleeding or cramping to appropriate health care personnel.

3. Additional individualized interventions: _____

Rationales

1. If the tail of the IUD is visible, removal may be medically indicated to lessen the risk of late abortion, infection, and prematurity.

2. Bed rest, associated with decreased bleeding and cramping, and abstinence are the only effective measures to minimize or prevent the progression of abortion. Increasingly severe symptoms warrant hospitalization and medical intervention.

3. Rationales: _____

COLLABORATIVE PROBLEM

Risk for fluid volume deficit related to hemorrhage (two expected outcomes)

Expected outcome 1

The patient will experience minimal risk for fluid volume deficit related to hemorrhage as evidenced by good skin turgor, good urine output, and serum (blood) chemistry levels within normal limits.

Interventions

1. Assess the patient for bleeding every hour or as the patient's condition warrants:

• Note vaginal bleeding, including the color; the number of perineal pads used, degree of saturation, and weight; and bleeding accompanied by gushes of fluid.

• Note passage of large or numerous clots and tissue; save all tissue passed.
• Monitor the patient for restlessness, tachycardia, hypotension, diaphoresis, and pallor.

2. Monitor Hb level and HCT.

3. Additional individualized interventions: _____

Rationales

1. In an incomplete abortion, partially retained placental tissue impedes uterine contraction and results in profuse bleeding. Severe hypovolemia may develop quickly.
• Accurate assessment helps evaluate blood loss. (*Note:* 1 g of blood by weight equals 1 ml; a saturated pad equals about 100 ml.)
• Examination of tissue assists in staging abortion. In complete abortion, abortus and full placenta have been passed.
• Deterioration into hemorrhagic shock warrants rapid intervention to reverse the process.

2. Decreasing Hb level and HCT signal blood loss; values provide a baseline for blood replacement needs.

3. Rationales: _____

Expected outcome 2

The patient will return to and maintain a normovolemic state as evidenced by stable vital signs, including blood pressure within normal limits.

Interventions

1. Monitor the patient's vital signs as her condition warrants.

2. Monitor blood study trends, including Hb level, HCT, and coagulation profile.

3. Type and crossmatch for 2 units of blood, as ordered.

4. Administer whole blood, packed red blood cells, or clotting factors, as ordered.

5. Monitor fluid intake and output.

6. Administer an oxytocin drip, as ordered. Monitor vital signs and uterine contractions, and assess fluid intake and output. Administer analgesics.

7. Prepare the patient for surgery.

8. Additional individualized interventions: _____

Rationales

1. Increasing pulse rate and falling blood pressure indicate continuing blood loss.

2. Clinical and laboratory profiles assist in the evaluation of the patient's needs and status and the effectiveness of treatment.

3. This procedure ensures that blood is readily available.

4. Replacement of blood or blood products may be necessary to restore adequate volume.

5. Output reflects renal perfusion.

6. Oxytocin is indicated in inevitable, incomplete, and missed abortion; it stimulates uterine contraction and facilitates complete expulsion of the products of conception. (*Note:* Discontinue oxytocin if tetanic uterine contractions occur.)

7. Surgical dilatation and curettage are indicated if complete passage of abortus and placenta has not been ascertained. Inevitable and incomplete abortions warrant complete evacuation of products of conception.

8. Rationales: _____

COLLABORATIVE PROBLEM

Risk for infection related to incomplete or self-induced abortion

Expected outcome

The patient will experience minimal signs of infection as evidenced by a normal temperature, no purulent or foul-smelling discharge, and no pain in the lower back, pelvis, or abdominal wall.

Interventions

1. Monitor for signs of infection, including:
• temperature higher than 100.4° F (38° C) and chills; foul, purulent vaginal discharge; elevated WBC count
• constant pain in lower back, pelvis, or abdominal wall.

2. Administer tetanus toxoid if the patient has previously been immunized or tetanus immune globulin (human) to an inadequately immunized patient.

3. Obtain anaerobic and aerobic blood cultures, including a smear for Gram stain, from the cervix or products of conception, if feasible.

Rationales

1. The retained products of conception or instrumentation (in self-induced abortion) may cause metritis, parametritis, or peritonitis. Profound sepsis, bacterial shock, acute renal failure, and death may occur if the condition goes unchecked.

2. Protection against *Clostridium tetani* is indicated in suspected or confirmed self-induced abortion.

3. Laboratory data identifies causative organisms.

4. Screen the patient for drug allergies. Administer broad-spectrum antibiotics after cultures are obtained. If self-induced abortion is suspected, administer prophylactic antibiotics, as ordered.

5. Prepare the patient for surgery.

6. Additional individualized interventions: _____

4. In confirmed septic abortion, drug therapy is initiated to combat infection. Prophylactic antibiotics can help prevent infection in self-induced abortion.

5. Complete evacuation of uterine contents is necessary to eliminate the infection source.

6. Rationales: _____

COLLABORATIVE PROBLEM

Risk for maternal injury related to fetal autolysis or Rh isoimmunization (two expected outcomes)

Expected outcome 1

The patient will not experience any maternal injury as evidenced by vital signs and laboratory values within normal limits.

Interventions

1. Note blood Rh factor of the patient and her partner.

2. Administer $Rh_o(D)$ immune globulin (RhoGAM) within 72 hours of abortion.

3. Additional individualized interventions: _____

Rationales

1. Rh-negative, nonsensitized patients with Rh-positive partners are candidates for treatment.

2. If the Rh of the products of conception is positive or unknown, RhoGAM must be given to prevent maternal isoimmunization.

3. Rationales: _____

Expected outcome 2

The patient will not experience maternal isoimmunization as evidenced by vital signs and laboratory values within normal limits.

Interventions

1. Monitor for signs of fetal death in the first half of pregnancy, including:
• history of normal early pregnancy: amenorrhea, possible nausea and vomiting, breast changes, and uterine enlargement
• possibly subsequent vaginal bleeding
• lack of change or decrease in uterine size
• mammary regression to prepregnancy state; weight loss.

Rationales

1. Most missed abortions terminate spontaneously and follow the sequence of any other spontaneous abortion.

2. Monitor for coagulopathy, including:
• multisite bleeding, including frank bleeding from slight trauma, ecchymoses, petechiae, hematomas, and bleeding from mucous membranes
• prothrombin time greater than 15 seconds (may vary widely)
• partial thromboplastin time greater than 60 seconds (may vary widely)
• fibrinogen levels less than 150 mg/dl
• platelet count less than 100,000/mm³ (rare in fetal death)
• fibrin degradation products greater than 100 µg/ml.

3. Prepare the patient for surgery.

4. Additional individualized interventions: _____

2. Prolonged retention of a dead fetus results in the release of thromboplastin, which may cause disseminated intravascular coagulation. Correction is directed at controlling the defect by possible heparin infusion followed by surgical intervention.

3. Uterine evacuation of the retained dead products of conception is necessary.

4. Rationales: _____

Nursing diagnosis

Pain related to uterine contractions

Expected outcome

The patient will experience minimal pain as evidenced by decreased verbalization of pain and decreased need for pain medications.

Interventions

1. Establish rapport with the patient and her partner. Call the patient by her preferred name. Do not leave her unattended for long periods.

2. Assess the patient for pain, including quality, frequency, location, and intensity.

3. Minimize distracting environmental stimuli.

4. Perform comfort measures, including position changes, relaxation techniques, and massage, and administer pharmacologic analgesia.

5. Additional individualized interventions: _____

Rationales

1. A positive relationship builds trust and decreases anxiety, which can in turn decrease regressive behavior, anger, resistance, and noncompliance.

2. The nature of the pain may help in determining the stage of labor or risk of an incomplete or inevitable abortion.

3. External stimuli may increase pain perception.

4. Increased tissue perfusion and stimulation of afferent fibers can decrease the perception of pain.

5. Rationales: _____

Nursing diagnosis

Anxiety related to pregnancy outcome and to uncertainty of future pregnancies

Expected outcome

The patient will express less anxiety as evidenced by verbalization of understanding of her status and use of positive coping strategies.

Interventions

1. Accept the patient's reaction to the loss. Do not minimize the loss or offer explanations, and do not offer false reassurances.

2. Provide information in a clear, forthright manner. As appropriate in the case of a spontaneous abortion, explain that an incompetent cervix is characterized by repeated spontaneous abortion, and habitual abortion is defined as three or more successive abortions. Explain the following as appropriate:
• Surgical repair of an incompetent cervix (cerclage) has a high success rate (85% to 90%).
• Death of the embryo early in pregnancy occurs before spontaneous abortion.
• Early abortion is commonly associated with chromosomal abnormalities.
• Risk of future abortion is only slightly higher than for the population as a whole.

• Late abortion may be associated with maternal abnormalities.

• Resumption of ovulation occurs as early as 2 weeks postabortion.

3. Additional individualized interventions: _____

Rationales

1. Silence, anger, bewilderment, denial, and regressive behaviors are possible reactions. Allowing the patient to act out can help her to cope and move toward resolution of her grief.

2. Providing understandable information helps reduce the patient's anxiety about her condition.

• The high success of this treatment option may decrease anxiety.
• Anxiety and guilt feelings associated with surgical uterine evacuation may be reduced or eliminated.
• This assures the patient that she is not at fault for having "caused" the abortion.
• The likelihood of a positive pregnancy outcome in the future may offer hope and decrease anxiety during an emotionally devastating period.
• Extensive history, hormonal assessment, endometrial biopsy, and hysterosalpingography of the woman and karyotyping of both parents may identify the cause of habitual abortion.
• Many doctors recommend delaying future pregnancy until two or three normal menstrual cycles have occurred. Contraceptive information is critical in cases of self-induced or selected therapeutic abortion.

3. Rationales: _____

NURSING DIAGNOSIS

Spiritual distress related to pregnancy outcome

Expected outcome

The patient will express less spiritual distress as evidenced by decreased use of self-blame and increased use of religious rituals.

Interventions

1. Accept the patient's response to loss in a calm, nonjudgmental manner.

2. Arrange for baptism of the dead fetus, if requested.

3. Provide the patient and her partner with referral to religious or counseling services.

4. Additional individualized interventions: _____

Rationales

1. Self-blame is frequently associated with abortion, whether spontaneous or induced.

2. Acknowledging religious beliefs and helping the patient to observe religious rites may offer consolation.

3. Dysfunctional grieving, impaired family relationships, and severe depression may require professional counseling.

4. Rationales: _____

Documentation checklist

During the hospital stay or clinic visit, document:
❐ patient status and assessment findings on admission or entry to the clinic
❐ any changes in patient status
❐ pertinent laboratory and diagnostic findings
❐ amount and color of blood loss
❐ pain characteristics — quality, location, frequency, and intensity
❐ the patient's response to treatment
❐ the patient's and family's response to threatened or complete abortion
❐ patient and family teaching guidelines
❐ discharge planning guidelines.

Associated plans and appendices

❐ Normal antepartum
❐ Preparing for nonemergency surgery (appendix E)
❐ Selected methods of family planning (appendix F)

Additional nursing diagnoses

❐ Altered sexuality patterns related to required pregnancy postponement
❐ Ineffective individual coping related to repeated loss of a desired pregnancy
❐ Powerlessness related to undiagnosed cause of habitual loss of a desired pregnancy

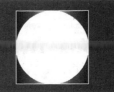

Abruptio placentae

DEFINITION

Abruptio placentae is the premature separation of the placenta from the uterus before delivery of the fetus. It usually occurs in the third trimester, taking place anywhere from 20 weeks' gestation to during second-stage labor. Severity ranges from marginal separation to life-threatening, complete detachment. Signs and symptoms correlate with the degree of separation and the amount of maternal blood lost. Minimal vaginal bleeding accompanied by strong fetal heart tones (FHT) of normal rate and rhythm indicates mild separation and may be treated conservatively with bed rest. Marked detachment may result in fetal distress, irreversible neurologic damage, or fetal death. Maternal complications include hemorrhage, shock, hypofibrinogenemia, disseminated intravascular coagulation (DIC), renal failure, Couvelaire uterus (uteroplacental apoplexy), and death.

Etiology and precipitating factors

• Etiology unknown
• Risk factors include maternal age greater than 35, parity of 5 or greater, history of chronic or pregnancy-induced hypertension, previous abruptio placentae, diabetes, vascular or renal disease, inferior vena cava compression, abdominal trauma, uterine anomaly or tumor, sudden decompression of uterus (after amniotomy in hydramnios or delivery of first twin), history of smoking or substance abuse (especially cocaine), and shortened umbilical cord.

Physical findings

Cardiovascular
• Tachycardia
• Hypotension
• Vertigo
• Syncope
• Diaphoresis
• Pallor
• Cyanosis

Genitourinary
• Uterine tenderness or tension, ranging from absent or minimal to boardlike (depending on degree of separation)
• Vaginal bleeding, ranging from none or scant to profuse and dark red
• Increased uterine size
• Increased uterine tone

• Proteinuria (in severe abruptio placentae)
• Oliguria or anuria
• High to engaged presenting part

Integumentary
• Cold, moist skin
• Dry mucous membranes

Neurologic
• Lethargy
• Confusion
• Somnolence

Respiratory
• Tachypnea
• Increasing shallow respirations

Subjective
• Feelings of thirst, cold, apprehension
• Marked pain in moderate to severe abruptio placentae
• Uterine pain that is localized or diffused, unrelenting, and excruciating

Diagnostic studies

• Accurate and complete history and physical examination may furnish data for a definitive diagnosis.
• Vaginal examination, which may be done by the doctor to rule out placenta previa, is performed only if delivery is imminent and if setups for both vaginal and cesarean section birth are immediately available.
• Ultrasonography reveals placental implantation site, fetal viability, gestational age, position and station and, possibly, hemorrhage site and retroplacental blood clots; it rules out placenta previa.
• Electronic fetal monitoring may reveal late deceleration related to uteroplacental insufficiency, fetal hypoxia, or the absence of FHT.
• Apt test of amniotic fluid may reveal maternal blood that turns amniotic fluid port wine in color.
• Hemoglobin (Hb) level and hematocrit (HCT) decrease.
• Coagulation factor may decrease.
• Fibrinogen degradation product may increase.
• Folic acid level may decrease.

COLLABORATIVE PROBLEM

Fluid volume deficit related to bleeding (three expected outcomes)

Expected outcome 1

The patient will experience minimal bleeding and fluid volume deficit as evidenced by moist mucous membranes, good skin turgor, and stable vital signs within normal limits.

Interventions

1. Assess bleeding every 30 minutes or as the patient's condition warrants:

• Record onset and amount of vaginal bleeding before admission.
• Monitor vital signs and compare with baseline; perform capillary blanch test and note pulse pressure.

• Note vaginal bleeding, including color of blood and number of perineal pads used and their degree of saturation and weight.

• Measure fundal height from the superior aspect of the symphysis pubis to the top of the uterine fundus.

2. Decreasing Hb level and HCT may signal blood loss.

• prothrombin time longer than 15 seconds (may be normal, prolonged, or shortened)
• partial thromboplastin time longer than 60 seconds (may be normal, prolonged, or shortened)
• fibrinogen levels less than 150 mg/dl
• platelet count less than 100,000/mm^3
• fibrinogen degradation products greater than 100 µg/ml
• multisite bleeding, including frank bleeding, ecchymoses, petechiae, hematomas, and bleeding from mucous membranes or sites of invasive procedures.

4. Additional individualized interventions: _____
_____

Rationales

1. Overt, retroplacental bleeding occurs when blood passes behind the membranes and exits externally through the cervix and vagina. Covert, internal bleeding occurs when blood is trapped behind the placenta.
• Blood loss may be as much as one-half the pregnant blood volume.
• A decreased refill time in the capillary blanch test indicates decreased peripheral circulation; a narrowing pulse pressure indicates early shock. The patient may lose 500 to 600 ml of blood before arterial blood pressure or cardiac output is significantly affected. Maternal hypervolemia, hypertension, and initial compensatory mechanisms may mask restlessness, tachycardia, hypotension, and tachypnea — all signs of shock.
• Accurate assessment helps estimate blood loss and replacement needs. (*Note:* 1 g of blood by weight equals 1 ml; a saturated pad equals approximately 100 ml.)
• Fundal height reflects gestational age. An increase may indicate covert bleeding.
2. Monitor Hb level and HCT.

3. Monitor coagulation factors, noting:

3. These signs and symptoms suggest DIC, which requires prompt blood replacement and correction of the underlying pathology.

4. Rationales: _____
_____

Expected outcome 2

The patient will return to and maintain a normovolemic state as evidenced by good urine output, good skin turgor, moist mucous membranes, normal central venous pressure, and urine specific gravity within normal limits.

Interventions

1. Maintain hydration.

• As ordered, start an I.V. infusion of crystalloid or balanced saline solution using a large-bore needle.

• Monitor fluid intake and output and urine specific gravity every hour.

2. Administer fresh whole blood, packed red blood cells, cryoprecipitate, plasma, or platelets, as ordered.

3. At postpartum, perform uterine massage; note uterine contractility.

4. Additional individualized interventions: _____

Rationales

1. Rapid fluid replacement is needed to correct hypovolemia.
• The patient should receive fluids while awaiting typing and crossmatching of blood products. If possible surgery is anticipated, she should not receive food or fluids.
• Fluid intake and output measurements allow assessment of kidney function. The minimum physiologically acceptable urine output is 30 ml/hour. Premature labor is associated with dehydration. Decreased kidney perfusion may result in renal failure. Decreased urine output, urine specific gravity, and creatinine clearance and increased blood urea nitrogen and creatinine levels indicate impending or actual renal failure.
• Monitor the central venous pressure (CVP) line.
• Normal CVP readings during pregnancy range from 8 to 10 cm H_2O. Readings of 15 to 20 cm H_2O indicate circulatory overload.

2. The patient may need a large amount of blood to replace lost volume. Plasma or cryoprecipitate may be given to correct decreasing fibrinogen levels.

3. Massage stimulates contraction. Decreased uterine contractility, coupled with blood between the myometrial fibers, is characteristic of Couvelaire uterus. Trapped blood makes the uterus feel deceptively firm.

4. Rationales: _____

Expected outcome 3

The patient will maintain optimal tissue perfusion as evidenced by positive capillary refill, pink nailbeds, and pink mucous membranes.

Interventions

1. Maintain bed rest in the left lateral position, if possible, or at least a left tilt. Elevate the feet 30 degrees.

2. Administer oxygen by mask at 7 to 10 L/minute as the patient's condition warrants.

3. Additional individualized interventions: _____

Rationales

1. Bed rest decreases physiologic and metabolic demands. The left lateral position decreases pressure on the vena cava, augmenting venous return and cardiac output. Elevating the feet increases blood flow to vital organs.

2. Supplemental oxygen enhances tissue perfusion at the alveolocapillary membrane.

3. Rationales: _____

(Text continues on page 28.)

•••••• **CLINICAL PATHWAY**

Abruptio placentae

	Admission: Triage
Tests	• Peripheral blood count • Coagulation studies • Type and screen • Type and crossmatch x 2 • Ultrasound • External fetal monitoring (expected outcome: fetal heart rate [FHR] within normal limits [WNL])
Assessment	• Take vital signs. • Assess contractions: – onset – frequency – duration. • Assess membrane status: – intact or ruptured – time of rupture – color. • Note amount and characteristics of bleeding. • Defer vaginal exam until site of bleeding determined. • Measure fundal height. • Check bracelet. • Make sure consents are signed, and note advance directives.
Medications	• Pain control medications as needed • Possibly Rho(D) immune globulin (RhoGAM) if patient Rh negative • Tocolytics if indicated
Treatments	• I.V. line placement
Therapies or other treatment considerations	• Support person • Check hepatitis screen. – If no results on chart, call lab to check for results. – If no results from lab, draw blood for hepatitis B surface antigen test. – If results positive or no results available by delivery, notify nursery.
Activities and safety	• Maintain strict bed rest.
Nutrition	• Nothing by mouth
Consults	• Resident doctor • Attending doctor
Patient teaching	• Teach about abruptio placenta. • Explain external fetal monitoring. • Go over plan of care with patient. • Determine if parents went to prenatal classes. • Review safety-related issues with patient.
Discharge planning	• Support system

Admission: Initial care	Stable
• External fetal monitoring (expected outcome: FHR WNL on reactive nonstress test)	• External fetal monitoring as scheduled and as needed (expected outcome: FHR WNL on reactive nonstress test)
• Take vital signs every 2 to 4 hours. • Measure intake and output every shift. • Assess bleeding by weighing perineal pads as needed. • Assess abdomen for pain, tenderness, and rigidity. • Assess for signs and symptoms of shock and disseminated intravascular coagulation (DIC). • Determine patient's ability to express concerns about her condition. • Assess contractions. *Expected outcomes* • Vital signs WNL • Urine output at least 30 ml/hour • Minimal vaginal bleeding • Minimal abdominal pain, tenderness, or rigidity • No signs or symptoms of shock or DIC • Expresses concerns appropriately • Contractions for less than 6 hours	• Take vital signs every 8 hours. • Measure intake and output every shift.
	• I.V. restart as scheduled and as needed • Convert I.V. line to saline well as scheduled
• Patient transferred _____	• Contact appropriate resources to plan for restrictions on activity or possible long-term hospitalization.
• Maintain strict bed rest or bed rest with bathroom privileges.	• Maintain bed rest with bathroom privileges.
• Ice chips	• Advance to regular diet.
• Regional neonatal intensive care unit • Obstetrics anesthesiology	
	• Teach signs and symptoms of preterm labor. • Teach about cesarean section. • Review pamphlet or video on cesarean section with patient.

Adapted with permission from Murray, Kathleen, 5th Medical Group/SGAL.

NURSING DIAGNOSIS

Pain related to uterine tonicity, fundal tenderness, and unrelenting, uncharacteristic uterine contractions

Expected outcome

The patient will experience minimal pain as evidenced by decreased complaints of pain, decreased use of pain medications, and vital signs within normal limits.

Interventions

1. Establish a rapport with the patient and her partner. Call the patient by her preferred name and check on her frequently.

2. Assess for pain, including quality, frequency, location, and intensity.

3. Minimize distracting environmental stimuli.

4. Perform comfort measures, including position changes, relaxation techniques, and massage and effleurage, and administer pharmacologic analgesia with caution.

5. Additional individualized interventions: _____

Rationales

1. A positive relationship builds trust and decreases anxiety, which can in turn decrease regressive behaviors, anger, resistance, and noncompliance.

2. A pain profile may indicate the degree and severity of the separation.

3. External stimuli may tend to increase the perception of pain, and interruptions of rest periods sap the patient's emotional reserves.

4. Increased tissue perfusion and stimulation of afferent fibers can decrease the perception of pain. Analgesics are given cautiously because they may compromise fetal status.

5. Rationales: _____

NURSING DIAGNOSIS

Fear related to fetal distress and possible fetal death

Expected outcome

The patient will express less fear.

Interventions

1. Provide information in a clear, forthright manner, and allow the patient to ask questions. Ascertain the patient's understanding of the information.

2. Additional individualized interventions: _____

Rationales

1. Open communication gives the patient a sense of control and helps decrease her fear. Infant survival depends on gestational age and maturity and the extent or severity of abruption. A realistic appraisal of the deteriorating stability of the undeveloped fetus allows the patient to begin the grieving process.

2. Rationales: _____

COLLABORATIVE PROBLEM

Risk for fetal injury related to uteroplacental hemorrhage and compromised gas exchange (two expected outcomes)

Expected outcome 1

The patient will experience minimal risk for fetal injury as evidenced by positive fetal heart rate (FHR) pattern, positive fetal movement, and no signs of distress.

Interventions

1. Assess fetal status with each maternal assessment, including FHR patterns and variability, fetal activity, and uterine contractility. Compare with baseline.

2. Additional individualized interventions: _____
_____

Rationales

1. Indicators of fetal distress include hyperactivity; slow, irregular FHT that are clinically difficult to hear; late decelerations; and increased FHR with decreased variability.

2. Rationales: _____
_____

Expected outcome 2

The preterm infant will be safely delivered.

Interventions

1. Take steps to bring about labor; monitor its progress.

2. Notify pediatric and neonatal staff of the impending delivery. Obtain the necessary resuscitative equipment.

3. Additional individualized interventions: _____
_____

Rationales

1. Fetal distress, loss of fetal viability, or uncontrolled vaginal bleeding with a ripe cervix warrants delivery. Oxytocin infusion or amniotomy can be used to help bring about a vaginal delivery. Vaginal delivery is preferable if the fetus has died and DIC is probable. If the cervix is not ripe or if fetal distress occurs, the fetus should be delivered by cesarean section. Prompt delivery of a compromised fetus is critical to its survival.

2. The ability of the fetus to survive outside the uterus depends on its gestational age and respiratory, neurologic, thermoregulatory, and GI maturity. Survival of the preterm infant depends on aggressive resuscitation and sustained intensive care.

3. Rationales: _____
_____

Documentation checklist

During the hospital stay, document:
❏ patient status and assessment findings on admission
❏ any changes in patient status
❏ pertinent laboratory and diagnostic findings
❏ amount and color of bleeding
❏ pain characteristics — quality, location, frequency, and intensity
❏ the patient's response to treatment
❏ the patient's and family's response to the illness
❏ patient and family teaching guidelines
❏ discharge planning guidelines.

Associated care plans and appendices

❏ Inappropriate size or weight: small for gestational age

❏ Normal antepartum
❏ Pregnancy complicated by diabetes mellitus
❏ Pregnancy-induced hypertension
❏ Preterm infant
❏ Aspects of psychological care — maternal (appendix D)

Additional nursing diagnoses

❏ Ineffective individual coping related to fear of fetal distress or death
❏ Ineffective family coping (compromised) related to rear of fetal distress or death
❏ Knowledge deficit related to risk profile and recurrence ratio

Acquired immunodeficiency syndrome — maternal

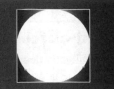

DEFINITION

Acquired immunodeficiency syndrome (AIDS) is the final stage of infection with the human immunodeficiency virus (HIV). AIDS begins when the patient is infected with HIV and generally progresses from an antibody-negative, asymptomatic carrier state; through seroconversion and, possibly, acute seroconversion syndrome; to an antibody-positive, asymptomatic carrier state; and finally to opportunistic infections or cancers.

AIDS is characterized by profound, irreversible immunosuppression that cannot be explained by maternal congenital conditions or by immunosuppressive or cytotoxic drug therapy. The disease affects both cell-mediated immunity and, to a lesser extent, humoral (antibody-mediated) immunity. Helper T lymphocytes or CD4 lymphocytes are the primary targets of HIV. Loss of these cells accounts for much of the immunologic dysfunction in the AIDS patient, leading to opportunistic infections from bacteria, fungi, protozoa, and viruses. *Pneumocystis carinii* pneumonia (PCP) is the most common and serious of these infections.

Various cancers also occur in AIDS patients, including Kaposi's sarcoma and invasive cervical carcinoma. A broad range of AIDS indicator diseases are included in the surveillance definition for AIDS established by the Centers for Disease Control and Prevention (CDC).

Because the number of women diagnosed with AIDS has risen sharply and because AIDS carries a grim prognosis, preventing HIV transmission is crucial. Management includes counseling women about disease prevention and the benefits of delaying pregnancy in HIV-infected women until more is known about perinatal transmission and control. Virus transmission from mother to fetus may occur during pregnancy or during labor and delivery. The CDC reports that from 1992 to the present, there has been a sharp decline in the vertical transmission of HIV. This decline is probably the result of increased awareness of the dangers of HIV, increased use of precautions (such as condoms) to prevent infection, increased voluntary testing, and better treatments for HIV infection — in particular, the use of zidovudine (Retrovir) before or during pregnancy. Breast-feeding has been implicated in HIV transmission. This plan focuses solely on women who are at high risk for acquiring HIV or are already infected and who are or may become pregnant.

Etiology and precipitating factors

• The causative agent of HIV-1 is a spherical, enveloped, single-stranded ribonucleic acid (RNA) retrovirus. Viral RNA is converted to deoxyribonucleic acid by the enzyme reverse transcriptase and incorporated into the host cell.
• Patients at risk include I.V. drug users; heterosexual, homosexual, or bisexual women with current or previous multiple sex partners; prostitutes; recipients of blood or blood products; women with a history of or who currently have sexually transmitted diseases (STDs) or HIV-related illnesses; and women with partners who:
   – are I.V. drug abusers
   – have hemophilia and received blood or blood products before 1985
   – are seropositive and asymptomatic
   – have AIDS
   – are bisexual
   – have multiple sex partners
   – engage in high-risk homosexual or heterosexual activity, including unprotected vaginal or anal intercourse, fellatio, cunnilingus, fisting (insertion of hand or fist into the rectum), or rimming (rectal-oral contact).

Physical findings

• Acute seroconversion syndrome: fever, malaise, raised red rash on trunk, sore throat, arthralgia, lymphadenopathy
• AIDS-related complex: malaise, fatigue, weight loss, intermittent fever, chronic diarrhea, and generalized lymphadenopathy
• Early manifestations of HIV infection: persistent generalized lymphadenopathy lasting longer than 3 months; painless nodules measuring ¾" (2 cm) or more in diameter found at two or more sites outside the groin; thrush and candidiasis; and herpes simplex
• Later manifestations of AIDS: findings vary greatly and depend on the opportunistic infection, cancer, or neurologic dysfunction manifested

Diagnostic studies
HIV antibody detection
• Enzyme-linked immunosorbent assay (ELISA) to detect HIV antibodies. This sensitive and specific test usually becomes reactive within 6 to 12 weeks of HIV infection. Seroconversion may be delayed 6 to 18

months. Usually, a repeat test is performed if initial results are positive.
• Western blot test: a positive result confirms a repeatedly reactive ELISA result.

HIV antigen detection
• Direct identification of HIV in host tissue by viral culture (used mainly in research)
• Positive results of any other highly specific, licensed test for HIV
• Detection of p24 antigen (aids diagnosis in patients with indeterminate Western blot tests)
• Detection of HIV antigen by polymerase chain reaction (test has shorter waiting period and is more readily available than the other test for p24 antigen).

Other laboratory data
• CD4 count yields a decreased absolute number per microliter of blood (normal count is 1,000 to 1,300 µl) or decreased percentage.
• CD4-CD8 ratio is decreased (normal ratio is 2:1).
• Beta-2 microglobulin increases during acute phase of infection, decreases during antibody production, and then rises again with clinical diagnosis.
• Neopterin increases at a rate inversely proportional to CD4 count.
• Soluble interleukin-2 receptors, immunoglobulin A, and delayed hypersensitivity skin test reactions are useful, although less specific and predictive.

COLLABORATIVE PROBLEM

Risk for maternal HIV infection related to sexual practices, illicit drug use, or exposure to infected blood products or carrier (three expected outcomes)

Expected outcome 1

The patient will experience minimal risk for maternal HIV infection as evidenced by no positive HIV cultures or tests.

Interventions

1. Obtain the patient's gynecologic history, including menstrual and obstetric histories and status of offspring, use of contraceptives and STD prophylaxis, history of STDs as well as vaginal and pelvic infections, sexual activities (including multiple sex partners), health and lifestyle of sex partners, and drug use. Review previous Papanicolaou (Pap) test results.

2. Perform a gynecologic examination. Examine vaginal and rectal areas, noting any lesions or signs of infection. Obtain a Pap smear and laboratory screen for STDs.

3. Counsel the patient and refer her for HIV testing.

4. Initiate substance abuse counseling for the patient.

5. Additional individualized interventions: _____

Rationales

1. A lag exists between the time of HIV infection and the appearance of HIV antibodies. During this interval, the patient is a seronegative, asymptomatic HIV carrier. (However, asymptomatic women may be seropositive.) Comprehensive evaluation of all women helps identify high-risk patients and determines the potential for exposure to HIV.

2. The examination may reveal gynecologic manifestations of HIV. Cervical dysplasia or neoplasia, human papillomavirus infection, ulcerative genital disease, recurrent *Candida* vaginitis, and pelvic inflammatory disease (PID) have been associated with HIV infection.

3. Counseling should help the patient understand the relationship between her test results and behavioral risk factors, disease control, and pregnancy prevention or management. Seronegative patients should be counseled about high-risk behaviors that put them at risk for HIV infection and referred for testing. Seropositive patients should be counseled to develop an individualized plan to prevent HIV transmission and on the need for health care and social services.

4. Counseling should decrease risk factors associated with HIV infection and increase the chances for a good pregnancy outcome.

5. Rationales: _____

Expected outcome 2

The high-risk patient will have minimal risk for infection as evidenced by normal temperature, WBCs within normal limits, and no localized redness or pain.

Interventions

1. Review results of ELISA and Western blot tests; integrate the results with the patient's history, looking for a pattern of high-risk behaviors. Women who go to prenatal clinics and those who live in areas where HIV infection is prevalent should receive ongoing testing, exclusive of self-described histories and risk behaviors.

2. If the pregnancy test is negative, advise the patient about family planning methods.

3. Advise the patient to use safer sex practices (see "Knowledge deficit related to modes of HIV transmission," page 36) to minimize the risk of infection.

4. Advise the patient not to share personal items that may have come in contact with blood or body fluids, such as razors and toothbrushes.

5. Refer an I.V. drug user to professional counselors and a detoxification center. Strongly discourage the sharing of needles and syringes. If the patient continues to inject I.V. drugs, instruct her to clean "works" with bleach and to use only clean, unused paraphernalia.

6. Follow standard precautions as well as institutionally prescribed infection-control measures. (See appendix K, Overview of isolation precautions.)

7. Advise the patient to avoid eating undercooked meats, raw or undercooked eggs, and unpasteurized dairy products; to stay away from people who might be ill; and to avoid cleaning fish tanks and cleaning and emptying cat litter boxes. Teach good hand-washing technique.

Rationales

1. Seronegativity may indicate that antibodies have not yet developed. Women whose sex partners are HIV positive (whether symptomatic or not) or whose behaviors put them at risk for HIV are at high risk for acquiring the disease.

2. Most women with HIV are in their childbearing years (ages 15 to 44). They should delay pregnancy as long as they remain at high risk. Except for condoms, family planning methods do not prevent transmission of HIV and other STDs. Oral contraceptives do not prevent STDs and may have multiple drug interactions. An intrauterine device may increase the risk of disease transmission by the HIV-positive woman and may promote susceptibility to ascending genital infection.

3. HIV has been isolated from blood, semen, vaginal secretions, saliva, tears, urine, cerebrospinal fluid, amniotic fluid, and breast milk. Only blood, semen, vaginal secretions and, possibly, breast milk have been associated with disease transmission.

4. Blood and body fluids are sources of infection. Contact with infected body fluids is required for disease transmission. HIV is not transmitted through casual contact or close, nonsexual contact.

5. Sharing drug paraphernalia, the practice of aspirating and reinjecting venous blood during I.V. drug use, and the high incidence of exchanging sex for drugs increase the chances for HIV transmission in I.V. drug users. Destructive, drug-abusing behaviors and the effects of mind-altering drugs foster noncompliance and make HIV transmission likely.

6. Health care workers should consider AIDS prophylaxis when caring for all patients, not just those who are HIV positive, diagnosed, or symptomatic.

7. Avoiding potentially infectious agents and washing hands decreases the chance of infection.

8. Limit the practice of HIV-positive health care providers during exposure-prone invasive gynecologic and obstetric procedures. The CDC recommends that such workers:
• follow standard precautions when using and disposing of needles and other sharp instruments; these workers also should comply with guidelines for disinfecting and sterilizing reusable devices used in invasive procedures
• refrain from all direct patient care and from handling patient care equipment and devices used in invasive procedures when they have exudative lesions or weeping dermatitis
• refrain from performing exposure-prone procedures until they have been advised by an expert review panel. (Practitioners who perform invasive procedures should know their HIV antibody status.)

9. Additional individualized interventions: _____
_____

8. The risk of HIV transmission by an HIV-infected health care provider is small. HIV-infected caregivers who do not perform invasive procedures and who adhere to standard precautions pose no transmission risk.

9. Rationales: _____
_____

Expected outcome 3

The patient will not experience AIDS-associated manifestations during pregnancy, such as secondary opportunistic infections, lympadenopathy, night sweats, or a falling CD4 count.

Interventions

1. Determine the estimated date of confinement, and correlate it with the patient's history and clinical profile. Perform routine prenatal testing as well as hepatitis B, cytomegalovirus, and toxoplasmosis tests.

2. Evaluate the patient's CD4 count.

3. Assess for fatigue, malaise, heartburn, anorexia, weight loss, increased temperature, night sweats, bleeding and swollen gums, nasal congestion, shortness of breath, and emotional lability. Relate your findings to the patient's CD4 count.

Rationales

1. Cell-mediated immunity is somewhat suppressed during normal pregnancy. HIV-infected patients may become symptomatic at any point. The benefits of HIV treatment must be balanced against possible health risks to the fetus. Except during advanced stages of HIV disease, pregnancy does not appear to influence the course of HIV infection or hasten its progression. HIV infection in seropositive, asymptomatic women does not seem to increase the risk of complications during pregnancy or result in preterm or low-birth-weight infants. Little data exists on the risks of fetal HIV infection. The rates of vertical perinatal transmission of HIV from mother to infant range from 13% to 30%. Infants of HIV-positive women may test positive for HIV antibodies for up to 18 months.

2. CD4 counts drop dramatically (by up to 50%) within months of initial HIV infection, although great variation exists among patients. As the CD4 count decreases, the risk and severity of opportunistic infection increase.

3. These signs and symptoms are associated both with normal pregnancy and with HIV-associated illnesses, possibly complicating assessment and diagnosis. CD4 counts are indicators of immune dysfunction and HIV progression. Clinical manifestations and CD4 counts serve as guides to management.

4. Assess the patient's history for a 1- to 2-week episode of fever, malaise, rash, arthralgia, and generalized lymphadenopathy; correlate the results with physical findings.

5. Review dates and results of Pap smears, colposcopic examinations, and colposcopically directed biopsy.

6. Review symptoms and perform a complete physical examination. Include eyes, ears, nose, and throat and respiratory, integumentary, neurologic, GI, and gynecologic systems.

7. Assess for pyrexia, chest tightness, shortness of breath, cough, and dyspnea on exertion.

8. Assess for genital discomfort, lesions, discharge, erythema, edema, excoriation, and fissures as well as for abdominal and pelvic pain. Obtain culture specimens for gonorrhea and *Chlamydia*. Perform the Venereal Disease Research Laboratory test for syphilis.

9. Assess the patient's cognition, emotional condition, and motor and sensory function. Note complaints of headache, lethargy, confusion, weakness, and paresthesia and any motor or sensory deficits.

10. Perform a tuberculin skin test (purified protein derivative), and obtain smears and culture specimens, as indicated. Relate response time to anergy and HIV status.

11. Refer the HIV-infected pregnant patient to a facility with staff expertise in HIV disease management.

12. Additional individualized interventions: _____

4. These signs and symptoms may indicate acute retroviral seroconversion syndrome. After the syndrome resolves, the patient typically becomes a seropositive, asymptomatic HIV carrier. Generalized lymphadenopathy persists and the CD4 count continues to fall. A patient with a CD4 count below 500 µl is a candidate for PCP prophylaxis. The patient with a CD4 count below 200 µl or a CD4 percentage below 14% has severe immunosuppression and should receive PCP prophylaxis. All HIV-infected women should receive zidovudine, regardless of their CD4 count, because it decreases the risk of transmitting HIV to the fetus and slows the progression of maternal HIV. Aerosolized pentamidine (NebuPent) generally is effective, and its low therapeutic serum levels make it relatively safe for the fetus. Oral trimethoprim-sulfamethoxazole (Bactrim) may be given, but adverse effects include fetal malformations. No antiviral drug is safe during pregnancy.

5. False-negative cytologic findings are more common in HIV-infected women than in those who are not infected. Colposcopic testing is indicated if the patient has abnormal or inconclusive Pap test results. The prevalence of cervical dysplasia is higher and the course of cervical neoplasia more aggressive in HIV-infected women. Invasive cervical carcinoma is an AIDS indicator disease.

6. HIV infection leads to a wide range of pathologic conditions, as indicated by the conditions listed in the CDC case definition.

7. Recurrent acute pneumonia or pulmonary tuberculosis may indicate AIDS. PCP is the most common serious opportunistic infection in HIV-positive women.

8. Herpes, syphilis, and other STDs may promote sexual transmission of HIV. Manifestations of PID may be atypical. Recurrent candidiasis is common and highly resistant to treatment; its presence portends severe opportunistic infection. HIV-related thrush and unexplained fever may increase the risk of PCP.

9. Neurologic manifestations may indicate HIV infection or be associated with late-stage syphilis. Altered sensorium and emotional lability also may indicate drug use.

10. Tuberculosis (TB) is an AIDS indicator disease. The risk of developing active TB increases when TB and HIV coexist.

11. Health care management for HIV disease is highly specialized and requires a focused multidisciplinary team to address a broad range of physical and psychosocial problems.

12. Rationales: _____

NURSING DIAGNOSIS

Knowledge deficit related to modes of HIV transmission

Expected outcome

The patient will receive information about HIV transmission.

Interventions

1. Review the patient's medical history, sexual orientation and practices, drug use, educational background, and cultural influences.

2. Help the patient develop a personalized risk assessment.

3. Provide information in a clear, nonjudgmental manner. Use language that is comfortable and familiar to the patient. Allow time for questions. Clarify written materials, and repeat instructions as often as necessary.

4. Provide the following information on sexual options:
• Sexual abstinence or a long-term monogamous relationship with a faithful, uninfected partner is the best protection against AIDS. Emphasize that neither partner can have a history of I.V. drug abuse and that both must refrain from subsequent I.V. drug abuse.
• Safer sexual practices include dry kissing and nongenital touching and masturbation.
• Possibly safer sex practices include consistent and correct use of a latex condom throughout vaginal or anal intercourse and during oral sex.
• Risky sexual practices include wet (open-mouth) kissing, oral sex on females, oral sex on males without a condom, and the use of alcohol, marijuana, amyl nitrate, amphetamines, or other mind-altering substances during sexual relations.
• High-risk practices include vaginal or anal intercourse without a condom; recipient role in anal sex; rimming; fisting; sharing of sex toys; any practice in which body fluids come in contact with the partner or with open or abraded skin; and sharing of I.V. needles and syringes.

5. Discourage high-risk or HIV-positive women from breast-feeding.

6. Discourage high-risk women from donating blood or organs for transplantation.

Rationales

1. This information helps create a physiologic profile and database for patient teaching. A patient-centered approach promotes receptivity to learning.

2. The patient who actively participates in developing her own risk assessment is more likely to comply with risk-reduction behaviors.

3. The devastating implications of an AIDS diagnosis may impede the patient's receptivity to health teaching. Providing complete, carefully explained information on HIV disease progression and control, behavior modification, and human sexuality and taking into account the patient's cultural influences and local mores can help the patient begin to understand and cope with the disease.

4. This information clearly defines various sexual practices and their consequences. Modification of sexual behavior is critical to reducing the risk of HIV transmission.

5. HIV has been isolated in breast milk and may be implicated in disease transmission.

6. Blood and tissues may harbor HIV. Blood and blood products are the most efficient agents of viral transmission.

7. Explain to the HIV-positive patient the importance of taking zidovudine as ordered during pregnancy and delivery to decrease the chance of passing HIV to her child.

8. Additional individualized interventions: _____
_____

7. Understanding that taking zidovudine can significantly decrease the chance of passing on HIV may increase compliance.

8. Rationales: _____
_____

Nursing diagnosis

Ineffective individual coping related to AIDS diagnosis and its implications

Expected outcome

The patient will exhibit positive coping, such as actively asking questions, using a support network, and discussing her HIV status.

Interventions

1. Assess the patient's coping abilities, taking into account verbal and nonverbal responses and the patient's interaction with family, friends, and health care workers.

2. Explore the patient's understanding of her condition and (if applicable) of pregnancy.

3. Maintain a nonjudgmental approach. Accept the patient's response to her illness. Ensure confidentiality.

4. Provide the patient with options for care and, as appropriate, help her make choices about care. Make referrals, as appropriate.

5. Additional individualized interventions: _____
_____

Rationales

1. Assessment identifies sources of strength and possible avenues of reinforcement.

2. The rates for pregnancy termination and repeat pregnancies are similar in HIV-infected and uninfected women. The meaning of pregnancy, the patient's health status, drug use, cultural and religious influences, perception of risk, and access to health care are factors in decisions about health care.

3. Fear of abandonment, violence from one's partner, family disruption, debilitation, disfigurement, and impending death may trigger various emotional reactions.

4. Confusion, denial, passivity, dependency, powerlessness, and low frustration tolerance — when coupled with great anxiety — may signal limited coping ability. Support groups, family counselors, and financial and religious or pastoral counselors may provide significant support.

5. Rationales: _____
_____

Documentation checklist

During clinic visits, document:
❒ patient status and assessment findings
❒ changes in patient status since the last clinic visit
❒ pertinent laboratory and diagnostic findings
❒ nutritional intake
❒ the patient's response to treatment
❒ the patient's and family's reaction to illness or threat of illness
❒ patient and family teaching guidelines
❒ follow-up planning guidelines.

Associated plans and appendices

❒ Acquired immunodeficiency syndrome — infant
❒ Aspects of psychological care — maternal (appendix D)
❒ Selected methods of family planning (appendix F)
❒ Overview of isolation precautions (appendix K)

Additional nursing diagnoses

❒ Hopelessness related to projected mortality associated with AIDS diagnosis
❒ Noncompliance with sexual prophylaxis related to denial of condition, fear of abandonment, or altered sensorium secondary to illicit drug use
❒ Risk for maternal infection secondary to HIV status
❒ Spiritual distress related to perceived guilt associated with sexual practices

Ectopic pregnancy

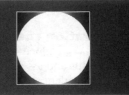

DEFINITION

Ectopic pregnancy is the implantation of the fertilized ovum outside the uterine cavity. The most common site of implantation is the fallopian tube, generally the right one. Other possible sites include the interstitium, the tubo-ovarian ligament, an ovary, the abdominal cavity, and the external cervical os.

Ectopic pregnancy is second only to spontaneous abortion as a primary cause of bleeding in the first trimester, and presenting symptoms and diagnosis typically occur within that period. After implantation, amenorrhea and the nausea and vomiting associated with pregnancy may occur. Slight vaginal bleeding (spotting), adnexal fullness, and unilateral or bilateral cramping and tenderness associated with an unruptured ectopic pregnancy may occur. When the thin, relatively inelastic fallopian tube can no longer accommodate the growing fetus, rupture becomes inevitable. The extent of bleeding depends on the size and number of ruptured vessels. Blood from eroded vessels and the products of conception spill into the pelvic or peritoneal cavity. Complications include hemorrhage, shock, and peritonitis. Ectopic pregnancy may require surgical intervention. Methotrexate is now given for ectopic pregnancies to arrest cell division in the embryo and allow the body to reabsorb it. Success is evidenced by a return to human chorionic gonadotropin (HCG) baseline levels.

Rarely, an abdominal pregnancy may be carried to term. Delivery is accomplished through a laparotomy; the umbilical cord is cut and the placenta left in place, where it will be absorbed by the viscera to which it is attached.

Etiology and precipitating factors
• Any condition that impedes or prevents the passage of the fertilized ovum from the ovary through the fallopian tube to the uterus may result in an ectopic pregnancy. Such conditions include endosalpingitis, pelvic inflammatory disease (PID), diverticula, adhesions (especially from endometriosis or puerperal infection), tumors, tubal surgery, hormonal factors, tubal infection, and scarring resulting from intrauterine devices (IUDs), sexually transmitted disease (STD), or induced abortion.

Physical findings
Cardiovascular
• Occasional tachycardia
• Hypotension
• Vertigo
• Syncope
• Diaphoresis
• Pallor
Gastrointestinal
• Diarrhea
• Possibly nausea and vomiting
• Cullen's sign (periumbilical ecchymoses)
Genitourinary
• Amenorrhea or abnormal menses followed by spotting or cramping; bleeding may be mistaken for menses
• Scant, dark brown vaginal bleeding
• Increased uterine size: nearly the same size as gestational age would warrant during first 3 months
• Unilateral or bilateral pelvic tenderness or pain, notably on movement of the cervix during pelvic examination ("chandelier effect")
• Palpable mass on the fallopian tube or in the cul-de-sac on pelvic examination
• Asymmetrical uterus in interstitial pregnancy
• Pelvic distention or feeling of fullness
• Sudden and acute abdominal or pelvic pain; referred shoulder or neck pain; rebound tenderness and guarding

Diagnostic studies
• Accurate and complete history and physical examination furnish enough data for a tentative diagnosis.
• Beta-subunit assay for HCG has low or falling levels.
• White blood cell (WBC) count may increase.
• Red blood cell (RBC) count decreases.
• Hemoglobin (Hb) level and hematocrit (HCT) decrease.
• Erythrocyte sedimentation rate (ESR) may increase.
• Ultrasonography may reveal extrauterine pregnancy or absence of intrauterine pregnancy.
• Culdocentesis (fluid aspirate from the vaginal cul-de-sac) reveals nonclotting blood.
• Laparoscopy visualizes extrauterine pregnancy and enlarged or ruptured fallopian tube.

COLLABORATIVE PROBLEM

Fluid volume deficit related to bleeding (two expected outcomes)

Expected outcome 1

The patient will experience no fluid volume deficit as evidenced by good urine output, good skin turgor, moist mucous membranes, and urine specific gravity within normal limits.

Interventions

1. Assess bleeding every 30 minutes or as the patient's condition warrants:
• Monitor vital signs.

• Assess vaginal bleeding, including color of blood and number of perineal pads used, their degree of saturation, and odor; confirm date of last menstrual period.

2. Monitor blood studies.

3. Additional individualized interventions: _____
_____

Rationales

1. Blood loss affects fluid balance.

• Vital signs may remain within normal limits initially. Careful evaluation of vital signs and cardiopulmonary status is critical because bleeding is internal and the extent of actual blood loss is not evident. Tachycardia, hypotension, tachypnea, and restlessness signal intense blood loss and resulting shock.
• Scant, dark red vaginal blood in suspected or confirmed early pregnancy, accompanied by abdominal or pelvic pain and a palpable mass on the fallopian tube or in the cul-de-sac, is consistent with a diagnosis of ectopic pregnancy. (*Note:* One saturated pad equals about 100 ml of blood loss.)

2. A falling RBC count, Hb level, and HCT are consistent with blood loss. Accurate assessment helps determine replacement needs.

3. Rationales: _____
_____

Expected outcome 2

The patient will return to and maintain a normovolemic state.

Interventions

1. Administer an I.V. infusion of a prescribed solution using a large-bore needle; draw blood for typing and crossmatching and Rh determination.

2. Administer blood products, as ordered.

Rationales

1. The patient should receive fluids while waiting for typing and crossmatching of blood products. Before surgery, she should not receive food and oral fluids. An Rh-negative, nonsensitized mother with an Rh-positive or unknown Rh conceptus will require an injection of $Rh_o(D)$ immune globulin (RhoGAM) within 72 hours of abortion to prevent isoimmunization.

2. Large volumes of blood products may be required to replace loss.

3. Prepare the patient for surgery:
• Monitor trends of vital signs and results of laboratory testing, and refer to the doctor as necessary.
• Assist in obtaining informed consents.
• Assist with physical preparation.

4. Additional individualized interventions: _____

3. Continual monitoring screens for and rules out other disorders that share similar signs and symptoms, such as appendicitis, salpingitis, ovarian torsion, ruptured corpus luteum, ovarian cyst, and uterine abortion. Laparotomy may be necessary to confirm the diagnosis of ectopic pregnancy. Surgical intervention varies with the location of the gestational sac; a salpingectomy — removal of the affected tube — may be performed as part of laparotomy. Every attempt is made to conserve the ovaries. The products of conception are removed and the bleeding controlled.

4. Rationales: _____

NURSING DIAGNOSIS

Risk for infection related to the trauma of tubal rupture and peritoneal inflammation

Expected outcome

The patient will show no signs of infection as evidenced by temperature and vital signs within normal limits, WBC count and ESR within normal limits, and no increase in pain or discomfort.

Interventions

1. Monitor the patient's vital signs.

2. Monitor WBC count and ESR.

3. Assess for pain trends and their characteristics. Administer analgesics cautiously, but do not withhold.

4. Additional individualized interventions: _____

Rationales

1. The patient's temperature may be low, normal, or elevated to 100.4° F (38° C). Pyrexia is consistent with generalized infection, and a temperature greater than 100.4° F may distinguish salpingitis from ruptured tubal pregnancy. The patient should receive prophylactic antibiotic therapy before and after surgery and appropriate antibiotics for any actual infection.

2. An ESR within normal limits is consistent with early or unruptured ectopic pregnancy. Increases occur in ruptured ectopic pregnancy. A transient, moderately elevated WBC count is associated with the trauma of rupture. Levels usually return to normal within 24 hours. Persistently elevated WBC count may signal infection as well as PID.

3. Analgesics may mask as well as alleviate the pain of intraperitoneal rupture and subsequent peritonitis. Scrupulous attention should be paid to abdominal size and tension and guarding. Cullen's sign may be visible.

4. Rationales: _____

NURSING DIAGNOSIS

Pain related to disruption of pelvic tissue

Expected outcome

The patient will experience less pain as evidenced by verbalization of decreasing pain levels and reduced need for pain medication.

Interventions

1. Assess for pain, including its quality, frequency, location, and intensity.

2. Establish a rapport with the patient and her partner. Call the patient by her preferred name, and do not leave her unattended for long periods.

3. Minimize distracting environmental stimuli.

4. Perform comfort measures, including position changes, relaxation techniques, and massage and effleurage, and administer pharmacologic analgesia, as ordered.

5. Additional individualized interventions: _____

Rationales

1. A pain profile may help in forming the medical diagnosis.

2. A positive relationship builds trust and decreases anxiety, which can in turn decrease regressive behaviors, anger, resistance, and noncompliance.

3. External stimuli may tend to increase the perception of pain, and interruptions of rest periods sap the patient's emotional reserve.

4. Increased tissue perfusion and stimulation of afferent fibers decrease sensation or perception of pain.

5. Rationales: _____

NURSING DIAGNOSIS

Fear related to loss of pregnancy and threat to fertility

Expected outcome

The patient will express less fear.

Interventions

1. Provide information in a clear, forthright manner, and ascertain the patient's understanding of the information.

2. Be supportive and nonjudgmental. Accept the patient's emotional response, and allow her to cope in the manner she has established for herself.

3. Teach the patient how to minimize the risk of ectopic pregnancy:
• Seek prompt treatment for genital infections and PID (the risk of ectopic pregnancy increases in a patient with confirmed PID or a history of fallopian tube surgery).
• Avoid IUD use (IUDs may contribute to the development of ectopic pregnancy).

Rationales

1. Open communication gives the patient a sense of control and helps decrease her fear. Understanding that rupture of the ectopic pregnancy leads to fetal death can help the patient begin the grieving process.

2. Because ectopic pregnancy may result from STD and resulting PID, the patient may perceive it as a punishment for dysfunctional relationships or sexual indiscretions.

3. The patient needs to understand how to decrease the risk of a future ectopic pregnancy. Discussion of these measures to reduce (not prevent) the incidence of ectopic pregnancy should be deferred until the patient's condition stabilizes, her pain is controlled, and her receptivity to teaching is demonstrated.

4. Additional individualized interventions: _____ | **4.** Rationales: _____

_____ | _____

Documentation checklist

During the hospital stay, document:
- ☐ patient status and assessment findings on admission
- ☐ any changes in patient status, especially signs of infection
- ☐ pertinent laboratory and diagnostic findings
- ☐ amount and color of blood loss
- ☐ pain characteristics— quality, location, frequency, and intensity
- ☐ the patient's response to treatment
- ☐ the patient's and family's response to pregnancy loss and future fertility
- ☐ patient and family teaching guidelines
- ☐ discharge planning guidelines.

Associated plans and appendices

- ☐ Normal antepartum
- ☐ Sepsis neonatorum and infectious disorders
- ☐ Aspects of psychological care — maternal (appendix D)
- ☐ Preparing for nonemergency surgery (appendix E)

Additional nursing diagnoses

- ☐ Ineffective breathing pattern related to abdominal incision
- ☐ Ineffective family coping, compromised, related to loss of fetus and possible infertility
- ☐ Ineffective individual coping related to loss of fetus and possible infertility
- ☐ Powerlessness related to loss of fetus and possible infertility
- ☐ Sexual dysfunction related to pelvic tenderness

Hyperemesis gravidarum

DEFINITION

Hyperemesis gravidarum is pernicious or malignant nausea or vomiting associated with pregnancy. Unlike morning sickness — transient nausea or vomiting that typically occurs during the first trimester — hyperemesis gravidarum is severe and unremitting and may persist past the first trimester. Left untreated, it can progress to dehydration, starvation, electrolyte and acid-base imbalances, liver damage, and hemorrhagic retinitis, which carries a high maternal mortality risk. The disorder must be treated before fetal or significant maternal injury results. With appropriate treatment, the prognosis is usually good.

Etiology and precipitating factors

• Coincident with elevated human chorionic gonadotropin levels of pregnancy as well as even higher levels associated with multiple pregnancy or hydatidiform mole
• Hypoglycemia resulting from altered carbohydrate metabolism early in pregnancy
• Hyperthyroidism
• Psychological factors

Physical findings
Cardiovascular
• Tachycardia
• Hypotension
• Vertigo
• Syncope
Gastrointestinal
• Severe nausea
• Marked emesis
• Mucosal bleeding
• Ptyalism

Genitourinary
• Oliguria
• Ketonuria
Integumentary
• Pale, dry skin; decreased turgor
• Dry mucous membranes and lips
• Sunken eyeballs
• Jaundice
Metabolic
• Low-grade fever
• Weight aberration (failure to gain weight or actual weight loss)
• Fruity breath
Neurologic
• Lethargy
• Confusion
• Somnolence
• Polyneuritis or peripheral neuropathy
Subjective
• Sour taste in mouth
• Sensation of thirst

Diagnostic studies
• An accurate and complete history and a physical examination are necessary to differentiate from the transient discomfort of early pregnancy and to rule out other conditions that may cause vomiting.
• Potassium, sodium, chloride, and protein levels decrease.
• Blood urea nitrogen, nonprotein nitrogen, and uric acid levels increase.
• Hemoglobin (Hb) level and hematocrit (HCT) increase.
• Urinalysis reveals ketones and, possibly, protein; urine specific gravity increases.
• Vitamin levels decrease.
• Thyroid-stimulating hormone, thyroxine, and triiodothyronine levels increase.

NURSING DIAGNOSIS

Altered nutrition: less than body requirements related to nausea, emesis, and subsequent inconsistent or insufficient food intake (four expected outcomes)

Expected outcome 1

The patient will exhibit no signs of altered nutritional status as evidenced by no weight loss, positive weight gain, and use of all four food groups and calorie intake guidelines during pregnancy.

Interventions

1. Weigh the patient at each prenatal clinic visit; if she is hospitalized, weigh her daily. Use the same scale, weigh her at same time of day, and make sure she is wearing the same type of clothing. Note patterns of weight gain.

2. Monitor the patient's intake by asking her to recall her diet over the past 24 hours.

3. Assess the patient for edema, noting tight or constrictive shoes, reports of feeling bloated, and benign, dependent leg edema.

4. Assess for ketones in urine.

5. Additional individualized interventions: _____
_____

Rationales

1. Consistency ensures accurate measurements and minimizes diurnal variation. A total gain of 25 to 35 lb (11 to 16 kg) is optimal for fetal growth and maternal changes. The patient should gain from 2 to 4 lb (1 to 2 kg) for the first trimester and about 9/10 lb (0.4 kg) per week for the remainder of the pregnancy.

2. A 24-hour diet recall provides a database for assessment.

3. Edema may mask a true failure to gain weight. Weight gain should reflect maternal and fetal growth, not retained excess fluid.

4. Ketonuria is a sign that stored reserves are being used for all growth and is associated with fetal brain damage.

5. Rationales: _____
_____

Expected outcome 2

The patient will express minimal discomfort from the nausea and vomiting of morning sickness.

Interventions

1. Monitor the patient for morning sickness, which typically causes nausea that lasts from the first missed period to the end of the 3rd month. The nausea may be accompanied by vomiting and may be more intense on arising and aggravated by fatigue. It usually resolves spontaneously at the beginning of the 4th month.

2. Provide nonmedical methods to minimize symptoms, including:
• a high-protein bedtime snack
• dry carbohydrates 30 minutes before rising
• a delay in mealtime until nausea has subsided, but no skipping of meals
• no fluids with meals
• frequent small meals rather than three large ones
• no greasy, spicy, gas-forming foods or foods that have a strong aroma
• no periods of more than 12 hours without eating.

3. Use all prescription and over-the-counter antiemetic drugs with caution.

4. Additional individualized interventions: _____
_____

Rationales

1. Morning sickness may result from hormonal changes, maternal hypoglycemia, and decreased gastric motility as well as from fatigue, emotional factors, and cultural expectations.

2. Palliative treatment focuses on minimizing both stressors and maternal hypoglycemia.

3. Many drugs have teratogenic effects in pregnancy, notably early in pregnancy.

4. Rationales: _____
_____

Expected outcome 3

The patient will report signs of pronounced or protracted emesis to a health care provider.

Interventions

1. Assess emesis, noting its onset, frequency, and duration; the time of day it occurs; its relation to intake; and precipitating and alleviating factors. For each occurrence, also note the color, amount, and consistency of the vomitus and the presence of undigested food, mucus, blood, or bile.

2. Assess the patient's abdomen every 2 hours or as her condition warrants, including size, contour, and bowel sounds; note pain, tenderness, and guarding. Also assess vital signs.

3. Additional individualized interventions: _____

Rationales

1. Vomiting may result in loss of acidic gastric contents or lower GI alkaline products; proper assessment is essential to reverse developing acid-base and electrolyte imbalances.

2. Accurate assessment can help diagnose various disorders that cause vomiting, including liver disease, kidney infection, pancreatitis, GI obstruction or lesions, drug toxicity, and intracranial lesions.

3. Rationales: _____

Expected outcome 4

The patient will achieve and maintain adequate nutrition as evidenced by no weight loss, positive weight gain, and serum (blood) chemistries within normal limits.

Intervention

1. Administer peripheral parenteral nutrition (PPN) through a peripherally inserted central catheter (PICC) line, as ordered.

2. Weigh the patient daily if hospitalized, or at each visit. Using the same scale, weigh her at the same time of day, making sure she is wearing the same type of clothing. Note patterns of weight gain.

3. Additional individualized interventions: _____

Rationale

1. When needed, PPN allows the GI tract to rest while the patient receives adequate nutrition. Inserting a PICC line is less invasive than inserting a central line, and administering PPN through a PICC line poses less risk of such complications as sepsis and clots.

2. Consistent weighing protocol ensures adequate measurement and minimizes diurnal variation.

3. Rationales: _____

COLLABORATIVE PROBLEM

Fluid volume deficit related to protracted emesis (two expected outcomes)

Expected outcome 1

The patient will experience no fluid volume deficit as evidenced by positive urine output, moist mucous membranes, urine specific gravity within normal limits, and good skin turgor.

Interventions

1. Monitor the patient for signs and symptoms of fluid volume deficit, including:
• dry skin with poor turgor and dry mucous membranes
• sunken eyeballs
• concentrated urine and oliguria
• malaise
• hypotension, vertigo, and syncope.

2. Assess Hb level and HCT.

3. Additional individualized interventions: _____

Rationales

1. Fluid volume deficit interferes with homeostatic mechanisms and threatens maternal and fetal well-being.

2. Increased Hb level and HCT may indicate hemoconcentration.

3. Rationales: _____

Expected outcome 2

The patient will return to and maintain a normovolemic state, have fewer episodes of vomiting, and maintain optimal nutrition.

Interventions

1. Restrict all oral intake for 24 to 48 hours.

2. Administer a balanced I.V. solution that contains electrolytes, glucose, and vitamins.

3. Permit the patient to progress to a normal diet after she has not vomited for 24 hours. If she starts vomiting after any of the following steps, revert to the previous step:
• Begin with clear fluids (an electrolyte solution, not plain water), not to exceed 100 ml, alternated every 1 to 1½ hours with dry toast or crackers.
• Progress to a soft diet.
• Progress to a regular diet; all portions should be small (six or seven meals per day) and well prepared.

4. Additional individualized interventions: _____

Rationales

1. Restriction allows the patient's stomach to rest and irritated gastric mucosa to heal.

2. This solution provides fluids to reverse fluid deficits and corrects acid-base imbalances, altered electrolyte levels, and hypovitaminosis.

3. Careful and slow introduction of food is usually effective.

4. Rationales: _____

NURSING DIAGNOSIS

Fear related to hospitalization and pregnancy outcome

Expected outcome

The patient will express less fear.

Interventions

1. Accept the patient's verbal and nonverbal responses to illness.

2. Provide information in a clear, forthright manner, and allow the patient to ask questions.

3. Be supportive and nonjudgmental. Accept the patient's emotional response, and allow her to cope in the manner she has established for herself.

4. Provide information on counseling, and refer the patient to the appropriate health care professionals, if necessary.

5. Inform the family and the patient's partner of her condition, especially because visitors are limited in early hospitalization.

6. Additional individualized interventions: _____

Rationales

1. Acceptance promotes communication and trust.

2. Open communication gives the patient a sense of control and helps decrease her fear. The severity and duration of the disorder helps determine the outcome of the pregnancy; once controlled, the disorder usually does not recur.

3. The patient may need to initiate anticipatory grieving over the pregnancy, which may result in a low-birth-weight infant.

4. Counseling may help the patient deal with reactions to stress or ambivalence she may feel about the pregnancy, both of which may play a significant role in the cause of the disorder.

5. Family interaction bolsters the patient's established support systems.

6. Rationales: _____

NURSING DIAGNOSIS

Pain related to repeated episodes of vomiting

Expected outcome

The patient will express less pain.

Interventions

1. Provide a clean, odor-free environment. Keep an emesis basin and bedpan out of sight but within reach. Keep the dietary food cart away from the patient's room. Remove the patient's tray as soon as possible after she has finished her meal.

2. Provide mouth care before each meal and snack and after each episode of vomiting.

3. Place the patient in high Fowler's position or seated upright for 30 minutes after each meal.

4. Additional individualized interventions: _____

Rationales

1. Some odors may trigger vomiting.

2. Good oral hygiene contributes to the patient's comfort and sense of well-being. Mouth care after emesis minimizes acid contact with teeth.

3. This position minimizes gastric reflux.

4. Rationales: _____

Documentation checklist

During the hospital stay or clinic visit, document:
❑ patient status and assessment findings on admission or entry to the clinic
❑ any changes in patient status, especially in fluid volume
❑ pertinent laboratory and diagnostic findings
❑ nutritional intake
❑ weight changes
pain characteristics — quality, location, frequency, and intensity
❑ the patient's response to treatment
❑ the patient's and family's response to pregnancy outcome
❑ patient and family teaching guidelines
❑ discharge planning guidelines, if applicable.

Associated plans and appendices

❑ Normal antepartum
❑ Selected daily dietary allowances — maternal (appendix B)
❑ Aspects of psychological care — maternal (appendix D)

Additional nursing diagnoses

❑ Constipation related to inadequate food intake
❑ Impaired home maintenance management related to debilitating emesis and subsequent generalized paresis
❑ Sensory/perceptual alterations (gustatory) related to persistent emesis

Multiple gestation

DEFINITION

Multiple gestation is the concurrent development of two or more embryos in utero. The fertilization of two separate ova results in dizygotic, or fraternal, twins; the fertilization of a single ovum that splits and gives rise to two embryos results in monozygotic, or identical, twins. Concurrent development of more than two fetuses involves either or both of the fertilization processes. Zygosity is usually established by postpartum examination of the placenta and membranes. Management of multiple gestation—primarily bed rest—aims to delay the onset of labor and the delivery of preterm infants, at least until the fetal lungs have sufficiently matured. Nontraumatic delivery of viable infants is of prime concern. Maternal complications include exaggerated discomforts of pregnancy, anemia, hydramnios, pregnancy-induced or pregnancy-aggravated hypertension, placenta previa, abruptio placentae, umbilical cord accidents, preterm delivery with a complicated labor, postpartum hemorrhage, possible coagulopathy, and spontaneous abortion and death of the fetus or the mother. Implications for the fetus include congenital malformation (more common in monozygotic twins), death in utero of one fetus, shunting of blood between placentas, restricted intrauterine growth or discordant growth, premature birth and subsequent low birth weight, and respiratory impairment.

Etiology and precipitating factors

• Monozygotic twinning is a random occurrence essentially unrelated to heredity, age, race, parity, or treatment for infertility.
• Dizygotic twinning is affected by these factors, revealed by a frequency profile:
  – race (higher rates in Blacks; lower rates in Asians)
  – women who were dizygotic twins carry an autosomal recessive genotype
  – increased maternal age and parity (age 35 or older; parity of more than four)
  – elevated level of endogenous follicle-stimulating hormone implicated
  – use of agents to treat infertility, such as gonadotropin or clomiphene citrate (Clomid), commonly results in ovulation of multiple ova.

Physical findings
Genitourinary
• Uterine size greater than gestational age would warrant
• Palpation of a large number of fetal parts on all sides of the abdomen
• Distinct, asynchronous fetal heart tones (FHT) at or after 20 weeks' gestation

Diagnostic studies
• Ultrasonography reveals separate gestational sacs.

NURSING DIAGNOSIS

Risk for maternal and fetal injury related to physiologic demands of a multifetal pregnancy (two expected outcomes)

Expected outcome 1

The patient will experience no maternal or fetal injury related to the multiple pregnancy as evidenced by positive prenatal care, stable vital signs, and no signs of fetal distress.

Interventions

1. Note date of last menstrual period and maternal history. Monitor weight, fundal height, FHT, and multiple areas of fetal activity at each clinic visit.

2. Additional individualized interventions: _____

Rationales

1. Early management of a multifetal pregnancy can decrease perinatal mortality and morbidity.

2. Rationales: _____

Expected outcome 2

The patient will experience minimal physiologic stress from the multifetal pregnancy as evidenced by positive fetal growth, positive maternal weight gain, and no complaints of excessive fatigue or other problems.

Interventions

1. Counsel the patient about increased dietary requirements, including:
• an intake of 300 kcal/day more than the typical intake of a woman pregnant with one fetus
• an increased protein intake up to 1.5 g/kg of body weight
• iron supplementation of 60 to 100 mg/day
• vitamin and mineral supplementation.

2. Encourage multiple small meals.

3. Weigh the patient at each clinic visit.

4. Counsel the patient about increased rest needs, suggesting that she get 10 hours of sleep per night and 2 hours per afternoon. The patient may be hospitalized as early as the beginning of the third trimester.

5. Additional individualized interventions: _____

_____

Rationales

1. Increased resting metabolic rate, fetal mass, and maternal changes require additional calories to support growth and activity. Extra protein is needed for fetal growth and accessory maternal tissue, especially uterine and placental tissue. Maternal blood volume is about 500 ml greater with twins than with a single-fetus pregnancy.

2. Pressure of the expanding uterus on the stomach may decrease the patient's appetite. Small, frequent meals may promote intake of required foods.

3. Progressive weight gain, uncomplicated by edema, usually indicates an adequate diet. Failure to gain suggests a poor prognosis.

4. Bed rest has been linked to promoting fetal growth, increasing birth weight, and preventing prematurity.

5. Rationales: _____

_____

COLLABORATIVE PROBLEM

Discomfort related to increased uterine size (two expected outcomes)

Expected outcome 1

The patient will express minimal discomfort.

Interventions

1. Counsel the patient on ways to minimize discomfort, such sleeping on her left or right side and placing pillows behind her back, under her stomach, and between her legs to provide support; using a maternity girdle; and wearing thromboembolic stockings.

2. Additional individualized interventions: _____

_____

Rationales

1. Bed rest minimizes mechanical pressure on the lower back. Lying on one's side increases uterine and kidney perfusion, reducing the hypertension to which the patient is prone. The maternity girdle provides muscle support. Pressure of the enlarged uterus on pelvic vessels impedes blood flow to and from the legs; thromboembolic stockings compress superficial leg veins and increase venous return from deep leg veins.

2. Rationales: _____

_____

Expected outcome 2

The patient will be able to verbalize recognition of signs of excessive accumulation of amniotic fluid and the importance of reporting these to a health care provider.

Interventions

1. Monitor fundal height, weight gain unrelated to intake or edema, onset of dyspnea or orthopnea, and signs of obstructive uropathy (oliguria and azotemia) at each clinic visit.

2. Make sure sonography is scheduled every 4 weeks after 20 weeks' gestation. Plot head and chest circumferences.

3. Additional individualized interventions: _____

Rationales

1. Hydramnios may result in preterm labor. Amniocentesis can provide dramatic relief of the patient's symptoms, but the fluid quickly reaccumulates.

2. Serial assessment helps in the recognition of discordant growth.

3. Rationales: _____
_____

NURSING DIAGNOSIS

Risk for injury related to preterm labor and delivery (two expected outcomes)

Expected outcome 1

The patient will exhibit no signs of preterm labor as evidenced by no contractions or bleeding.

Interventions

1. Reinforce the need for rest. Bed rest and hospitalization may be required during the third trimester.

2. Instruct the patient to avoid coitus, nipple stimulation, enemas, and cathartics during the third trimester.

3. Additional individualized interventions: _____

Rationales

1. Bed rest may increase uterine perfusion. Decreased mechanical force on the cervix may delay dilation.

2. These activities may trigger uterine contractions.

3. Rationales: _____
_____

Expected outcome 2

The preterm infant will be delivered safely.

Interventions

1. Confirm the number of fetuses evidenced in sonography.

2. Prepare the patient for vaginal delivery or cesarean section.

Rationales

1. Duration of gestation is inversely proportionate to the number of fetuses. Preparation for delivery includes expert care for each of the infants delivered.

2. Vaginal delivery may be attempted if a cephalic presentation of the presenting twin exists. Cesarean section is indicated with fetal distress, hypotonic uterine dysfunction, placental anomalies, severe hypertension, or marked difference between the size of the fetuses.

3. Notify obstetric and neonatal teams. Have on hand routine delivery room equipment as well as resuscitative equipment for each of the deliveries anticipated. Make sure the equipment is functioning correctly and that supplies are stocked.

4. Additional individualized interventions: _____

_____

3. Preterm delivery of multiple infants requires coordinated, aggressive treatment.

4. Rationales: _____

_____

Nursing diagnosis

Ineffective individual coping related to dramatic increase in family size

Expected outcome

The patient will demonstrate effective coping strategies such as verbalizing concerns and using a support network.

Interventions

1. Accept the patient's response to the pregnancy outcome. Answer any questions she may have directly and honestly. Include the patient's partner in interactions.

2. Provide an opportunity as soon as feasible for handling infants. During the pregnancy, arrange for child care classes that include the care of twins.

3. Assess the patient's support systems. Refer her to social service, as indicated.

4. Refer the patient to a Multiple Mothers support group.

5. Additional individualized interventions: _____

_____

Rationales

1. Each person responds to a pregnancy outcome in her own way. Accepting the patient's response and including her partner increase her ability to cope.

2. Handling promotes maternal-infant bonding. Child care classes help the patient and her partner learn ways to care for multiple infants, providing practice and opportunities for reinforcement.

3. Increased or unexpected family needs may trigger a financial crisis.

4. Members of a Multiple Mothers support group can give the new mother practical tips from their own experiences.

5. Rationales: _____

_____

Documentation checklist

During prenatal visits, document:
❏ family history, including a genetic risk assessment for multigestational pregnancy, a history of previous pregnancies and their outcomes, and assessment findings
❏ patient status of each visit, especially weight and signs of edema or preterm labor
❏ any changes in patient status since the last visit
❏ fundal height, weight, and FHT
❏ pertinent laboratory and diagnostic findings
❏ discomfort characteristics — quality, location, frequency, and intensity
❏ the patient's response to treatment
❏ the patient's and family's response to multifetal pregnancy
❏ follow-up guidelines.

Associated plans and appendices
❏ Cesarean section birth
❏ Inappropriate size or weight: small for gestational age
❏ Normal antepartum
❏ Preterm infant
❏ Aspects of psychological care — maternal (appendix D)
❏ Preparing for nonemergency surgery (appendix E)

Additional nursing diagnoses
❏ Activity intolerance related to anatomic and physiologic demands of multifetal pregnancy
❏ Ineffective breathing pattern related to uterine pressure against the lungs

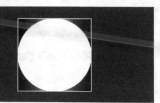

Placenta previa

DEFINITION

In placenta previa, the placenta is attached low in the uterus over or near the internal cervical os. The degrees of placental placement, from least to greatest severity, are:
• low implantation or low-lying placenta, in which the placenta is implanted in the lower uterine segment close to the os
• marginal placenta previa, in which the placenta encroaches on but does not occlude the os
• partial or incomplete placenta previa, in which the placenta partially occludes the os
• total or central placenta previa, in which the placenta completely occludes the os.

Uterine segment differentiation later in pregnancy causes the lower section to lengthen and thin. Placental villi tear, and bleeding occurs from open uterine sinuses. Maternal complications include hemorrhage and shock and may necessitate preterm delivery. There is no associated pain in this third-trimester event unless it is concurrent with the onset of labor.

Confirmed placenta previa associated with minimal vaginal bleeding early in the third trimester may be treated conservatively with bed rest to allow the fetus time to mature. Uncontrolled vaginal bleeding, fetal distress, or loss of fetal viability warrants delivery. Labor may be spontaneous or induced by amniotomy. The mother may deliver vaginally if gestational age is 37 weeks or more, or fetal lung maturity has been established by lecithin-sphingomyelin ratio, the cervix is partially dilated, there is a low presenting fetal part, and bleeding is minimal or controlled. Cesarean section delivery is necessary if the placenta is felt on cervical examination; if the mother has massive, uncontrolled bleeding; or if the fetus is in distress.

Etiology and precipitating factors
• Etiology unknown
• Risk increases with parity, advancing age, multiple gestation, uterine scarring associated with surgery, and erythroblastosis fetalis

Physical findings
Cardiovascular
• Tachycardia
• Hypotension
• Vertigo
• Syncope
• Diaphoresis
• Pallor
• Cyanosis
Genitourinary
• Painless, bright red, scant to profuse vaginal bleeding in third trimester
• Normal uterine tone
• Soft, nontender uterus
• Fetal malpresentation: oblique, breech, or transverse
• Fundal height greater than gestational age would warrant; placenta hindering fetal descent
• Oliguria or anuria
Integumentary
• Cold, moist skin
• Dry mucous membranes
Neurologic
• Restlessness
• Lethargy
• Confusion
• Somnolence
Respiratory
• Tachypnea
Subjective
• Sensation of thirst, cold, apprehension

Diagnostic studies
• Ultrasonography reveals placental implantation site, fetal viability, gestational age, position, and station.
• X-ray studies may reveal soft-tissue density in front of presenting fetal part.
• Isotope scanning or localization locates the placenta.
• Vaginal or rectal examination is contraindicated because manipulation of the cervix may initiate massive bleeding. If patient is at or near term, if labor has begun, or if bleeding threatens maternal welfare, the doctor may perform a vaginal examination in an operating room in which setups for both vaginal and cesarean section deliveries are immediately available.
• Hemoglobin (Hb) level and hematocrit (HCT) decrease.
• Coagulation factors are usually within normal limits.

COLLABORATIVE PROBLEM

Fluid volume deficit related to bleeding (three expected outcomes)

Expected outcome 1

The patient will exhibit no signs of excessive bleeding as evidenced by no large volume of blood passed vaginally and no sharp decrease in Hb level or HCT.

Interventions

1. Assess bleeding every 15 minutes or as the patient's condition warrants:
• Note onset and amount of vaginal bleeding before admission.
• Monitor vaginal bleeding, including color of blood and the number of perineal pads used and their degree of saturation and weight.
• Assess vital signs, capillary refill time, and pulse pressure; compare with baseline.

• Assess fetal heart tones (FHT).

• *Don't* perform vaginal examination.

2. Monitor Hb level and HCT.

3. Additional individualized interventions: _____

Rationales

1. Blood loss may occur at rest or during activity; it may be characterized as spotting, gushing, or continuous.
• Painless, bright red vaginal bleeding in the third trimester characterizes placenta previa.
• Accurate assessment helps estimate blood loss and replacement needs. (*Note:* 1 g of blood by weight equals 1 ml; a saturated pad equals about 100 ml.)
• A decreased refill time in the capillary blanch test indicates decreased peripheral circulation. A narrowing pulse pressure indicates early shock. Maternal hypervolemia and initial compensatory mechanisms may mask signs of shock: tachycardia, hypotension, tachypnea, and restlessness.
• FHT can indicate fetal distress consistent with blood loss.
• Vaginal examination may trigger severe hemorrhage.

2. Decreasing Hb level and HCT are consistent with blood loss.

3. Rationales: _____

Expected outcome 2

The patient will return to and maintain a normovolemic state.

Interventions

1. Maintain hydration.

• Administer an I.V. infusion of lactated Ringer's solution, using a large-bore needle.

• Monitor hourly fluid intake and output.

• Perform central venous pressure (CVP) monitoring.

2. Administer blood products, as ordered.

3. Additional individualized interventions: _____

Rationales

1. Rapid fluid replacement is necessary to correct hypovolemia.
• Fluids and venous access are provided while awaiting typing and crossmatching of blood products. Food and water are withheld in anticipation of delivery.
• The minimum physiologically acceptable urine output is 30 ml/hour. Output reflects renal perfusion.
• Normal CVP readings during pregnancy are 8 to 10 cm H_2O. Readings of 15 to 20 cm H_2O indicate circulatory overload. Monitoring trend response and adjusting I.V. flow rates aid safe, accurate replacement therapy.

2. The patient may need large volumes to replace loss.

3. Rationales: _____

Expected outcome 3

The patient will maintain optimal tissue perfusion as evidenced by good capillary refill, pink nailbeds, no skin mottling, and no complaints of painful or cold extremities.

Interventions

1. Maintain bed rest in the side-lying position.

2. Administer oxygen by mask at 7 to 10 L/minute, as the patient's condition warrants.

3. Additional individualized interventions: _____
_____

Rationales

1. Bed rest decreases physiologic and metabolic demands. The side-lying position promotes blood flow to the uterus and fetus.

2. Supplemental oxygen enhances tissue perfusion at the alveolocapillary membrane.

3. Rationales: _____
_____

COLLABORATIVE PROBLEM

Risk for fetal injury related to uteroplacental insufficiency (two expected outcomes)

Expected outcome 1

The patient will exhibit no signs of fetal distress as evidenced by positive fetal heart rate (FHR) pattern and good variability.

Interventions

1. During each maternal assessment, assess fetal status with electronic fetal monitoring (EFM) and a nonreactive stress test (NST). Note FHR patterns and variability as well as fetal activity; compare with baseline. *Don't* perform a vaginal examination.

2. Additional individualized interventions: _____

Rationales

1. Indications of fetal distress include fetal tachycardia and decreased long-term variability with late decelerations. Continued ominous FHR patterns may lead to cessation of FHR, warranting immediate surgical intervention. (See the "Cesarean section birth" plan, page 96.)

2. Rationales: _____
_____

Expected outcome 2

The preterm infant will be safely delivered.

Interventions

1. Prepare for cesarean section delivery.

2. Notify perinatal team of impending delivery and have operative and resuscitative equipment at hand.

3. Additional individualized interventions: _____
_____

Rationales

1. Prompt delivery of a compromised fetus is critical to its survival.

2. Survival of the preterm infant depends on aggressive resuscitation and sustained intensive care.

3. Rationales: _____
_____

NURSING DIAGNOSIS
Fear related to unknown fetal outcome

Expected outcome
The patient will express less fear.

Interventions

1. Provide information in a clear, forthright manner; ascertain the patient's understanding of the information given.

2. Encourage the presence of significant others. Keep them informed of the patient's progress, and allow phone calls and visits as appropriate.

3. Additional individualized interventions: _____

Rationales

1. Open communication gives the patient a sense of control and helps decrease her fear. Infant survival depends on gestational age and maturity and the amount of blood lost.

2. Interaction with family and friends can give the patient support.

3. Rationales: _____

Documentation checklist
During the hospital stay, document:
❑ patient status and assessment findings on admission
❑ any changes in patient status
❑ pertinent laboratory and diagnostic findings
❑ amount and color of blood loss
❑ fetal status, including signs of fetal distress
❑ patient's and family's response to the diagnosis in relation to fear of fetal outcome
❑ patient and family teaching guidelines
❑ discharge planning guidelines.

Associated plans and appendices
❑ Cesarean section birth
❑ Inappropriate size or weight: small for gestational age
❑ Labor and vaginal birth
❑ Preterm infant
❑ Aspects of psychological care — maternal (appendix D)

Additional nursing diagnoses
❑ Knowledge deficit related to impending emergency surgery
❑ Self-esteem disturbance related to inability to give birth vaginally and to preterm delivery

Pregnancy complicated by cardiac disease

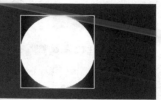

DEFINITION

Anatomic and physiologic changes occur in the cardiovascular system throughout pregnancy. Normal compensatory mechanisms of pregnancy include — but are not limited to — increases in cardiac output, heart rate, and total blood volume. A pregnant patient with a normal, uncompromised cardiovascular system can withstand the stresses of pregnancy, labor, delivery, and the postpartum state. However, the cardiovascular system of a pregnant patient that is already stressed by cardiac disease lacks the reserve to adapt to these changes.

Normal changes of pregnancy — such as functional systolic murmurs, dyspnea, and edema — make diagnosing cardiac disease more difficult. The cardiac disorders most frequently seen during pregnancy are rheumatic heart disease and congenital defects. Ideally, surgical correction of underlying defects takes place before conception, although they may be performed during pregnancy. Obstetric care aims to prevent or minimize complications.

A standardized patient classification system is based on the patient's increasing disability (ranging from class I to class IV) and reflects the functional capacity of the heart. Regardless of the cause of the cardiac disorder, management depends on the patient's classification, taking into account the implications of each classification and the potential for progression from one classification to the next.

The most serious complication, cardiac decompensation may result in spontaneous abortion, fetal growth retardation, preterm delivery, and intrauterine or maternal death. The prognosis is usually good but depends on the functional capacity of the heart, complications that would further stress the already compromised heart, aggressive treatment, and the ability of the patient to comply with the rigid prescribed regimen.

Etiology and precipitating factors
• Rheumatic heart disease; congenital heart defects; syphilis; arteriosclerosis; coronary occlusion; renal, pulmonary, and thyroid disorders; skeletal defects of the spine; and peripartal cardiomyopathy

Physical findings
Cardiovascular
• Vertigo
• Syncope
• Tachycardia
• Pulse irregularities*
• Progressive generalized edema*
• Diastolic, presystolic, or continuous murmur†
• Loud, harsh, systolic murmur, especially if associated with a thrill†
• Severe arrhythmia†
• Unequivocal cardiac enlargement†
Integumentary
• Cyanosis*
Respiratory
• Dyspnea
• Orthopnea*
• Cough, with or without hemoptysis*
• Basilar crackles*
Subjective
• Fatigue, palpitations, feelings of smothering

Diagnostic studies
• X-ray studies may reveal abnormalities in cardiac or vessel size, contour, outline, position, or density; unequivocal cardiac enlargement confirms a diagnosis of cardiovascular disease in pregnancy. (*Note:* The need for X-ray studies must be carefully evaluated; if studies are performed, a lead shield should cover the abdomen and pelvis.)
• Electrocardiography may reveal hypertrophy, arrhythmias, ischemia, conduction defects, heart block, pericarditis, and electrolyte abnormalities.
• Echocardiography may reveal valvular abnormalities, ventricular dysfunction, or other cardiac disorders.
• Phonocardiography may reveal valvular abnormalities and other cardiac disorders.
• Hemoglobin (Hb) level and hematocrit (HCT) may decrease in response to expansion of blood volume (normal ranges from 12 to 15 g/dl and 35% to 45%, respectively); HCT may increase from constant hypoxia.
• White blood cell count increases (normal ranges from 5,000 to 10,000/mm³ in first trimester; 10,000 to 12,000/mm³ by term).
• Clotting factors decrease; depression of fibrinolytic activity occurs during normal pregnancy and postpartum period.
• Serum electrolyte, sodium, and potassium levels increase (normal range of sodium level is 136 to 145 mEq/L and potassium level is 3.5 to 5 mEq/L).

*Presenting signs and symptoms of cardiovascular disease in pregnancy, with other findings normal
†Confirms the diagnosis of cardiovascular disease in pregnancy

COLLABORATIVE PROBLEM

Increased cardiac output related to the physiologic demands of pregnancy on an already-compromised heart (three expected outcomes)

Expected outcome 1

The patient will exhibit no signs of cardiac compromise as evidenced by edema, changes in vital signs outside expected parameters, shortness of breath, or cyanosis.

Interventions

1. Note at each clinic visit and compare with baseline of nonpregnant state:
- blood pressure

- heart rate

- respiratory rate.

2. Assess for benign physiologic edema, including dependent leg edema.

3. Assess for anemia, including decreased Hb level and HCT, pallor, and disproportionately decreased activity tolerance.

4. Coordinate consultation with a cardiologist.

5. Additional individualized interventions: _____

_____

Rationales

1. Ongoing assessment permits timely interventions, if required.
- A decrease of 5 to 10 mm Hg in both systolic and diastolic arterial pressure occurs in the first half of pregnancy and is related to peripheral vasodilation; by the third trimester, values return to earlier levels.
- A gradual increase of 10 to 20 beats/minute occurs between the 14th and 20th week of pregnancy; the increase persists for the remainder of the pregnancy, resulting from increased cardiac output.
- An increase in respiratory rate of about 2 breaths/minute occurs along with increased volume or depth of respiration and is related to increased oxygen demands; a lowered carbon dioxide threshold in response to hormonal changes contributes to feelings of dyspnea.

2. Pooling of fluid in the legs occurs later in pregnancy and results from pressure of the gravid uterus on blood vessels.

3. Hb level and HCT of 10 g/dl and 35%, respectively, indicate anemia. Symptoms result from decreased oxygen availability. Activity intolerance may indicate heart failure.

4. Care of the high-risk pregnant patient requires medical as well as obstetric management.

5. Rationales: _____

_____

Expected outcome 2

The patient will experience fewer stressors that place further demands on cardiac function as evidenced by no signs of infection, increased activity intolerance, or excessive weight gain.

Interventions

1. Advise the patient to get adequate rest. Minimum requirements include:
• 10 hours of sleep every night
• half hour rest period after each meal
• light housework only, with some easy walking permitted
• no lifting or straining
• rest periods after any activity.

2. Teach the patient how to control her diet:

• Make sure weight gain does not exceed the recommended 25 to 35 lb (11 to 16 kg) during the course of pregnancy.
• Limit sodium intake: avoid high-sodium foods, and don't add salt to food or during food preparation.
• Monitor potassium intake, and watch for symptoms of hypokalemia, such as thirst, vertigo, confusion, hypoventilation, muscle weakness, twitching, tetany, and pulse irregularities.
• Monitor iron intake, and know which foods are high in iron.

3. Promote infection control, including prevention of respiratory and urinary tract infections. Take a drug sensitivity history; as ordered, administer penicillin G benzathine (Bicillin L-A), 1.2 million units I.M. each month, to the patient who has a history of rheumatic fever or rheumatic heart disease.

4. Monitor anticoagulant (heparin) therapy, if prescribed, including the following:
• activated partial thromboplastin time (APTT)
• signs of bleeding: petechiae, ecchymosis, hematuria, tarry stools, and bleeding from any orifice.

5. Additional individualized interventions: _____

Rationales

1. Activity intolerance is normal in pregnancy, but rest requirements increase in a pregnancy compromised by cardiac disease. Requirements progress from class I to class IV. A class III or class IV patient requires bed rest and hospitalization for the duration of pregnancy. A class IV patient has decompensation at rest and requires aggressive medical and obstetric care.

2. Dietary control decreases stress on the cardiovascular system.
• Appropriate weight gain promotes optimal fetal growth and maternal changes.

• Excess weight from retained fluid increases the cardiac workload. Sodium intake can increase fluid retention.
• Erratic or decreased potassium levels may be associated with cardiac dysfunction or be an adverse reaction to digitalis therapy.

• Dietary iron requirements of pregnancy are about 18 mg/day with supplementary preparations of 200 mg of simple iron compounds recommended.

3. Infection is implicated in triggering decompensation because it may increase metabolism and contribute to the spread of organisms to cardiac structures. Prophylactic antibiotics may be given to minimize the risk of bacterial endocarditis.

4. Heparin is the drug of choice antepartum because it does not cross the placenta.
• APTT from 1½ to 2½ times the control indicates an acceptable therapeutic anticoagulant range.
• These signs may require decreasing or stopping heparin administration or giving protamine sulfate.

5. Rationales: _____

Expected outcome 3

The patient will exhibit no signs of cardiac decompensation as evidenced by no generalized edema, pulse irregularities, increasing fatigue, or vertigo.

Interventions

1. Assess the following at each clinic visit, every 8 hours during hospitalization, or as the patient's condition warrants:
• patient's perceptions of increasing fatigue, vertigo, difficulty breathing, palpitations, and chest pain
• generalized edema
• persistent basilar crackles, hemoptysis
• pulse irregularities.

Rationales

1. Continual assessment is imperative because the onset of signs and symptoms may be gradual or abrupt. Cardiac decompensation warrants immediate medical intervention; correction is necessary for safe delivery with satisfactory maternal and fetal outcomes.

3. Additional individualized interventions: _____
_____

3. Rationales: _____
_____

COLLABORATIVE PROBLEM

Risk for maternal injury related to increased cardiac workload during labor and delivery

Expected outcome

The patient will experience minimal or no injury and will safely deliver a healthy infant.

Interventions

1. Monitor labor, and take these steps:

• Administer oxygen by mask at 8 to 10 L/minute.

• Withhold heparin just before delivery.

• Administer epidural anesthesia or morphine if delivery is not imminent.
• Administer aqueous penicillin G, gentamicin (Garamycin), or other antibiotics, as ordered.
• Place the patient in a side-lying position, preferably on the left side. Elevate her head and shoulders with pillows.

2. Monitor for cardiac decompensation with each labor assessment, noting a pulse rate greater than 100 beats/minute or a respiratory rate greater than 24 breaths/minute or dyspnea.

3. Assist with treatments for cardiac decompensation, including the following:
• Place the patient in Fowler's position, and administer oxygen by way of intermittent positive pressure.
• Administer furosemide (Lasix) I.V., as ordered.
• Administer digoxin I.V., as ordered.

4. Assist with delivery, including these steps:
• Place the patient in the left lateral or semirecumbent position.
• Do not use stirrups.

• Assist with the administration of anesthesia, possibly epidural anesthesia.
• Teach the patient how to avoid Valsalva's maneuver by using open-glottis pushing.
• Monitor blood pressure.

5. Additional individualized interventions: _____

Rationales

1. Vaginal delivery is the procedure of choice; cesarean section is usually limited to correction of an obstetric emergency.
• Supplemental oxygen enhances perfusion at the alveolocapillary membrane. Oxygen demand increases about 300% during labor.
• The increased risk of hemorrhage associated with labor and delivery precludes anticoagulant use.
• Pain and anxiety increase cardiac workload.

• Antibiotics minimize the risk of bacterial endocarditis and infective arteritis.
• Lying on the side minimizes the risk of supine hypotensive syndrome and facilitates uterine perfusion.

2. These signs, when accompanied by a completely dilated cervix and engaged presenting part, are indicators of delivery. With only partial dilation, cardiac decompensation is diagnosed and will increase with delivery.

3. Fowler's position enhances oxygenation and decreases the potential for pulmonary edema. Stimulation of diuresis will ultimately reduce pulmonary congestion. A rapid-acting cardiac glycoside, such as digoxin, increases the force and effectiveness of the myocardial contraction.

4. Assistance promotes safe delivery.
• These positions enhance cardiac function.

• Venous compression from the stirrups impedes circulation.
• Anesthesia decreases stress from pain.

• Valsalva's maneuver stresses the heart.

• Hypotension associated with anesthesia poses grave maternal risks.

5. Rationales: _____

NURSING DIAGNOSIS

Risk for fetal injury related to uteroplacental insufficiency

Expected outcome

The patient will exhibit no signs of fetal injury as evidenced by positive fetal activity, a reactive nonstress test (NST), and positive fetal heart rate (FHR) patterns.

Interventions

1. Starting in the last half of pregnancy, instruct the patient to count daily fetal movements and to report any sudden decreases in or cessation of movement.

2. Starting at 32 weeks' gestation, perform a NST with each clinic visit.

3. Assess fetal status with each maternal assessment, including FHR patterns and variability and fetal activity. Compare with baseline.

4. Additional individualized interventions: _____

Rationales

1. Fetal activity is highly variable. Consistent movement later in pregnancy is one indicator of fetal health. Sudden decreases in activity may signal fetal jeopardy.

2. A reactive NST (fetal activity with an increase in FHR) is one indicator of fetal well-being and is associated with fetal development and maturity.

3. Indications of fetal distress include hyperactivity; fetal heart tones that are slow, irregular, and clinically difficult to hear; late decelerations; and increased FHR with decreased variability.

4. Rationales: _____

Documentation checklist

During the hospital stay or clinic visit, document:
❏ patient status and assessment findings on admission to the hospital or entry to the clinic
❏ any changes in patient status since the last visit, especially in cardiac function
❏ pertinent laboratory and diagnostic findings
❏ the patient's response to labor
❏ the patient's response to treatment
❏ the patient's and family's responses to the pregnancy outcome and long-term maternal health
❏ patient and family teaching guidelines
❏ discharge planning guidelines, if applicable.

Associated plans and appendices

❏ Inappropriate size or weight: small for gestational age
❏ Normal antepartum
❏ Preterm infant
❏ Aspects of psychological care — maternal (appendix D)

Additional nursing diagnoses

❏ Activity intolerance related to cardiovascular stresses of pregnancy on a compromised heart
❏ Altered sexuality patterns related to need for family planning of future pregnancies
❏ Impaired home maintenance management related to decreased ability to perform usual homemaker functions
❏ Powerlessness related to conflicting maternal role and rigid health restrictions

Pregnancy complicated by diabetes mellitus

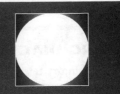

DEFINITION

Diabetes mellitus is a disorder of carbohydrate, protein, and fat metabolism. It results from abnormal insulin secretion or use and is characterized by fasting hyperglycemia and decreased glucose tolerance. Because pregnancy places additional stressors on carbohydrate metabolism, it may actually trigger diabetes. It may also aggravate preexisting diabetes and increase the risk of certain complications associated with pregnancy. Gestational diabetes is a classification that includes glucose intolerance, either induced by pregnancy or discovered during pregnancy.

In general, the diabetic patient is at risk for ketoacidosis associated with hyperglycemia, macrovascular and microvascular diseases, and neuropathy. Hypoglycemia and resulting shock may result from variable insulin regulation. During pregnancy, the diabetic patient is at greater risk for more frequent and more severe infection, pregnancy-induced hypertension, abruptio placentae, spontaneous abortion, hydramnios, dystocia and vaginal injuries associated with macrosomia (large-for-gestational-age [LGA] infants), postpartum hemorrhage, and death.

The infant of a diabetic mother is at risk for being small for gestational age (SGA), if the mother has advanced diabetes complicated by vascular disease; lung immaturity; respiratory distress syndrome; macrosomia, if the mother has mild diabetes without vascular disease; multiple birth traumas related to macrosomia and difficult vaginal delivery; multiple congenital anomalies; hypoglycemia; hypocalcemia; hyperbilirubinemia; a predisposition to diabetes; and death. Medical management, ranging from dietary modifications alone to control with insulin, seeks to maintain maternal euglycemia throughout pregnancy to ensure maternal health, minimize complications, and improve the chances for a good fetal outcome.

Etiology and precipitating factors
• Results from a complex interplay of heredity and environment
• Risk increases with a close familial history of diabetes, including twin concordance; obstetric history of hydramnios or fetal demise; previous delivery of an LGA neonate (weighing 9 lb [4,000 g] or more); and congenital anomalies.
• Disorder suggestive in patient with recurrent, resistant candidal vaginitis; hydramnios; LGA fetus; and persistent glycosuria

Physical findings
Findings represent early diabetes not complicated by impending ketoacidosis or by vascular neurologic changes.
Genitourinary
• Fundal height greater than gestational age would warrant
• Urinary frequency after the first trimester
• Persistent glycosuria
Subjective
• Excessive thirst or hunger

Criteria for diagnosing gestational diabetes using 100-g oral glucose tolerance tests

All pregnant women should undergo the 50-g screening test for gestational diabetes at 24 to 28 weeks. A patient who has risk factors for diabetes (such as family history of diabetes mellitus or a prepregnancy weight of more than 200 lb [90.7 kg]) should undergo screening at the first prenatal visit. Normal levels at 1 hour should range between 130 and 140 mg/dl. A patient whose level is more than 140 mg/dl should undergo the 100-g diagnostic test.

Several tests are now in use. In the Carpenter and Coustan criteria for the 100-g oral glucose tolerance test, gestational diabetes is confirmed when two or more of the following plasma glucose oxidase levels are met or exceeded.

Fasting level ≥ 95 mg/dl
1-hour level ≥ 180 mg/dl
2-hour level ≥ 155 mg/dl
3-hour level ≥ 140 mg/dl

Some institutions base a diagnosis of gestational diabetes on the National Diabetes Data Group conversion of the O'Sullivan and Mahan criteria. A diagnosis is made when two or more of the following venous plasma levels are met or exceeded.

Fasting level ≥ 105 mg/dl
1-hour level ≥ 190 mg/dl
2-hour level ≥ 165 mg/dl
3-hour level ≥ 145 mg/dl

Diagnostic studies
• All patients are screened for diabetes at 28 weeks; a suspicious patient history or clinical profile warrants a laboratory workup to confirm diagnosis.
• Sonography confirms fetal age and identifies hydramnios, fetal macrosomia, and intrauterine growth restriction.
• Fasting plasma glucose (FPG) increases.

• Glycosylated hemoglobin (HbA$_{1C}$) increases (values represent mean blood glucose level over previous 4 to 8 weeks; accurate only after 7th week of gestation).
• Postprandial plasma glucose increases.
• Oral glucose tolerance test (OGTT) increases (see *Criteria for diagnosing gestational diabetes using 100-g oral glucose tolerance tests*).

COLLABORATIVE PROBLEM

Alteration in carbohydrate metabolism related to normal gestation or to pregnancy-induced or overt dysfunction (three expected outcomes)

Expected outcome 1

The patient will exhibit no alterations in carbohydrate metabolism as evidenced by serum glucose levels within normal limits, or euglycemia.

Interventions

1. Teach the patient to monitor glucose levels at home four times each day: once fasting, before and after a meal, and at bedtime. Show her how to use the home glucose test kit to collect a capillary blood sample on a reagent strip coated with glucose oxidase and read the change in color against a glucose meter. A patient with gestational diabetes needs to test only once a day. If the patient is hospitalized, monitor blood and urine glucose levels, as ordered.

2. Additional individualized interventions: _____

Rationales

1. Home test kits make it easy to monitor capillary glucose levels at home. More sensitive than urine tests, they reflect changes in blood glucose levels in relation to enteral intake. Patients hospitalized for diabetes management may require more frequent testing.

2. Rationales: _____

Expected outcome 2

The patient will maintain adequate nutrition as evidenced by positive weight gain within normal limits, use of all four food groups in diet as recommended for pregnant women, and no signs of diabetic complications.

Interventions

1. Coordinate with the dietitian to regulate the patient's diet, including adequate daily intake of high-quality foods, specifically:
• protein: 1.3 to 1.7 g/kg of pregnant body weight; add 1 oz (30 g) to current diet
• carbohydrate: 5 to 7 oz (150 to 200 g) of complex starches; avoid concentrated sweets
• fat: 2 to 3 oz (60 to 80 g).

Rationales

1. A balanced diet promotes fetal growth and maternal changes. Control of maternal glucose levels early in pregnancy minimizes the risk of congenital fetal anomalies.

2. Regulate the patient's weight gain:
• Recommend 13.5 to 18 kcal/lb (30 to 40 kcal/kg).
• Do not recommend weight reduction or calorie restriction in obese patient.
• Pattern of weight gain should be 2 to 4 lb (1 to 2 kg) during first trimester and ⁹⁄₁₀ lb (0.4 kg) per week afterward
• Suggest three meals per day with three equally spaced snacks.

3. Monitor the patient's exercise regimen; tell her to avoid spurts of activity or sporadic exercising. Individualize her exercise program based on prepregnancy endurance levels, trimester, glucose levels, and insulin requirements.

4. Monitor the patient for signs of:
• upper respiratory tract infection, including sore throat, nasal congestion, sneezing, rhinorrhea, and watery eyes
• urinary tract infection, including urinary frequency and nocturia combined with urgency and dysuria
• candidiasis, including scant white or yellow vaginal discharge; vulval edema, erythema, and pruritus; possibly white, cheesy patches on vaginal walls; and dyspareunia.

5. Teach the patient how to manage diet and exercise to maintain euglycemia.

6. Additional individualized interventions: _____
_____

2. Caloric intake supports fetal growth, enlargement of the breasts and uterus, and production of amniotic fluid, blood, and extracellular fluid. Inadequate caloric intake may result in nutritional deficiencies and catabolism of maternal tissue. Food intake should parallel peaks of insulin activity. Spacing of meals minimizes the risk of hypoglycemia and promotes euglycemia.

3. Blood glucose levels usually decrease with exercise, reducing the need for insulin. The patient's insulin dose may need to be altered to parallel maternal glucose levels. Complex carbohydrate intake before exercise reduces the risk of hypoglycemia. Sporadic, inconsistent exercise causes fluctuations in blood glucose levels that are difficult to control.

4. Infections in the pregnant diabetic patient are more frequent, severe, and resistant to treatment. The physiologic stressors of infection, compounded by insulin resistance that can result from infection during pregnancy, may trigger hyperglycemia.

5. Maintaining euglycemia helps to prevent diabetic complications and to ensure a positive pregnancy outcome; understanding this can help motivate the patient.

6. Rationales: _____
_____

Expected outcome 3

The patient will receive exogenous insulin based on her physiologic demands and blood glucose levels. (*Note:* Most patients with gestational diabetes will not require insulin.)

Interventions

1. Monitor the patient's blood glucose levels, as ordered, and administer insulin accordingly.

2. Regulate the insulin dose based on the patient's physiologic needs, which vary with trimester demands. In the first trimester, requirements are low; in the second and third trimesters, the requirements increase and become highly individualized.

Rationales

1. A blood glucose profile reflects the patient's glycemic state more accurately than a urine test. Lowered renal threshold may result in glycosuria with blood glucose levels as low as 130 mg/dl.

2. Proliferation of placental hormones, human placental lactogen, estrogen, and progesterone results in insulin resistance; insulinase, a placental enzyme, increases the degradation of insulin. Hormone production peaks between weeks 18 and 20.

3. Monitor the patient for the sudden onset of:
- nervousness
- shaking, trembling
- weakness
- hunger
- moist, pale skin
- shallow respirations
- full, bounding pulse
- headache
- diplopia, blurred vision
- disorientation
- seizures, coma.

4. Monitor for the gradual onset of:
- polyuria, polydipsia
- thirst
- nausea and vomiting
- abdominal pain
- flushed, dry skin
- weak, rapid pulse and low blood pressure
- fruity, acetone breath
- drowsiness, headache.

5. Additional individualized interventions: _____

3. These are signs and symptoms of hypoglycemia, which may result from insufficient food intake or excessive insulin administration. Blood glucose levels drop below 60 mg/dl, no glucose appears in the urine, and ketones are absent (negative) or only trace amounts are present in the blood and urine. To prevent maternal cerebral hypoglycemia, which may jeopardize the fetus's life, prompt treatment with a readily absorbable oral carbohydrate in the conscious patient or I.V. glucagon or glucose in the unconscious patient is crucial.

4. These are signs and symptoms of diabetic ketoacidosis, which may result from normal or excessive food intake and insufficient insulin. Blood glucose levels rise above 250 mg/dl, urine glucose levels increase, and ketone levels in blood and urine are high.

5. Rationales: _____

NURSING DIAGNOSIS

Anxiety related to maternal diagnosis

Expected outcome

The patient will express less anxiety.

Interventions

1. Provide information on diabetes and diabetes control in a clear, forthright manner. Ascertain the patient's comprehension of information, and introduce new information slowly and sequentially.
- Include information on diet, blood testing, insulin administration and glucose monitoring, hypoglycemic reactions and remedies, and infection control; stress prevention.
- Demonstrate blood testing and insulin administration.

- Ask the patient to give return demonstrations of blood testing and insulin administration.

2. Refer the patient to a diabetes support group.

3. Additional individualized interventions: _____

Rationales

1. Open communication helps establish trust and good rapport.

- Accurate information gives the patient a sense of control over the disorder.

- The patient needs these skills to maintain consistent blood levels.
- Demonstrations allow the nurse to assess the patient's competency.

2. A support group allows patients with similar problems to share information and offer support.

3. Rationales: _____

NURSING DIAGNOSIS

Powerlessness related to fetal outcome

Expected outcome

The patient will express feelings of empowerment.

Interventions	Rationales
1. Accept the patient as part of the health care team; keep her informed of fetal status.	**1.** Providing information on test results and options for self-care gives the patient a sense of control.
2. Reinforce teaching on diabetes control.	**2.** Control of blood glucose level early in pregnancy lowers the risk of congenital anomalies.
3. Additional individualized interventions: _____	**3.** Rationales: _____

COLLABORATIVE PROBLEM

Ineffective breathing pattern related to uterine enlargement and excessive amniotic fluid

Expected outcome

The patient will breathe normally and effectively.

Interventions	Rationales
1. Monitor the patient's color, activity tolerance, and vital signs.	**1.** Comprehensive assessment rules out other causes of dyspnea.
2. Maintain the patient in an upright position.	**2.** The upright position decreases the mechanical pressure of the uterus on adjacent organs.
3. Assist the doctor with amniocentesis.	**3.** Release of fluid provides immediate relief.
4. Additional individualized interventions: _____	**4.** Rationales: _____

COLLABORATIVE PROBLEM

Risk for fetal injury related to dependence on maternal glycemic states (two expected outcomes)

Expected outcome 1

The fetus will exhibit no injury as evidenced by positive fetal heart rate (FHR) patterns, fetal activity, and a positive or reactive nonstress test (NST).

Interventions	Rationales
1. Monitor maternal insulin requirements and glucose level control; correlate with trimester.	**1.** Initial decreases in insulin requirements followed by increases in the second and third trimesters imply placental function.

2. Starting in the second half of the pregnancy, instruct the patient to count daily fetal movements and to report any sudden decrease in or cessation of movements.

3. Explain to the patient that she will undergo an NST at each clinic visit, starting at 32 weeks' gestation.

4. Additional individualized interventions: _____

_____

2. Fetal activity is highly variable. Consistent movement later in pregnancy is one indicator of fetal health; a sudden decrease in activity portends fetal jeopardy.

3. A reactive NST (fetal activity with an increase in fetal heart rate) is one indicator of fetal well-being and is associated with adequate placental function.

4. Rationales: _____

_____

Expected outcome 2

The infant will be safely delivered.

Interventions

1. Assess fetal lung maturity, based on the lecithin-sphingomyelin (L/S) ratio and the phosphatidyglycerol (PG) level. To obtain the L/S ratio rapidly, use the TDx instrument (automated fluorescence polarized assay); the Amino-Stat-FLM test measures the PG level.

2. Assist with labor induction, augmentation, vaginal delivery, or cesarean section, as follows:

• Withhold food and beverages.

• Administer an I.V. of dextrose 5% in lactated Ringer's solution with 10 units of regular insulin at 100 ml/hour or as ordered.
• Monitor the patient's blood glucose level hourly.

• Administer regular insulin I.V.; do not give long- or intermediate-acting insulins.

3. Notify the neonatal unit of the impending delivery. Have the necessary resuscitative equipment on hand.

4. Additional individualized interventions: _____

_____

Rationales

1. An L/S ratio of 2:1 or greater indicates fetal lung maturity in normal pregnancy; the ratio should be at least 3:1 in a diabetic pregnancy. A more sensitive indicator, a positive PG level is also a sign of lung maturity. The two tests together provide a highly reliable result. PG normally appears in amniotic fluid by 35 weeks.

2. Safe delivery requires precise nursing actions based on the expected type of delivery. The delivery date is determined by estimating fetal age and maturity and evaluating the potential risks of acidosis or placental insufficiency.

Vaginal delivery is attempted when cephalopelvic disproportion has been ruled out, a vertex presentation is fixed in the pelvis, and the cervix is ripe, soft, moderately effaced, and dilated.

Cesarean section delivery is indicated in macrosomia or when complications require preterm delivery.

• Vomiting and resulting aspiration are a significant cause of maternal morbidity and mortality.
• I.V. infusion is a source of fluid and calories.

• Euglycemia during the work of labor or the stress of surgery can be maintained by frequently evaluating blood glucose levels and individualizing insulin doses.
• Regular insulin is the drug of choice because it acts rapidly and has a short duration of effect; it is the only insulin that can be administered I.V.

3. The infant of a diabetic mother, even if near term, may be subject to various complications or congenital malformation. Sustained, coordinated aggressive care may be warranted.

4. Rationales: _____

_____

Documentation checklist

During the clinic visit, document:

❏ patient status and assessment findings on entry to the clinic

❏ any changes in patient status since the last visit

❏ pertinent laboratory and diagnostic findings, especially glucose levels

❏ the patient's response to the diabetes and fear of fetal outcome

❏ discomfort characteristics—quality, frequency, location, and intensity (include breathing discomfort)

❏ fetal status—activity, size, fetal heart tones, response to NST, and fetal maturity rating based on L/S ratio

❏ the patient's response to treatment

❏ patient and family teaching guidelines

❏ follow-up planning guidelines.

Associated plans and appendices

❏ Abortion

❏ Abruptio placentae

❏ Cesarean section birth

❏ Hemorrhage

❏ Hyperbilirubinemia

❏ Hypocalcemia

❏ Hypoglycemia

❏ Inappropriate size or weight: large for gestational age

❏ Inappropriate size or weight: small for gestational age

❏ Labor and vaginal birth

❏ Normal antepartum

❏ Oxytocin-induced or oxytocin-augmented labor

❏ Pregnancy-induced hypertension

❏ Aspects of psychological care—maternal (appendix D)

❏ Preparing for nonemergency surgery (appendix E)

Additional nursing diagnoses

❏ Risk for trauma associated with delivery of large fetus

❏ Knowledge deficit related to preconception diabetic regulation before future pregnancies

Pregnancy-induced hypertension

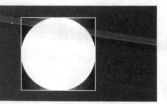

DEFINITION

Also called preeclampsia, pregnancy-induced hypertension (PIH) is a syndrome characterized by hypertension, proteinuria and, frequently, edema. Pathophysiologic processes include — but are not limited to — vascular constriction and vasospasm, increased pressor responses to angiotensin II, decreased normal hypervolemia (hypovolemia), hemoconcentration, coagulopathy, and renal and hepatic dysfunction. PIH may be mild or severe. The preeclamptic condition usually appears at or after the 20th week of gestation and continues into the postpartum period; it may occur later in pregnancy, during labor, or during the first 48 hours postpartum. Symptoms may be present earlier with proliferating chorionic villi, as is found in hydatidiform mole, or marked molar degeneration. Preeclampsia may progress until eclampsia (seizure) occurs. Maternal complications include cerebrovascular accident, cerebral edema, coagulopathy, abruptio placentae, renal and hepatic dysfunction, and a fetus that is small for gestational age or stillborn. Management aims to control preeclampsia, minimize the risk of eclampsia, deliver a viable fetus as close to term as possible, and restore maternal homeostasis.

Etiology and precipitating factors
• The cause of vasospasm and hypertension in response to chorionic villi is unknown.
• Risk factors include being a primigravida, maternal age less than 17 or greater than 35, family history of PIH, presence of multiple fetuses or hydramnios, diabetes mellitus, chronic vascular or renal disease, hydatidiform mole, and hydrops fetalis.

Physical findings
Cardiovascular
• Systolic blood pressure of 140 mm Hg or more or any increase of 30 mm Hg or more over predetermined baseline; diastolic blood pressure of 90 mm Hg or more or any increase of 15 mm Hg or more over predetermined baseline
• Edema of hands and face present on arising
Genitourinary
• Proteinuria (+1 or more)
• Oliguria (severe PIH)
Neurologic
• Headache (severe PIH)
• Visual disturbances (severe PIH)
• Hyperreflexia (severe PIH)
• Seizures (severe PIH)
Subjective
• Epigastric or right upper abdominal pain (severe PIH)

Diagnostic studies
• Ultrasonography may reveal intrauterine growth restriction (IUGR).
• Urinalysis reveals presence of protein.
• Serum total protein and albumin levels decrease.
• Hematocrit (HCT) increases.
• Uric acid level increases (thiazide therapy may cause independent hyperuricemia).
• Blood urea nitrogen (BUN) and creatinine levels increase in severe PIH.
• Aspartate aminotransferase (AST) and lactate dehydrogenase levels increase in severe PIH.
• Bilirubin levels increase in severe PIH.
• Platelet count decreases in severe PIH.

NURSING DIAGNOSIS

Risk for maternal injury related to organ or system dysfunction as a sequela of vasospasm and increased blood pressure (five expected outcomes)

Expected outcome 1

The patient will exhibit no signs of maternal injury as evidenced by blood pressure within normal limits, no proteinuria, and no edema.

Interventions

1. Monitor the patient's blood pressure at each clinic visit.

• Use the same arm and ensure that the patient is in the same position each time you take her blood pressure.

• Confirm prepregnant baseline values and monitor trends; integrate the risk profile with clinical findings.

• Monitor the patient's mean arterial blood pressure (MAP).

2. Monitor the patient for proteinuria, defined as 300 mg or more of protein in a 24-hour urine specimen or 1 g/L concentration or greater in a minimum of two random urine specimens taken 6 or more hours apart. Use a clean-catch, midstream urine specimen.

3. Monitor the patient for nondependent pathologic edema, especially of the hands and face, and integrate findings into a complete clinical profile.

4. Additional individualized interventions: _____
_____

Rationales

1. Blood pressure normally doesn't change during pregnancy, but slight decreases can occur in the second and early in the third trimesters. Psychosocial variables that may increase blood pressure (clinic visit, noise, young children, lack of support system) should be evaluated. Hypertension exists if blood pressure is elevated on two separate readings at least 6 hours apart.
• Position affects blood pressure readings. Brachial readings vary as follows: highest (patient sitting), intermediate (patient supine), lowest (patient lying in left lateral position).
• A differential diagnosis of a hypertensive state helps direct management. The patient may have chronic, pre-existing hypertension. Eclampsia may develop rapidly in pregnancy-aggravated hypertension; significant increases in blood pressure without any other symptom may trigger eclampsia.
• A MAP > 90 mm Hg in the second trimester signals an increased risk of developing PIH; a MAP ≥ 105 mm Hg indicates PIH.

2. Proteinuria is seen in about 20% of all pregnant patients. It develops later in the course of PIH and may be the last of the triad of symptoms to appear. Proteinuria from hypertension is associated with a significant rate of fetal demise. A clean-catch specimen avoids a false-positive reading from vaginal secretions or the presence of red blood cells.

3. Dependent edema is a common finding in uncomplicated pregnancies. Generalized edema is the first of the triad of symptoms to appear. The severity bears little relation to fetal outcome.

4. Rationales: _____
_____

Expected outcome 2

The patient will experience minimal or no progression of PIH as evidenced by no sudden weight gain, no signs of edema, and no headache or changes in visual patterns.

Interventions

1. Closely monitor the patient's weight gain:

• Instruct the patient to weigh herself daily at home. Confirm her weight at bimonthly or weekly clinic visits; note dramatic as well as progressive changes.

• Tell the patient to increase her protein intake from the suggested pregnancy diet of 1 g/kg/day to 1.5 g/kg/day.

• Instruct the patient to maintain a normal sodium intake (2 to 6 g daily) and to avoid excessive intake and use of diuretics.

Rationales

1. A gradual total weight gain of 25 to 35 lb (11 to 16 kg) is optimal for fetal growth and maternal changes.
• A sudden increase of more than 2 lb (0.9 kg)/week or 6 lb (2.3 kg)/month suggests sodium and water retention related to PIH. Sudden and pronounced weight gain usually precedes overt nondependent edema.
• Protein deficiency has been hypothesized as a cause of PIH; dietary increase may replace urinary loss of protein.
• Body fluid loss may exacerbate PIH hemoconcentration and decreased placental perfusion. Diuretics have been implicated in decreased renal and uteroplacental perfusion. Potassium and sodium depletion may occur as a result of thiazide therapy.

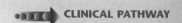

CLINICAL PATHWAY

Pregnancy-induced hypertension (preeclampsia)

	Acute stage	Postpartum stage (after vaginal or cesarean section delivery)
Tests	• Complete blood count • Clotting and chemistry studies • Sequential multiple analysis of 20 chemical constituents (SMAC-20) • Liver enzyme levels stat • Magnesium levels as ordered • Urine protein levels every 1 to 4 hours	• Magnesium levels as needed • Peripheral blood count
Assessment	• Take vital signs per protocol. • Assess reflexes per protocol, noting seizure activity. • Assess breath sounds every 2 to 4 hours. • Measure intake and output hourly. • Assess for indications of magnesium toxicity (visual changes, edema, headache, epigastric pain). *Expected outcomes* • Vital signs stable; blood pressure ≤ 160/110 • No seizure activity • Normal breath sounds • Urine output ≥ 30 ml/hr • No signs or symptoms of magnesium toxicity (magnesium levels range from 4 to 7 mEq/L)	• Take vital signs per routine postpartum protocol and every hour until stable. • Assess reflexes every 1 to 2 hours. • Assess breath sounds every 2 to 4 hours. • Measure intake and output hourly. *Expected outcomes* • Same as for acute stage.
Medications	• Magnesium sulfate per protocol • Calcium gluconate available at bedside • Antihypertensives if indicated	• Magnesium sulfate per protocol; wean after 24 hours or as ordered • Calcium gluconate available at bedside • Antihypertensives if indicated
Treatments	• Indwelling urinary catheter with urimeter • I.V. intake restricted to 125 ml/hr	• Indwelling urinary catheter with urimeter
Therapies or other treatment considerations	• Maintain quiet environment and limit visitors.	• Allow infant to visit mother if both are stable. • Contact nursery or regional neonatal intensive care unit for infant updates, as appropriate.
Activities and safety	• Maintain strict bed rest. • Keep side rails up.	• Maintain strict bed rest until stable. • Keep side rails up.
Nutrition	• Nothing by mouth (NPO) or ice chips	• NPO or ice chips until stable; then advance as tolerated.
Consults	• Perinatology • Neonatology or pediatrics	
Patient teaching	• Teach about pregnancy-induced hypertension. • Explain effects of magnesium sulfate.	
Discharge planning		

Adapted with permission from Murray, Kathleen, 5th Medical Group/SGAL.

2. Assess edema at each clinic visit, keeping these guidelines in mind:
• 1+ (2 mm)—minimal edema of pedal and pretibial areas
• 2+ (4 mm)—marked edema of lower extremities
• 3+ (6 mm)—edema of hands, face, lower abdominal wall, and sacrum
• 4+ (8 mm)—severe generalized edema with ascites (anasarca).

2. Decreased renal perfusion and glomerular filtration as well as fluid volume shifts from vascular to interstitial spaces cause sudden, excessive weight gain and edema.

3. Institute bed rest measures at home, recommending the lateral recumbent position when appropriate.

3. Bed rest decreases metabolic and physiologic demands. Lateral positioning improves uterine and renal perfusion.

4. Teach the homebound patient and her family to report signs of increased PIH severity, including:
• headache, often frontal or occipital and unrelieved by common analgesics
• visual disturbances, from blurring to overt blindness
• hyperreflexia
• markedly decreased urine output
• epigastric or right upper abdominal pain
• altered sensorium
• vaginal bleeding, abdominal or uterine tenderness or pain, and significant changes in fetal activity.

4. These signs indicate worsening of the condition, requiring immediate hospitalization and intensive management to prevent eclampsia.

5. Additional individualized interventions: _____

5. Rationales: _____

Expected outcome 3

The patient will receive appropriate treatment for progressing indications of PIH, such as I.V. fluids, urinary catheterization, and close monitoring of her physical condition.

Interventions

1. Take the patient's blood pressure every 4 hours or as her condition warrants, using the same size cuff on the same arm and with the patient in the same position.

2. Start an I.V. line, using a large-gauge needle; infuse a balanced saline solution.

3. Weigh the patient daily, and monitor for edema.

4. Insert an indwelling urinary (Foley) catheter with a urometer.

Rationales

1. A diastolic pressure of 110 mm Hg or greater indicates severe PIH. A systolic pressure of 140 mm Hg or greater or a diastolic pressure of 90 mm Hg or greater warrants hospitalization. Rapid fluctuations may occur.

2. An I.V. line provides immediate venous access. Fluids may be given to correct hypovolemia associated with PIH. Some patients may need fluids restricted or minimized to prevent fluid shift.

3. Sudden weight gain indicates water and sodium retention.

4. Catheterization allows for frequent renal assessment, which is critical in advanced dysfunction.

5. Monitor renal function hourly, noting the following:

• urine output

• specific gravity

• protein level, measured by dipstick:
1+: 30 mg/dl
2+: 100 mg/dl
3+: 300 mg/dl
4+: 2,000 mg/dl or greater.

6. Monitor laboratory values, including creatinine, BUN, and AST levels; platelet count; and HCT.

7. Monitor for ominous signs of deteriorating condition, including:
• headache
• visual disturbances
• hyperreflexia (3+ or 4+) of brachial, wrist, patellar, or Achilles tendons
• markedly decreased urine output
• epigastric or right upper abdominal pain
• crackles, rhonchi, dyspnea
• vaginal bleeding, abdominal or uterine tenderness or pain, significant change in fetal activity, and coagulopathy.

8. Monitor fetal well-being with nonstress tests and a biophysical profile.

9. Administer the vasodilator hydralazine (Apresoline) I.V., and monitor fetal heart tone and maternal blood pressure and pulse rate.

10. Additional individualized interventions: _____

5. Renal function is evaluated by the following measures:
• An output < 400 ml/day indicates severe PIH. The minimum acceptable physiologic urine output is 30 ml/hour.
• Increased urine specific gravity is consistent with oliguria.
• Persistent protein level measurements of 2+ or greater indicate severe PIH.

6. An increase in HCT signals increased hemoconcentration; a decreased platelet count indicates coagulopathy. Increases in creatinine and BUN levels indicate reduced renal perfusion and glomerular filtration; an increased AST level indicates altered hepatic function.

7. These indications characterize a deteriorating condition.
• The first episode of eclampsia is commonly preceded by headache.
• Visual disturbances are thought to result from retinal arteriolar spasm (visible on funduscopic examination), ischemia, and edema.
• Brisk, hyperactive neurologic responses may be related to cerebral edema or hemorrhagic lesions.
• Decreased urine output indicates compromised renal function.
• Edema or bleeding may engorge the hepatic capsule.
• These symptoms indicate pulmonary edema.
• Abruptio placentae, disseminated intravascular coagulation, and HELLP syndrome (*H*emolysis, *E*levated *L*iver enzymes, and *L*ow *P*latelet count) are potential complications of PIH.

8. These tests can help identify fetal compromise or distress.

9. Vasodilation results in lowered blood pressure. Small, incremental doses of hydralazine should have few untoward effects on the fetus. Uteroplacental blood flow is adequate with diastolic levels of 90 to 100 mm Hg. Tachycardia may result from drug therapy.

10. Rationales: _____

Expected outcome 4

The patient will experience no seizures.

Interventions

1. Administer a bolus dose of I.V. magnesium sulfate followed by a continuous or an intermittent piggyback infusion per protocol or doctor's order.

Rationales

1. Magnesium sulfate blocks neuromuscular transmission and prevents or stops seizures.

2. Monitor the following during magnesium sulfate therapy:
• blood pressure—every minute or continuously during I.V. administration
• magnesium sulfate blood levels

• patellar or brachial reflexes; if absent, do not give drug

• respiratory rate; if depressed (less than 16 breaths/minute), do not give drug
• urine output.

3. Have these items ready for immediate use:
• 1.5 ml of 10% solution I.V. calcium gluconate
• oxygen and suctioning equipment
• resuscitative equipment.

4. Maintain seizure precautions:
• Place the patient in a quiet, dimly lit room; limit visitors
• Secure and pad side rails.

• Have an artificial airway available.

5. Additional individualized interventions: _____
_____

2. Assessment helps evaluate therapeutic response and adverse reactions.
• Vasodilation may cause marked hypotension.

• Magnesium blood levels between 4 and 7.5 mEq/L indicate therapeutic values and may prevent seizures.
• Magnesium blood levels of 8 to 10 mEq/L indicate toxicity, manifested by loss of deep tendon reflexes.
• Respiratory depression and, possibly, cardiac arrest develop with magnesium blood levels of 12 to 15 mEq/L.
• Renal function must be determined because the drug is excreted almost exclusively by the kidneys; 30 ml/hour is the minimum acceptable level.

3. Calcium acts as an antagonist to magnesium sulfate and is the treatment of choice for respiratory depression. Administer it slowly for about 3 minutes concurrently with oxygen. Endotracheal intubation and artificial ventilation are necessary in cases of respiratory or cardiac arrest.

4. Seizure precautions ensure patient safety.
• A quiet room reduces stimuli that may trigger a seizure.
• This precaution reduces the potential for trauma or injury during tonic-clonic seizure or during the combative stage.
• An airway is inserted only before the patient's jaw is clenched. It may prevent injury to the mouth and tongue and help maintain the patient's airway.

5. Rationales: _____
_____

Expected outcome 5
The patient will remain safe during and after a seizure.

Interventions

1. Position the patient on her side, if possible. Do not restrict activity; administer oxygen, and suction, as necessary.

2. Remain with the patient after a seizure.

3. Monitor the patient for crackles, rhonchi, dyspnea, and hemoptysis; note the amount of I.V. fluid infused.

4. Additional individualized interventions: _____

Rationales

1. The side-lying position reduces the risk of airway occlusion and aspiration. Restriction of forceful, almost violent muscular movement may result in injury. Supplemental oxygen is necessary to reverse hypoxia, and suctioning removes secretions.

2. After a tonic-clonic seizure ends, the patient may experience varying degrees of consciousness, combativeness, impaired vision, further seizures, or coma.

3. These symptoms stem from pulmonary edema, which may be compounded by fluid overload from I.V. fluids used to correct hemoconcentration.

4. Rationales: _____
_____

NURSING DIAGNOSIS

Risk for fetal injury related to impaired maternal-placental perfusion (two expected outcomes)

Expected outcome 1

The patient will exhibit no signs of fetal injury as evidenced by positive FHR, fetal activity, fetal growth, and appropriate fundal height.

Interventions

1. At each clinic visit, assess:
• fundal height; correlate findings with the mother's last menstrual period and estimated date of confinement
• fetal activity; compare findings with the mother's diary of fetal movement and with FHR.

2. Assist with maternal ultrasonography.

3. Assist with a nonstress test.

4. Additional individualized interventions: _____
_____

Rationales

1. Lack of appropriate growth or smaller uterine growth than gestational age would indicate may suggest intrauterine growth retardation (IUGR). A significant decrease in fetal activity may indicate uteroplacental insufficiency.

2. Ultrasonography identifies fetal and placental size and may reveal IUGR or grade III placenta (acceleration of the maturational process of the placenta) associated with PIH.

3. An FHR that accelerates in response to fetal movement indicates fetal well-being.

4. Rationales: _____
_____

Expected outcome 2

A viable infant will be safely delivered.

Interventions

1. Continue maternal assessments. If preeclampsia is severe, prepare for and assist with amniotomy and oxytocin-induced labor and delivery if the patient's cervix is ripe.

2. Prepare for cesarean section birth if induction is not successful.

3. Notify obstetric and neonatal teams of anticipated delivery. Have resuscitative equipment immediately available for use.

4. Additional individualized interventions: _____
_____

Rationales

1. In severe preeclampsia, continuing the pregnancy may put the fetus at greater risk than inducing preterm delivery.

2. An unfavorable cervix or failure to progress in labor requires surgical intervention.

3. The preterm, immature infant will need aggressive and protracted treatment for survival.

4. Rationales: _____
_____

Documentation checklist

During the clinic or home visit or hospital stay, document:
- [ ] patient status and assessment findings
- [ ] any changes in patient status
- [ ] pertinent laboratory and diagnostic findings
- [ ] any changes in fetal status — activity, heart tones, ultrasound changes
- [ ] the patient's response to treatment
- [ ] patient and family teaching guidelines
- [ ] discharge or follow-up planning guidelines.

Associated plans and appendices

- [ ] Abruptio placentae
- [ ] Cesarean section birth
- [ ] Labor and vaginal birth
- [ ] Multiple gestation
- [ ] Normal antepartum
- [ ] Preterm infant
- [ ] Aspects of psychological care — maternal (appendix D)

Additional nursing diagnoses

- [ ] Altered nutrition: less than body requirements related to low protein intake
- [ ] Fluid volume deficit related to fluid shift from intravascular to extravascular spaces
- [ ] Sensory/perceptual alterations (visual) related to retinal edema

Premature rupture of membranes

DEFINITION

Premature rupture of membranes (PROM) is the usually spontaneous rupture of the amniochorionic sac before labor begins. Preterm premature rupture of membranes (PPROM) refers to this action occurring before 37 weeks' gestation. Labor frequently begins within 24 to 48 hours, and delivery is effected within days, whether or not attempts at labor suppression occur. Complications may include maternal or fetal infection, prolapsed cord resulting from fetal malpresentation or small presenting part, and delivery of a preterm infant.

Etiology and precipitating factors

• Etiology is usually related to infection, possibly from a sexually transmitted disease.
• Risk factors include a history of sexually transmitted infections, maternal smoking and substance abuse, poor nutrition, multiple gestation, hydramnios, a history of incompetent cervix or cervical manipulation before pregnancy, fetal malpresentation, abruptio placentae, and placenta previa.

Physical findings
Genitourinary
• Amniotic fluid in the vagina
Subjective
• Feeling of fluid gushing or leaking from the vagina

Diagnostic studies

• Fern test is positive, showing a crystalline frondlike or fern pattern that indicates amniotic fluid; urine, blood, or vaginal secretions do not elicit this configuration.
• pH of vaginal secretions (nitrazine paper test) is 7 to 7.5; blood, cervical mucus, and some vaginal infections are also alkaline and may invalidate this test. (See also *pH test for intact membranes.*)
• Urinalysis — for signs of infection
• White blood cell (WBC) count with differential, C-reactive protein — for signs of infection
• Blood and vaginal cultures — for signs of infection

pH test for intact membranes

	pH	Color
Membranes probably intact	5	Yellow
	5.5	Olive-yellow
	6	Olive-green
Membranes probably ruptured	6.5	Blue-green
	7	Blue-gray
	7.5	Deep blue

COLLABORATIVE PROBLEM

Risk for intrauterine infection related to disruption of amniochorionic barrier (two expected outcomes)

Expected outcome 1

The patient will exhibit no signs of PROM as evidenced by the presence of leaking amniotic fluid.

Interventions

1. Review and document the time of rupture, color of fluid, estimation of amount, odor, and patient's subjective sensations.

2. Review the patient's menstrual history, including regularity, duration, characteristics of each menses, and the date of her last menstrual period.

Rationales

1. An accurate database helps formulate a diagnosis and plan subsequent treatment.

2. An accurate history helps establish gestational age and fetal maturity.

3. Measure fundal height.

4. Assist the doctor, nurse-midwife, or practitioner with sterile speculum vaginal examination, taking the following steps:

• Use sterile water as lubricating fluid.
• Confirm the presence of amniotic fluid, and identify its characteristics, especially pH.

5. Additional individualized interventions: _____
_____

3. Fundal height is used to estimate gestational age; however, fetal size does not necessarily correspond with fetal age.

4. Vaginal inspection should be kept to a minimum. If PPROM has occurred, then the vaginal examination may be omitted. Sterile speculum examination minimizes the introduction or spread of organisms.
• Water will not alter pH of secretions.
• Urine and vaginal secretions are acidic. Amniotic fluid is neutral or mildly alkaline (as evidenced by turning a nitrazine strip blue). Microscopic crystalline fern configuration confirms amniotic fluid. Bloody show may render a false-positive reading because blood is alkaline.

5. Rationales: _____
_____

Expected outcome 2

The patient will receive home management if she exhibits no signs of infection as evidenced by a normal temperature and no purulent vaginal drainage.

Interventions

1. Determine if the patient is a candidate for home management. She should be afebrile with a normal WBC count, absence of labor, gestational age of less than 37 weeks, and absence of maternal or fetal dysfunction or disease that would warrant immediate delivery.

2. Begin conservative home treatment. Tell the patient to:

• avoid coitus and douching

• immediately report signs of infection, including a temperature greater 100.4° F (38° C) and thick, foul-smelling vaginal discharge
• take prophylactic antibiotics as prescribed, if her doctor orders antibiotic therapy.

3. If gestational age is greater than 33 weeks, prepare for delivery. Induced labor or cesarean section birth may be necessary.

4. Additional individualized interventions: _____
_____

Rationales

1. If no infection is present, conservative management may allow time for the fetus to develop and mature in utero.

2. The patient whose condition is managed at home needs specific guidelines.
• Vaginal penetration of any kind may be a source of infection.
• Pyrexia or thick, foul-smelling discharge indicates active infection.

• Although the effectiveness of prophylactic antibiotics is suspect, the doctor may prescribe them as a precaution.

3. Greater gestational age and consequent fetal maturity are associated with lower neonatal mortality. If spontaneous labor has not begun 6 hours after PROM, the patient may need oxytocin to induce labor. Once membranes rupture, delivery is optimal in 18 to 20 hours. Cesarean section birth is indicated if labor cannot be induced or if the fetus is in a breech presentation or transverse lie.

4. Rationales: _____
_____

NURSING DIAGNOSIS

Fear related to PROM and possible fetal jeopardy

Expected outcome

The patient will express less fear.

Interventions

1. Speak calmly and deliberately. Explain procedures and examinations before they are done, and keep the patient and her partner informed of their outcomes.

2. Additional individualized interventions: _____

_____

Rationales

1. Fear of fetal jeopardy is real, and fetal outcome may be compromised. A realistic appraisal of maternal condition and the implications for the fetus may give the patient some sense of control, decrease fear, and allow for possible anticipatory grieving for preterm infant.

2. Rationales: _____

_____

Documentation checklist

During the hospital stay, document:
- ❏ patient status and assessment findings, especially the appearance of vaginal secretions, time membranes ruptured, and gestational age
- ❏ any changes in patient status, especially the onset of labor
- ❏ pertinent laboratory and diagnostic findings, pH test for intact membranes, fern test results, WBC count with differential, and culture results
- ❏ any changes in fetal status, including activity, heart tones, and ultrasound changes
- ❏ the patient's response to treatment, especially to prophylactic antibiotics
- ❏ patient and family teaching guidelines
- ❏ discharge or follow-up planning guidelines.

Associated plans and appendices

- ❏ Cesarean section birth
- ❏ Inappropriate size or weight: small for gestational age
- ❏ Labor and vaginal birth
- ❏ Normal antepartum
- ❏ Oxytocin-induced or oxytocin-augmented labor
- ❏ Preterm infant
- ❏ Preterm labor
- ❏ Sepsis neonatorum and infectious disorders
- ❏ Aspects of psychological care — maternal (appendix D)

Additional nursing diagnoses

- ❏ Altered sexuality patterns related to medically prescribed sexual abstinence
- ❏ Risk for fetal trauma related to cord compression
- ❏ Self-esteem disturbance related to inability to carry fetus to term

Preterm labor

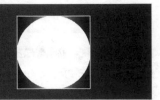

DEFINITION

Preterm labor is the onset of the first phase of labor before the 38th week of gestation and after the 20th week. Delivery before the 20th week is considered a spontaneous abortion. A good fetal outcome is more likely when delivery occurs after the 37th week and the infant weighs 5.5 lb (2,500 g) or greater. Preterm infants are at increased risk for mental and physical impairment and death. Every effort should be made to continue the pregnancy as long as it does not jeopardize maternal well-being and as long as the uterine environment is more favorable to the fetus than delivery.

Etiology and precipitating factors

• Etiology is unknown in most instances.
• Maternal risk factors include preterm premature rupture of membranes, incompetent cervix, preeclampsia or eclampsia, cardiovascular or renal disease, substance abuse, diabetes, infection, injury, abdominal surgery, uterine anomalies, history of previous preterm labor and delivery, and retained intrauterine device (IUD).
• Placental risk factors include abruptio placentae, placenta previa, placental malformation, and malnutrition.

• Fetal risk factors include multiple gestation, hydramnios, fetal anomaly or infection, and fetal death.

Physical findings
Gastrointestinal
• Diarrhea
Genitourinary
• Uterine contractions before the 37th week of gestation that occur at least every 10 minutes and last for 30 or more seconds for 1 or more hours
• Cervical dilation and effacement
• Possibly ruptured membranes
Subjective
• Pain or pressure in lower back and abdomen
• Sensation of baby "balling up"

Diagnostic studies
• Accurate and complete history and physical examination may furnish enough data for a definitive diagnosis.
• Ultrasonography may reveal gestational age of fetus or fetuses, fetal maturity, presentation, position, viability, placental abnormalities, hydramnios, or retained IUD.

COLLABORATIVE PROBLEM

Risk for preterm labor and delivery (two expected outcomes)

Expected outcome 1

The patient will exhibit no signs of preterm labor as evidenced by absence of regular contractions, increasing frequency, and intensity; no cervical dilation; and no back and abdominal discomfort.

Interventions

1. Review the patient's menstrual history, including regularity, duration, characteristics of each menses, and date of last menstrual period.

2. Measure fundal height.

3. Monitor for signs of false labor, including contractions that occur at irregular, long intervals and do not increase in regularity, intensity, or duration; localized lower abdominal discomfort; nondilated cervix; and contractions that are unaffected or relieved by walking and usually relieved by sedatives.

Rationales

1. An accurate history helps establish a precise gestational age.

2. Fundal height is used to estimate gestational age; however, fetal size does not necessarily correspond with fetal age.

3. False labor is a common phenomenon and requires no interventions.

4. Recognize signs of true labor, including regular con tractions that increase in frequency and intensity; back and abdominal discomfort; cervical dilation; and contractions that are usually intensified by walking and not halted by sedatives.

5. Teach the patient to recognize the signs and symptoms of preterm labor and to report any indications at once.

6. Encourage adequate hydration.

7. Additional individualized interventions: _____

_____

4. Correctly identifying labor early on allows for successful tocolysis (suppression of labor).

5. The patient needs to understand the importance of recognizing and reporting preterm labor so that she can receive appropriate treatment.

6. Dehydration can trigger preterm labor.

7. Rationales: _____

Expected outcome 2

The patient's spontaneous, preterm labor will stop.

Interventions

1. Enact conservative treatment methods, including bed rest, with the head of the bed slightly elevated and, if possible, the patient lying on her side. Explain to the patient that she must not use enemas and must avoid coitus.

2. Determine if the patient and fetus are candidates for tocolytic therapy. Tocolytic therapy may be effective in the following:
• viable fetus of 20 to 35 weeks' gestation with good fetal heart tones and no distress or disease
• true labor
• intact membranes with no bulging
• cervix dilated no more than 4 cm
• cervical effacement of less than 50%
• absence of maternal bleeding and outstanding medical disorders.

3. Start an I.V. line. Maintain hydration and strict fluid intake and output monitoring.

4. Have I.V. magnesium sulfate available.

• Monitor for intact deep tendon reflexes, respiratory rate greater than 12 breaths/minute, and urine output greater than 30 ml/hour; note serum magnesium levels.
• Have I.V. calcium gluconate on hand.

5. Have I.V., S.C., and oral terbutaline available. Assess the patient for severe preeclampsia and eclampsia, cardiac dysfunction, hypertension, thyroid dysfunction, and chorioamnionitis as well as diabetes mellitus and concurrent glucocorticoid therapy. Note restlessness, dyspnea, cyanosis, sense of suffocation, and crackles; also note chest pain or tightness, tachycardia, hypotension, widened pulse pressure, hypokalemia, hyperglycemia, hyperinsulinism, acidosis, decreased hematocrit, and subsequent headache, nausea, and vomiting.

Rationales

1. In the absence of bleeding and ruptured membranes, bed rest effectively arrests labor in 50% of cases by minimizing the gravitational pull of the fetus on the cervix. Side-lying positions improve uterine perfusion. Coitus and enema administration may initiate or stimulate labor.

2. Tocolytic agents, given early on, inhibit labor, allowing the fetus to continue to grow and develop. If spontaneous preterm labor advances too far, labor becomes difficult to stop. Tocolytics are contraindicated in conditions where continuing the pregnancy would jeopardize maternal or fetal health, such as in hemorrhage.

3. An I.V. line provides venous access. Premature labor may result from dehydration.

4. As a tocolytic agent, magnesium sulfate decreases myometrial contractility.
• Depressed respirations and hyporeflexia indicate magnesium toxicity. Intact renal function is needed to excrete magnesium.
• Calcium is the antagonist of magnesium.

5. As a tocolytic agent, terbutaline is beta-adrenergic agonist that relaxes the smooth muscle of the uterus. It is contraindicated in patients with hypertensive conditions, cardiac and thyroid dysfunction, and chorioamnionitis; it should be used with caution in those with diabetes mellitus and those receiving glucocorticoid therapy. After administering, watch for signs of pulmonary edema, which may indicate toxicity. The other symptoms may warrant discontinuing terbutaline.

6. Have I.V. ritodrine hydrochloride available. Evaluate the patient for severe preeclampsia and eclampsia, cardiac dysfunction, pulmonary hypertension, thyroid dysfunction, hemorrhage, chorioamnionitis, and asthma (requiring medication) as well as diabetes mellitus and concurrent corticosteroid therapy. Monitor for signs of pulmonary edema and cardiovascular response, including tachycardia, chest pain or tightness, palpitations, shortness of breath, restlessness, dyspnea, and cyanosis. Also monitor for hypokalemia, hyperglycemia, acidosis, headache, nausea, and vomiting.

6. As a tocolytic agent, ritodrine is a beta-adrenergic agonist that inhibits contractions of uterine smooth muscle. It is contraindicated in patients with hypertensive conditions, cardiac and thyroid diseases, and chorioamnionitis; it should be used cautiously in patients with diabetes and in those receiving concurrent corticosteroids and other sympathomimetic agents. Its action can be potentiated by magnesium sulfate, diazoxide, meperidine, and potent general anesthetics. After administering ritodrine, watch for signs of impending pulmonary edema, which sometimes occurs after delivery. Monitor hydration status closely; symptoms may warrant discontinuing the drug.

7. Have a beta-blocking agent, such as propranolol (Inderal), on hand.

7. A beta blocker may be needed to antagonize drug action.

8. Additional individualized interventions: _____

8. Rationales: _____

_____

_____

COLLABORATIVE PROBLEM

Risk for fetal injury related to maternal preterm labor status and imminent delivery

Expected outcome

The fetus will experience no fetal injury as evidenced by positive fetal lung maturity, no meconium staining, and no fetal tachycardia.

Interventions

1. Review the maternal history and confirm gestational age.

2. Review amniotic fluid analysis for fetal lung maturity, noting results of the rapid surfactant test (shake, bubble, or foam test) and the following:
• lecithin-sphingomyelin (L/S) ratio

• phosphatidylglycerol (PG) level

• creatinine level

• bilirubin level
• lipids

• color.

Rationales

1. Preterm birth is implicated in more than two-thirds of all neonatal deaths.

2. In this practical, bedside version of L/S analysis, if bubbles are present 15 minutes after vigorous shaking, fetal lung maturity is indicated.
• The L/S ratio can be used to determine fetal lung maturity: a 1:1 ratio indicates immaturity; 2:1, maturity; and 3:1, maturity in a diabetic patient. The TDx instrument (automated fluorescence polarized assay) allows for rapid testing of the L/S ratio.
• Absence of bubbles indicates immaturity. Determining both the PG level (with the Amnio-Stat-FLM test) and the L/S ratio provides a more reliable result. Both tests are faster and more reliable than the rapid surfactant test.
• Creatinine levels of 1.8 to 2 mg/dl indicate maturity (more than 36 weeks). Note maternal hypertensive and renal status because these diseases can cause deceptive increases.
• Bilirubin is not present after 36 weeks.
• A level greater than 20% indicates maturity (more than 36 weeks).
• Meconium staining may indicate fetal hypoxia.

3. Monitor fetal heart rate, and report a rate greater than 160 beats/minute.

4. Prepare for glucocorticoid drug therapy:

• Assess for the patient for diabetes, hypertension, infection, peptic ulcer, and imminent delivery.
• Review hospital and drug manufacturer's protocols for administration, including fetal age of less than 34 weeks; administer on initiation of tocolytic therapy and again in 24 hours. The patient may need treatment repeated if she does not deliver within 7 days.

5. Prepare for vaginal delivery or cesarean section; alert the obstetric and neonatal teams. Have resuscitative equipment ready for use. If necessary, the infant can be transferred to a tertiary care center with a neonatal intensive care unit.

6. Additional individualized interventions: _____
_____

3. Fetal tachycardia is associated with the use of to-colytics; the drug dose may be reduced or the drug discontinued, depending on the patient's response.

4. Betamethasone (Betatrex), dexamethasone (Decadron), or hydrocortisone (Hydrocortone) administered to the mother may stimulate fetal lung maturity and decrease the risk of respiratory distress syndrome. The drug should be given 6 to 12 hours before delivery.
• Adrenocorticosteroids are contraindicated under these conditions.
• Increased surfactant levels associated with steroid use are transitory; return to uncorrected levels occurs in 8 to 10 days.

5. If membranes rupture, labor will probably continue. The preterm infant will require intensive and long-term care. A tertiary care center can provide the specialized care a very premature or severely compromised infant needs.

6. Rationales: _____
_____

NURSING DIAGNOSIS

Pain related to uterine contractions

Expected outcome

The patient will experience less pain.

Interventions

1. Establish rapport with the patient and her significant others.

2. Assess the patient for pain and its characteristics.

3. Perform comfort measures, including position changes, relaxation techniques, and massage and effleurage, and provide pharmacologic analgesia cautiously.

4. Keep the patient informed of the status of her fetus. Allow her to listen to fetal heart tones during assessment.

5. Additional individualized interventions: _____
_____

Rationales

1. A positive relationship builds trust and decreases anxiety.

2. Typically, pain in the lower back radiates to the abdomen and increases in intensity, frequency, and duration.

3. Increased tissue perfusion plus stimulation of afferent fibers decrease pain perception. The depressive effects of analgesics may compromise fetal status.

4. Anxiety related to fetal outcome may intensify pain perception.

5. Rationales: _____
_____

Documentation checklist

During the hospital stay or home care visits, document:

❏ patient status and assessment findings, including history of previous pregnancies and their outcomes

❏ any changes in patient status

❏ characteristics of pain, including quality, location, frequency, and intensity

❏ fetal status, including activity, heart tones, and maturity

❏ the patient's response to treatment

❏ the patient's and family's response to possible premature birth

❏ patient and family teaching guidelines.

Associated plans and appendices

❏ Abruptio placentae

❏ Cesarean section birth

❏ Inappropriate size or weight: small for gestational age

❏ Labor and vaginal birth

❏ Multiple gestation

❏ Placenta previa

❏ Pregnancy complicated by diabetes mellitus

❏ Pregnancy-induced hypertension

❏ Premature rupture of membranes

❏ Preterm infant

❏ Aspects of psychological care — maternal (appendix D)

❏ Parent teaching guides (appendix J)

Additional nursing diagnoses

❏ Anxiety related to unknown fetal outcome

❏ Ineffective family coping, compromised, related to unknown fetal outcome

❏ Ineffective individual coping related to unknown fetal outcome

❏ Knowledge deficit related to preterm labor and use of tocolytic drugs

❏ Spiritual distress related to perception that some activity may have triggered preterm labor

Prolapsed umbilical cord

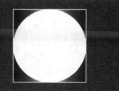

DEFINITION

Prolapsed umbilical cord is an emergency condition in which the umbilical cord is displaced between the presenting fetal part and the maternal bony pelvis or vagina or both. This results in cord compression, leading to fetal hypoxia. If not immediately corrected, the fetus can die.

Etiology and precipitating factors

• Any condition that prevents proper engagement of the presenting fetal part snugly into the maternal pelvis may result in prolapsed umbilical cord.
• Risk factors include fetal malpresentation, unengaged fetal head, contracted maternal inlet, premature rupture of the membranes, placenta previa, small fetus, multiple (and therefore smaller) fetuses, and a longer umbilical cord.

Physical findings
Genitourinary
• Bradycardia or absent fetal heart tones (FHT)
• Ruptured membranes
• Cord palpable on vaginal examination
• Cord protrusion from vagina
Subjective
• Sensation of cord passage

Diagnostic studies
• Ultrasonography may reveal the conditions that could predispose the patient to prolapsed umbilical cord.

NURSING DIAGNOSIS

Risk for fetal injury (hypoxia) related to cord compression (three expected outcomes)

Expected outcome 1

The patient will experience no fetal injury as evidenced by positive fetal heart rate patterns and no prolonged variable decelerations.

Interventions

1. Monitor fetal presentation and position.

2. Monitor FHT and electronic tracings throughout labor, especially when membranes rupture and immediately after amniotomy. Monitor for baseline bradycardia and prolonged variable decelerations.

3. Additional individualized interventions: _____

Rationales

1. Breech or shoulder presentation or transverse lie may result in cord prolapse.

2. Rupture of the membranes is commonly followed by prolapse when the presenting part is not complementary to maternal structure. Variable deceleration may indicate cord compression.

3. Rationales: _____

Expected outcome 2

The patient will experience no further cord compression.

Interventions

1. Call for assistance.

Rationales

1. At least two persons are needed in cases of cord compression.

2. Perform a sterile vaginal examination. If you feel the umbilical cord, position your fingers to move the presenting part off the cord. Do not handle the cord itself. Maintain this position until an emergency delivery can be performed.

3. Place the patient in the knee-chest or Trendelenburg position. Support her with pillows.

4. Administer oxygen by mask at a rate of 8 to 10 L/minute.

5. Do not reinsert the externally prolapsed umbilical cord.

6. Apply warm sterile saline solution compresses to the umbilical cord if it is externally prolapsed.

7. If the cord is not in the vagina, prepare for amnioinfusion, if ordered.

8. Additional individualized interventions: _____
_____

2. Moving the presenting part off the cord reduces compression and improves circulation through the cord. Handling the cord may trigger vasospasm.

3. Gravitational release of the presenting fetal part reduces cord compression.

4. This improves oxygenation, which may be compromised when fetal position changes further compress the uterus against ventilatory structures.

5. Reinsertion may twist or kink the cord and exacerbate the compression.

6. Compresses may help keep the cord pulsating unless it is completely compressed.

7. In amnioinfusion, instilled fluid holds the presenting part off the cord until a cesarean section can be completed.

8. Rationales: _____
_____

Expected outcome 3

The fetus will be safely delivered.

Interventions

1. Monitor the patient for ruptured membranes, ripe cervix (dilated fully, spontaneously, and progressively), cephalopelvic proportion, occiput presentation, and uteroplacental adequacy.

2. Do not administer oxytocin.

3. Prepare for cesarean section birth.

4. Additional individualized interventions: _____
_____

Rationales

1. Assessing for these conditions helps determine the risk for a prolapsed cord.

2. Forceful uterine contractions may bottleneck the fetus's head against the maternal bony pelvis, resulting in dire consequences for both the mother and the fetus.

3. Delivery must be accomplished rapidly to prevent fetal hypoxia, central nervous system impairment, and death.

4. Rationales: _____
_____

NURSING DIAGNOSIS

Risk for intrauterine infection related to exposure of externally prolapsed cord to perineal area

Expected outcome

The patient will exhibit no signs of infection, such as fever, redness, or alterations in vital signs.

Interventions

1. Do not reinsert the umbilical cord.

2. Completely cover the protruding cord with a warm sterile saline solution dressing or perineal pad.

3. Additional individualized interventions: _____

Rationales

1. The cord may be grossly contaminated with organisms or pathogens from the vulva, anus, skin, or bedclothes.

2. The dressing acts as a barrier, minimizing the risk of further contamination; the warm sterile saline solution minimizes the risk of cord vessel atrophy or chilling.

3. Rationales: _____

NURSING DIAGNOSIS

Fear related to fetal outcome

Expected outcome

The patient will express less fear.

Interventions

1. Calmly explain procedures and their rationale. Repeat as necessary. Keep the patient advised of fetal status.

2. Additional individualized interventions: _____

Rationales

1. Fear is realistic, and explanations may give the patient a sense of control, decrease her fear, and enhance compliance.

2. Rationales: _____

Documentation checklist

During the hospital stay, document:
❏ patient status and assessment findings, including history of previous pregnancies and their outcomes
❏ any changes in patient status
❏ pertinent laboratory and diagnostic findings
❏ fetal status — activity, heart tones, and reactivity
❏ the patient's and fetus's response to treatment
❏ the patient's and family's response to possible negative fetal outcome
❏ patient and family teaching guidelines
❏ discharge planning guidelines.

Associated plans and appendices

❏ Multiple gestation
❏ Placenta previa
❏ Premature rupture of membranes
❏ Aspects of psychological care — maternal (appendix D)

Additional nursing diagnoses

❏ Ineffective breathing pattern related to therapeutically imposed knee-chest position
❏ Knowledge deficit related to diagnosis and emergency procedures
❏ Powerlessness related to fetal outcome

Rh isoimmunization

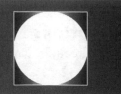

DEFINITION

Rh isoimmunization is an antigen-antibody sensitization response that causes the development of maternal antibodies to fetal red blood cells (RBCs). Placental transfer of antibodies to the fetus destroys fetal RBCs and produces hemolytic anemia and hyperbilirubinemia.

Several antigens may evoke this incompatibility response (ABO group; Rh D, C, c, e; other blood groups), but the Rh genotype D carries the most severe antigenic potential. If untreated, fetal effects include erythroblastosis fetalis, choreoathetosis, neurologic and sensory deficits, and death. The prognosis for the fetus or neonate used to be grim, but identification of nonsensitized patients and pharmacologic prophylaxis have dramatically improved this outcome.

Etiology and precipitating factors

• Rh production in the Rh-negative pregnant patient is stimulated by exposure to the Rh antigen during pregnancy with an Rh-positive conceptus, incompatible blood transfusion, and fetomaternal bleeding associated with abruptio placentae or placenta previa. The first pregnancy, whether full term, stillborn, aborted, ectopic, or molar, is usually unaffected. The risk of sensitization increases with each subsequent pregnancy.
• The patient at risk is Rh negative and has an Rh-positive sexual partner; Basque ethnicity increases the risk.

Physical findings
• None (maternal)

Diagnostic studies
• Rh and ABO screenings identify blood type and Rh.
• Maternal antibody titers: A positive indirect Coombs' test indicates maternal Rh-positive antibodies.

COLLABORATIVE PROBLEM

Risk for fetal injury related to fetomaternal blood incompatibility (four expected outcomes)

Expected outcome 1

The patient at risk for fetomaternal incompatibility will be identified as evidenced by ABO blood group or negative Rh factor.

Interventions

1. At the first clinic visit, review:
• ABO blood group and Rh of the patient and her sexual partner
• maternal history, including history of blood or blood product transfusion, plasmapheresis, or amniocentesis and previous Rh immune globulin injections after delivery or abortion.

2. Refer the Rh-negative patient and the fetus's Rh-positive father for analysis of blood group, Rh, and zygosity.

3. Additional individualized interventions: _____

Rationales

1. Determining whether the patient is at risk allows for early management. Introduction of fetal erythrocytes into the maternal circulation may occur at delivery, usually during separation of the placenta; ill-matched blood transfusions may introduce the antigen, as may any procedure or condition in which blood from the fetal circulation leaks into the maternal circulation.

2. Laboratory data confirms the history.

3. Rationales: _____

Expected outcome 2

The Rh$_o$(D)-negative, nonsensitized patient will not develop isoimmunization as evidenced by negative Coombs' test.

Interventions

1. Determine whether the patient is a candidate for immune globulin prophylaxis. Such a candidate would be an Rh$_o$(D)-negative, nonsensitized patient with an Rh-positive partner or one who delivered an Rh$_o$(D)-positive neonate with a negative direct Coombs' test (both determined from cord blood).

2. Administer RhoGAM I.M., using the following guidelines:
• Administer to the mother only (never to the father or infant).
• Administer 300 mcg within 72 hours of each delivery; administer a 50-mcg dose after an abortion.
• Administer 300 mcg per protocol or order at these times:
– 28 and 34 weeks' gestation
– when amniocentesis is performed
– with vaginal bleeding associated with placental abruption.
• Individualize the dose after heavy fetomaternal bleeding or a transfusion accident.

3. Additional individualized interventions: _____

Rationales

1. Rh$_o$(D) immune globulin (RhoGAM) provides temporary passive immunity by preventing the formation of maternal antibodies in the Rh-negative patient with an Rh-positive infant. If the Coombs' test is positive, then sensitization has already occurred and RhoGAM will not help.

2. I.M. administration of RhoGAM accomplishes the following:
• Administration to an Rh-positive person results in lysis of RBCs.
• One 300-mcg dose suppresses the maternal immune response to 15 ml of Rh-positive RBCs. Only a 50-mcg dose is needed after an abortion.
• Prenatal administration may reduce the incidence of isoimmunization associated with silent fetomaternal bleeding.
• Doses after bleeding can be determined by laboratory techniques, such as the Kleihauer-Betke acid elution technique.

3. Rationales: _____

Expected outcome 3

The Rh$_o$(D)-negative, sensitized patient with a jeopardized fetus will be identified as evidenced by antibody titers greater than 1:16 and increasing bilirubin levels.

Interventions

1. Continually monitor antibody titers to determine the degree of maternal sensitization monthly through the 24th week of gestation, biweekly for the 25th through 40th weeks, and 1 week before the estimated date of confinement.

2. Assist with amniocentesis if titers are greater than 1:16.

3. Monitor spectrophotometric measurements of the delta optical density of amniotic fluid.

4. Additional individualized interventions: _____

Rationales

1. Detecting sensitization is critical; untreated sensitization results in a 30% perinatal mortality rate.

2. Increased titers indicate that marked hemolytic disease of the fetus may exist.

3. Spectrophotometric readings indicate bilirubin levels; the severity of fetal hemolytic disease is indicated by the following zones:
A — mild or no disease
B — moderate
C — severe.

4. Rationales: _____

Expected outcome 4

The fetus will experience minimal, if any, injury as evidenced by minimal hemolysis, positive fetal heart rate (FHR) patterns, and no repetitive decelerations.

Interventions

1. Confirm zone A or B spectrophotometric readings of amniotic fluid.

2. Prepare for intrauterine fetal transfusions, as follows:

• Perform periumbilical blood sampling or cordocentesis with ultrasound.
• Infuse crossmatched, fresh, Rh-negative, type O packed RBCs into the umbilical cord, close to the junction of the placenta (X-ray visualization or a radiopaque contrast agent identifies the location).
• Repeat the transfusion procedure every 2 weeks.

3. Monitor FHR, noting sinusoidal FHR pattern and repetitive decelerations.

4. Prepare for induced delivery or cesarean section birth.

5. Notify the neonatologist.

6. Additional individualized interventions: _____

Rationales

1. Delivery can be delayed until the fetus matures, usually after the 36th week of gestation.

2. The immature fetus between 23 and 32 weeks' gestation with severe hemolysis (zone C) needs transfusions to correct anemia from RBC hemolysis.
• This procedure identifies the placental site, fetal position, and location of the umbilical cord.
• RBCs infused directly into the umbilical artery provide the fetus with the transfusion it needs.

• Treatment continues until the fetus matures.

3. Sinusoidal FHR pattern and repetitive decelerations have been associated in part with erythroblastosis fetalis; delivery is usually warranted.

4. Cesarean section birth is indicated when delivery is required before labor begins. Manual removal of the placenta is contraindicated.

5. If an emergency cesarean section becomes necessary during cordocentesis, the preterm infant may need resuscitation and will need support.

6. Rationales: _____

Documentation checklist

During the clinic visit or hospital stay, document:
❑ patient status and assessment findings
❑ any changes in patient status
❑ pertinent laboratory and diagnostic findings
❑ fetal status — activity, heart tones, and maturity
❑ the patient's and fetus's response to treatment
❑ the patient's and family's response to possible negative fetal outcome
❑ patient and family teaching guidelines
❑ discharge planning guidelines.

Associated plans and appendices

❑ Cesarean section birth
❑ Hyperbilirubinemia
❑ Inappropriate size or weight: small for gestational age
❑ Labor and vaginal birth
❑ Oxytocin-induced or oxytocin-augmented labor

❑ Preterm infant
❑ Aspects of psychological care — maternal (appendix D)

Additional nursing diagnoses

❑ Fear related to intrauterine blood transfusion and effects on fetus
❑ Ineffective individual coping related to bimonthly invasive procedure to gravid uterus
❑ Knowledge deficit related to blood type, Rh type, and zygosity of self and partner and implications for fetus

Sexually transmitted diseases

DEFINITION

Pathogenic invasion of a microorganism or virus into the pregnant patient may cause injury to the mother, fetus, or both. Invasion may occur before conception, during the insemination that causes pregnancy, or during pregnancy. Transmission to the fetus occurs by means of transplacental inoculation, fetal contact with the infected maternal genitalia, or both. Sexually transmitted diseases (STDs) include syphilis, gonorrhea, chlamydial infection, toxoplasmosis, rubella, cytomegalovirus (CMV) infection, and herpes simplex virus infection. Other diseases vary by geographic location but may include varicella and group B beta-hemolytic streptococcus.

Etiology and precipitating factors
- Syphilis: the spirochete *Treponema pallidum*
- Gonorrhea: the bacterium *Neisseria gonorrhoeae*
- Chlamydial infection: the bacterium *Chlamydia trachomatis*
- Toxoplasmosis: the protozoan *Toxoplasma gondii*
- Rubella: the virus rubella
- CMV infection: the virus *Cytomegalovirus*
- Herpes simplex virus type 2 (HSV-2) infection: the virus *Herpesvirus hominis*
- Risk factors include low socioeconomic status, high parity, previous urinary tract infection, sickle cell trait, undiagnosed obstructive lesions, congenital abnormalities of the genitourinary tract, substance abuse, and human immunodeficiency virus infection.

Physical findings
Syphilis
Primary
- Painless chancres at entry point
- Painless, single, enlarged lymph node
- Low-grade fever
- Weight loss
- Malaise
- ransient alopecia

Secondary
- Symmetrical, well-defined rash over body
- Condylomata on moist surfaces
- Malaise, headache, anorexia, nausea, myalgia, and fatigue

Tertiary
- Local or diffuse gummas
- Periostitis or osteitis
- Cardiovascular syphilis
- Neurosyphilis

Gonorrhea
Early
- Frequently asymptomatic
- Mucopurulent or purulent, foul-smelling cervical or rectal discharge
- Gray vulval exudate or condylomata; vulvovaginitis
- Cervical edema, erosion, and tenderness
- Urinary frequency and dysuria

Late
- Lower abdominal pain and distention and chronic pelvic pain
- Pyrexia, cervical tenderness, nausea, and emesis

Chlamydial infection
- Frequently asymptomatic
- Occasional cervicitis and urethritis with urinary frequency and dysuria
- Pelvic pain, dyspareunia

Toxoplasmosis
- Possibly asymptomatic
- Myalgia
- Malaise
- Diffuse maculopapular rash
- Splenomegaly
- Posterior, cervical lymphadenopathy

Active rubella
- Prodromal headache
- Malaise
- Anorexia
- Low-grade fever
- Coryza
- Lymphadenopathy
- Conjunctivitis
- Maculopapular rash on face, trunk, and extremities
- Forschheimer petechial macules on soft palate
- Photophobia

CMV infection
- Asymptomatic
- Possibly mononucleosis-like cluster of symptoms
- Cervical discharge

HSV-2 infection
- Painless vesicles rupture followed by:
  - recurrent itchy, purulent, painful vesicles on external genitalia, vagina, and cervix
  - pyrexia, malaise, and anorexia

- Genital irritation and pruritus
- Foul-smelling, profuse vaginal and urethral discharge
- Painful inguinal lymphadenopathy
- Dysuria

Diagnostic studies
- Syphilis: positive darkfield microscopy for *T. pallidum* from chancre exudate or secondary lesion; weakly reactive or reactive Venereal Disease Research Laboratory (VDRL) test; positive fluorescent treponemal antibody absorption (FTA-ABS) test
- Gonorrhea: identification of gonococcus by Gram stain of exudate and confirmation by bacterial culture
- Chlamydial infection: positive culture of *C. trachomatis*; Gram stain may reveal numerous leukocytes

- Toxoplasmosis: identification of protozoa with Wright or Giemsa stain; Sabin-Feldman dye titers greater than 1:1,000; presence of immunoglobulin M (IgM)-fluorescent antibodies to evaluate recent acquisitions
- Rubella: acute sample antibody titer greater than 1:10; previous infections and, therefore, immunity evidenced by hemagglutination inhibition (HAI) titer greater than 1:10 or positive complement fixation
- CMV infection: intranuclear inclusions in epithelial cells in urine sediment; complement fixation in sera during acute and convalescent phases
- HSV-2 infection: positive cytopathic effect on culture from exudate; smear may contain large, multinucleated cells with eosinophilic viral inclusion bodies; concurrent rise in antibody titer may be seen

COLLABORATIVE PROBLEM

Risk for maternal infection related to exposure to pathogens (two expected outcomes)

Expected outcome 1

The patient will exhibit no signs of infection as evidenced by negative cultures.

Interventions

1. Screen for syphilis. Administer the VDRL test on the patient's first clinic visit, to be confirmed by FTA-ABS test if it is positive. Repeat in the third trimester and on all umbilical cord blood tests in high-risk patients (those with infected, multiple, or casual sexual partners).

2. Screen for gonorrhea, noting cervical, urethral, or rectal discharge; cervical edema, tenderness, or erosion; urinary frequency, urgency, and dysuria; and pelvic or abdominal discomfort. Culture all exudates; repeat screenings in the third trimester in high-risk patients.

3. Screen for asymptomatic chlamydial infection, noting a history of PID or genital infection; those at risk include teens and pregnant women whose partners have a history of nongonococcal urethritis (NGU). Culture any exudates.

4. Screen for toxoplasmosis, noting rash, lymphadenopathy, constitutional symptoms, history of foreign travel, ingestion of raw or undercooked meats, and exposure to cats and cat excreta.

5. Screen for exposure to rubella, noting a confirmed history of disease, recent exposure to disease, rash, and constitutional symptoms.

6. Screen for CMV infection, noting mononucleosis-like or constitutional symptoms; complement fixation, IgM antibody titer, or a neutralization test may be recommended.

Rationales

1. Syphilis transmission to the fetus may cause midtrimester abortion, stillbirth, or preterm or term delivery of an infant with congenital syphilis. Maternal implications include progression to tertiary syphilis with cardiovascular and neurologic involvement.

2. Gonorrhea transmission to the fetus may cause ophthalmia neonatorum, gonococcal pneumonia, or neonatal sepsis. Maternal implications include salpingitis, chronic pelvic inflammatory disease (PID), gonococcal arthritis, and disseminated infection with bacteremia.

3. Transmission of chlamydial infection to the fetus may cause ophthalmia neonatorum, chlamydial pneumonia, preterm birth, stillbirth, or neonatal death. Maternal implications include PID and NGU.

4. Toxoplasmosis transmission to the fetus may cause preterm birth, stillbirth, or congenital toxoplasmosis. Maternal implications include localized or massive generalized infection.

5. Rubella transmission to the fetus during the first trimester may cause death or marked congenital anomalies of the heart, brain, eyes, or ears; second-trimester exposure is associated with hearing impairment.

6. Transmission of CMV infection to the fetus may result in abortion, stillbirth, or delivery of an infant who is small for gestational age and who has active disease.

7. Screen for HSV-2 infection, noting painful vesicles, genital irritation and pruritus, lymphadenopathy, dysuria, and pyrexia; culture active lesions.

8. Additional individualized interventions: _____

7. First-trimester transmission of HSV-2 infection to the fetus may result in abortion; later infection is associated with preterm birth, neonatal vesicular lesions, and overwhelming infection.

8. Rationales: _____

Expected outcome 2

The patient will develop minimal, if any, infection as evidenced by a positive response to treatment or negative cultures.

Interventions

1. To treat syphilis infection, have I.M. penicillin G benzathine (Bicillin L-A) or I.M. aqueous penicillin G procaine (Wycillin) on hand if the patient is not allergic to penicillin; if she is, have erythromycin stearate (Erythrocin Stearate), doxycycline (Vibramycin), or ceftriaxone (Rocephin) on hand. Monitor her progress. Recommend that her partner also receive treatment.

2. To treat gonorrhea infection, have amoxicillin (Wymox), probenecid (Benemid), spectinomycin (Trobicin), and ceftriaxone on hand. Recommend that the patient's partner also receive treatment.

3. To treat chlamydial infection, have erythromycin base (PCE Robimycin), erythromycin ethylsuccinate, or amoxicillin on hand. Culture any exudate, if possible. Recommend to the patient that her partner also receive treatment if he has positive cultures or exhibits signs of NGU.

4. To prevent toxoplasmosis, instruct the patient to avoid cats, never to handle litter boxes or cat excreta, and to eat only thoroughly cooked meats. For treatment of toxoplasmosis infection, have pyrimethamine (Daraprim) and sulfonamides on hand; discontinue sulfonamides before delivery.

5. To prevent rubella infection, have live rubella vaccine on hand for:
• postpartum mothers with HAI titers of less than 1:8
• prepubescent children older than 15 months
• sexually active, susceptible women who are not pregnant and are using contraceptives.

6. Tell the high-risk patient that CMV infection cannot be prevented or treated. The virus, present in urine, saliva, cervical mucus, semen, and breast milk, can be spread by close or intimate contact.

Rationales

1. These drugs are part of the protocols recommended by the Centers for Disease Control and Prevention. Continual monitoring detects recurrences. Treatment of the patient's partner minimizes the risk of reinfection.

2. Treatment of the patient's partner minimizes the risk of reinfection. Culture results indicate efficacy of drug therapy.

3. Cultures may not be widely available or the cost may be prohibitive. If the patient's partner is culture positive or exhibits symptoms of NGU, he should also receive treatment.

4. These instructions can help prevent infection. If the patient has an infection, pyrimethamine is the drug of choice, although its use is limited because of its teratogenic effects, most notably early in pregnancy. Sulfonamides can increase bilirubin levels.

5. No treatment exists for rubella; prophylaxis is the only way to control the disease. The vaccine is contraindicated in pregnancy because the fetus can be affected by it early in pregnancy. Pregnancy is not advised for 3 months after inoculation because of possible effects on the fetus.

6. Transmission of CMV infection to the fetus across the placenta or through contact with the genital tract mainly affects the fetal blood, brain, and liver.

7. To treat HSV-II infection, encourage the patient's partner to use condoms, whether he is symptomatic or not.
• Administer acyclovir (Zovirax) if the patient has severe disseminated infection.
• Prepare the patient for cesarean section if she has genital lesions or is suspected of having lesions in the genital tract or if cultures reveal the presence of the virus.

8. Additional individualized interventions: _____

7. Viral shedding persists even without overt symptoms.
• Acyclovir reduces maternal viral shedding time; it is not routinely recommended.
• Fetal contact with the infected genital tract is the major source of transmission. Delivery by cesarean section may prevent transmission.

8. Rationales: _____

Documentation checklist
During the clinic visit, document:
☐ patient status and assessment findings
☐ any changes in status since the last visit
☐ pertinent laboratory and diagnostic findings
☐ the patient's response to treatment
☐ patient and family teaching guidelines
☐ follow-up planning guidelines.

Associated plans and appendices
☐ Cesarean section birth
☐ Inappropriate size or weight: small for gestational age
☐ Normal antepartum
☐ Preterm infant
☐ Sepsis neonatorum and infectious disorders
☐ Aspects of psychological care — maternal (appendix D)

Additional nursing diagnoses
☐ Activity intolerance related to prodromal symptoms or subclinical disease
☐ Altered sexuality patterns related to required condom use or safer sex practices to reduce genital reinfection of partner
☐ Fear related to unknown fetal outcome
☐ Spiritual distress related to guilt for having acquired disease and its possible repercussion on fetus or infant

Part 2

Intrapartum

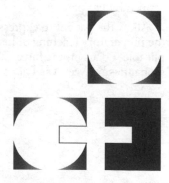

Cesarean section birth

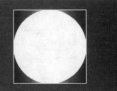

Definition

In cesarean section birth, the fetus is delivered through incisions made into the abdominal and uterine walls. This procedure is indicated for any condition that jeopardizes maternal or fetal health and for which postponement of delivery or vaginal birth itself would compromise the patient's safety. Indications for cesarean section birth include — but are not limited to — the following: a nonreassuring fetal heart rate (FHR) pattern (fetal distress); previous cesarean section; dystocia; cephalopelvic disproportion; breech, shoulder, or compound presentation; abruptio placentae; placenta previa; prolapsed umbilical cord; prolonged rupture of membranes; preeclampsia or eclampsia; insulin-dependent diabetes mellitus; spinal or pelvic fractures; pelvic tumors; gonorrhea; and genital herpes. For more detailed information on each condition, see the appropriate plans of care.

Cesarean section may be an emergency procedure or anticipated. If it is anticipated, the parents have greater latitude about birthing and anesthesia options and can receive comprehensive preoperative teaching. This plan of care includes physical findings associated with fetal distress, types and implications of cesarean section procedures, and postpartum considerations specific to cesarean section patients. Review of the normal postpartum experience is essential.

Physical findings

Common indications of fetal distress include:
• sudden decrease or cessation of fetal movement
• meconium-stained amniotic fluid (without breech presentation)
• FHR persistently less than 110 or greater than 160 beats/minute
• in the absence of short-term variability, repetitive early, late, or variable patterns of deceleration with slow recovery
• sinusoidal FHR pattern (rare)
• pH of fetal scalp (capillary) blood 7.25 or lower
• positive oxytocin challenge test
• absent or short-term variability of 0 to 2 beats/minute
• biophysical profile of 4 or less
(See *Clinical pathway for cesarean birth*, pages 98 to 101.)

NURSING DIAGNOSIS

Ineffective individual coping related to surgical intervention, perceived loss of the birthing experience, and fatigue

Expected outcome

The patient will exhibit positive coping as evidenced by verbalization of feelings and no signs of inconsolable crying.

Interventions

1. Accept the patient's reaction to cesarean section birth. Note isolation, lack of concentration, silence, regressive behaviors, or repeatedly asked questions. Integrate with prepregnancy and prenatal behavior described by her partner.

2. Allow the patient to express her feelings. Reinforce the preparatory teaching of her prenatal classes, if applicable. Focus on the birth experience and the commonalities between vaginal and cesarean section birth.

Rationales

1. An inability to cope may take various forms; subtle manifestations may signal an inability to cope as much as such overt behaviors as verbalizing, moaning, and crying.

2. Although prenatal classes include information on cesarean section birth, many patients do not want to apply that information to themselves. A patient completing her first pregnancy or who has had repeat cesarean sections may be especially disappointed if she will not be delivering vaginally. Focusing on the birth rather than the surgical experience is a positive activity and may lessen disappointment and guilt.

3. Cluster nursing assessments and activities. Allow intervals of inactivity.

4. Perform or review family and home assessments; include the patient and significant others in discharge planning.

5. Reassure the patient that she may deliver vaginally in the future.

6. Additional individualized interventions: _____

_____

3. Fatigue lessens the patient's ability to cope.

4. Caring for her infant and maintaining a home may be especially difficult if the patient has limited assistance and multiple responsibilities. Discharge planning that begins on admission may prevent, improve, or resolve home problems.

5. The patient may think that future deliveries must be by cesarean section; the resulting anxiety may interfere with her ability to cope with the current situation.

6. Rationales: _____

_____

COLLABORATIVE PROBLEM

Pain related to surgical incision

Expected outcome

The patient will experience less pain.

Interventions

1. Assess the patient's pain, including location, severity, duration, and defining characteristics. Ascertain that the incision site is not infected and the bladder not distended.

2. Administer meperidine (Demerol) I.M. or morphine I.V. or I.M. Alternatively, administer morphine (Duramorph) by way of an epidural at delivery and again 12 hours after delivery, or let the patient control the amount of medication she receives with patient-controlled analgesia (PCA). Later, the patient should switch to 800 mg of ibuprofen every 6 hours or a combination drug, such as acetaminophen and hydrocodone (Lortab), every 4 hours, as needed.

3. Monitor PCA.

4. Assess the patient's response to pharmacologic pain management.

5. Perform comfort measures and encourage relaxation techniques.

6. Additional individualized interventions: _____

_____

Rationales

1. Assessment confirms that pain is related to the surgical incision.

2. Pharmacologic analgesia is necessary for 48 hours or more because of surgical manipulation, unless the patient received a long-acting epidural anesthetic, which provides pain relief for 24 hours. Epidural morphine also increases the patient's ability to walk some of the soreness out, instead of becoming stiff from lying in bed. In either case, weaning to oral analgesics occurs afterward. The continued pain relief increases the patient's ability to cope and comply with activities and allows her to hold her infant easily, fostering bonding.

3. Monitoring allows assessment of the effectiveness of PCA.

4. Assessment confirms the effectiveness of pain relief.

5. These techniques enhance pharmacologic analgesia and give the patient a sense of control.

6. Rationales: _____

_____

(Text continues on page 102.)

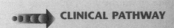

CLINICAL PATHWAY

Cesarean Birth

Patient problem	Preoperative	Intraoperative	Recovery
Fluid balance	• Patient receives an I.V. preload of at least 1,000 ml lactated Ringer's solution • Complete blood count (CBC) within normal limits	• Surgical blood loss < 1,000 ml • Urine output ≥ 30 ml/hour • Oxygen saturation ≥ 96% or unchanged from preoperative level	• Uterus firm; not more than 1 fingerbreadth above umbilicus • Small to moderate amount of vaginal bleeding • Incision drainage within normal limits • Skin warm, dry; capillary refill brisk • Urine output ≥ 30 ml/hour
Pain and discomfort	• Patient expresses understanding of pain-relief options and potential adverse effects. • Patient understands use of 0 to 10 pain scale.	• Patient expresses no pain during surgical procedures.	• Patient states pain or discomfort is controlled.
Family integration	• Family understands visitation opportunities.	• Family holds and touches infant.	• Family holds and touches infant. • Breast-feeding begins within 60 to 90 minutes of delivery (if breast-feeding).
Infection	• Body temperature within normal limits • Lungs clear on auscultation and examination		
Potential for ileus			• No increased surgical risk
Assessment	• Intake and output (I &O), including ice chips • Preanesthesia score • Admission interview • Vital signs, physical examination, laboratory results review • Electronic fetal monitoring (including central surveillance and recording) • Anesthesia interview	• Cardiopulmonary monitoring per anesthesia • I & O	• Vital signs (VS) every 15 minutes • Dressing, bleeding, fundus assessment every 15 minutes • Postanesthesia recovery score • I & O • Breast and nipple assessment and latch score (if breast-feeding)
Teaching	• Teach patient side-lying position. • Orient patient to room, procedures, and visitation. • Provide anesthesia information and instructions. • Teach patient to cough and deep breathe.	• Orient patient to OR. • Instruct father or significant other on garb and orient to OR.	

Day of delivery	Postoperative day 1	Postoperative day 2
• Uterus firm; not more than 1 finger-breadth above umbilicus • Small to moderate amount of vaginal bleeding • Incision drainage within normal limits • Skin warm, dry; capillary refill brisk • Urine output ≥ 30 ml/hour	• Uterus firm; at or below the umbilicus • Small to moderate amount of vaginal bleeding • CBC within normal limits • I & O within normal limits • No bladder distention; voiding every shift within 8 hours	• Uterus firm and below umbilicus • Small to moderate amount of vaginal bleeding
• Patient has periods of sleep during immediate postoperative period. • Patient states pain or discomfort is controlled. • Patient describes how to manage pain with increased activity.	• Patient progresses to oral pain management. • Patient states pain or discomfort is controlled with oral medication. • Patient describes how to manage pain with increased activity.	• Patient states pain or discomfort is controlled. • Patient describes how to manage pain with increased activity.
• Family holds and touches infant. • Milk production is stimulated.	• Patient achieves latch score greater than 7 (if breast-feeding). • Family holds infant. • Mother and infant make eye contact. • Family provides infant care.	• Family provides infant care. • Family responds to infant's needs. • Patient achieves latch score greater than 7 (if breast-feeding).
• Body temperature < 100.8° F (38.2° C) • Patient tolerates small amounts of clear liquids	• Body temperature <100.4° F (38° C) • Incision not extremely red; shows no purulent drainage	• Patient able to describe signs of infection
• VS on admission, at 2 hours, then every 6 hours for 24 hours • Physical examination and assessment • I & O (including ice chips) • Breast and nipple assessment and latch score (if breast-feeding)	• Tolerates soft diet • Bowel sounds present • Abdomen soft and minimally distended	• Flatulent • Has bowel sounds • Tolerates diet
• Prepare patient for self-care. • Instruct and review deep breathing and coughing. • Refer to neonatal pathway for care of infant.	• I & O (including ice chips) • Physical examination and assessment • Incision inspection • VS every 6 hours for first 24 hours, then every shift • Breast and nipple assessment and latch score (if breast-feeding)	• VS every shift • Physical examination and assessment • Breast and nipple assessment and latch score (if breast-feeding)
• Give patient discharge packet.	• Promote and reinforce self-care. • Review discharge packet. • Teach breast-feeding or bottle-feeding. • Provide health channel or video education.	• Review self-care. • Provide information on birth control or family planning. • Review discharge instructions, including signs and symptoms of infection. • Reinforce breast-feeding or bottle-feeding education.

(continued)

Cesarean birth *(continued)*

Patient problem	Preoperative	Intraoperative	Recovery
Discharge planning	• Identify pediatrician. • Note caregiver on admission record.		
Tests	• Rapid plasma reagent test • Blood type and screen • CBC (cell profile) • Ultrasonography		
Interventions	• Complete operative permission and operating room (OR) checklist. • Obtain informed consent permission. • Obtain signature for circumcision permission. • Make sure patient is registered, admitted, logged in book. • Determine OR availability. • Consider need for pediatric resuscitation team. • Prepare to support parent-infant contact.	• Begin regional anesthesia procedure. • Insert indwelling urinary (Foley) catheter. • Consider need for pediatric resuscitation team. • Support parent-infant contact.	• Maintain indwelling urinary catheter. • Provide perineal hygiene. • Remove epidural catheter. • Transport to postpartum unit pending postanesthesia record (PAR) score ≥ 8.
Consultations	• Consider neonatology and pediatric consult • Resident and 2nd option consult • Social service (SS) consult		
Medications	• Start I.V. for preload of 1,000 ml lactated Ringer's solution. • Administer preoperative medications. • Administer I.V. lactated Ringer's solution.	• Maintain I.V. fluids. • Administer prophylactic antibiotics after cord is clamped. • Maintain morphine. (Duramorph) administration through epidural.	• Administer I.M. or I.V. analgesics. • Maintain morphine administration through epidural. • Administer antiemetics. • Maintain I.V. fluids.
Nutrition	• Nothing by mouth (NPO)	• NPO	• NPO
Activities and safety	• Call light within reach	• Safety belt after insertion of indwelling urinary catheter • Bovie/grounding pad on • Suction for patient and neonate • Wedge to maintain patient in left lateral position	• Side rails up

Day of delivery	Postoperative day 1	Postoperative day 2
	• Identify support systems. • Help patient plan for home needs.	• Provide instructions for follow-up appointments and prescriptions.
	• CBC (cell profile) • Rh status • Rh$_o$(D) immune globulin given (if applicable) • Rubella status • Rubella vaccination given (if applicable)	• Rubella status • Rubella vaccination given (if applicable)
• Perform perineal hygiene. • Check sensation in legs and perform passive leg exercise. • Maintain indwelling urinary catheter. • Assist with coughing and deep breathing. • Have patient breast-feed or pump every 2 to 3 hours (unless bottle-feeding).	• Have patient breast-feed or pump every 2 to 3 hours (if breast-feeding). • Discontinue indwelling urinary catheter. • Assist with morning and hygiene care. • Encourage deep breathing and coughing four times a day. • Have doctor check circumcision permission. • Provide ice packs or support bra. • Have breast pump at bedside (if breast-feeding).	• Encourage patient to shower. • Encourage deep breathing and coughing four times a day. • Discontinue saline lock.
• Consider SS	• Consider SS • Consider lactation	
• Manage pain with morphine. • Maintain I.V. fluids for fluid balance. • Provide antiemetics.	• Provide oral analgesics. • Convert I.V. to saline lock or discontinue. • Administer antacids for gas control, as needed. • Administer laxative and stool softener, as needed.	• Provide oral analgesics, as needed. • Administer laxative and stool softener, as needed.
• Sips of water and ice chips • Clear liquids as tolerated	• Diet advances as tolerated	• Regular diet
• Out of bed with assistance as tolerated	• Up freely	• Up and ambulate freely

Adapted with permission fromTriHealth Health System, Cincinnati, Ohio.

Intrapartum

COLLABORATIVE PROBLEM

Risk for fluid volume deficit related to blood loss associated with surgery, underlying condition that necessitated surgery, and uterine hypotonicity

Expected outcome

The patient will have minimal or no fluid volume deficit as evidenced by stable vital signs, including blood pressure within normal limits, and no excessive blood loss.

Interventions

1. Assess the patient's vital signs every 15 minutes for the first hour, every 30 minutes for next hour, every hour for next 4 hours, and then every 4 hours as the patient's condition warrants. Correlate findings with prenatal levels. Note estimated blood loss during surgery and types of anesthetic administered.

2. Assess fundal contractility. Support the incision with your nondominant hand and palpate the fundus from the sides, using your dominant hand. Schedule an assessment, when possible (based on the patient's condition), after administration of analgesics.

3. Concurrently assess the number of perineal pads used, time interval before changing, and degree of saturation. Assess lochia for color, amount, odor, characteristics, and the presence and amount of clots. Differentiate lochia rubra from frank bleeding.

4. Assess the abdominal dressing for drainage, noting color. Circumscribe and date the drainage area with a pen.

5. Assess incision for active bleeding, seepage, approximation of edges, and hematoma formation.

6. Note hematocrit, comparing prenatal, intrapartum, and postpartum percentages.

7. Determine whether the patient is receiving sufficient fluids. Continue fluid administration initiated intrapartally.

8. Additional individualized interventions: _____

Rationales

1. If there is no hemorrhaging, blood pressure is essentially unchanged in the postpartum period and bradycardia is common. Early indications of hemorrhage include prolonged capillary refill times on the blanch test; initially, blood pressure and heart rate increase, then blood pressure decreases while heart rate remains somewhat elevated. Eventually, both return to within normal limits.

2. Hemorrhage is a significant source of maternal morbidity. Assessment of fundal height and contractility is commonly neglected or postponed because it causes discomfort to the patient.

3. Significant fluid loss may occur intrapartally. The postpartum course should be the same as for vaginal birth. Typically, cesarean section results in less lochia postpartum secondary to irrigation during surgery.

4. Telfa pads are often used as thick abdominal dressing. When they fall off (usually the next day), the incision is left with no dressing. Dressings that become saturated or soiled should be changed. Assessment technique must be modified but not eliminated.

5. Visualization is possible when the original dressing has been changed or removed.

6. A hematocrit of 33% or greater usually indicates maternal tolerance of blood loss.

7. Prolonged labor before surgical delivery may have caused hypovolemia. The administration of I.V. fluids enhances circulating blood volume and minimizes sequelae of loss.

8. Rationales: _____

NURSING DIAGNOSIS

Risk for maternal infection related to delivery and secondary to surgical incision, repeated vaginal examination, sequelae of anesthetic administration, bladder intubation, or I.V. lines

Expected outcome

The patient will not develop an infection as evidenced by stable vital signs, no fever, and no redness or edema at the incision site.

Interventions

1. Monitor the patient's vital signs every 4 hours and as her condition warrants.

2. Assess the patient's abdomen, incision, and abdominal dressing.

3. Assess the perineum, noting any foul-smelling lochia. Continue perineal care.

4. Assess bladder drainage; note color, amount, and odor of urine; presence of blood, clots, or sediment; and fluid intake and output. Catheter care should be incorporated into perineal care. Assess for dysuria and retention after the catheter is removed.

5. Assess breath sounds; note decreased or absent sounds, crackles, rhonchi, and cough. Schedule coughing and deep-breathing exercises after administration of analgesics.

6. Assess the I.V. site for erythema, edema, induration, and infiltration. Change the I.V. tubing and dressing once daily.

7. Additional individualized interventions: _____

Rationales

1. An initial low-grade fever (temperature less than 100.4° F [38° C]) is associated with parturition and the inflammatory changes associated with surgery. Protracted low-grade fever or actual pyrexia is associated with infection and warrants antibiotic therapy.

2. Indications of healing include no signs of *r*edness, *e*dema, *e*cchymosis, or *d*rainage, and the incision should have well-*a*pproximated edges — the REEDA parameters. The outer dressing should be clean, dry, and intact, and the abdomen should feel soft, with the uterus contracted below the umbilicus as involution progresses.

3. Ascending genital tract infection may result from repeated intrapartum vaginal examinations or questionable hygienic practices. Scrupulous perineal care is indicated, regardless of the type of delivery.

4. An indwelling urinary (Foley) catheter is usually inserted before surgery and remains in place for 24 hours postpartum; its presence contributes to the risk of infection. The urine should be clear, amber, odorless, and free of blood, sediment, or clots. Increased output is associated with diuresis secondary to intrapartum administration of oxytocin and to normal postpartum changes. Bloody urine may indicate trauma associated with delivery and warrants immediate attention.

5. General anesthesia and voluntary immobility secondary to pain may result in accumulation of secretions and decreased ventilatory function.

6. Infection at the I.V. site can cause significant maternal morbidity.

7. Rationales: _____

Intrapartum

NURSING DIAGNOSIS

Activity intolerance related to delivery and secondary to anesthetic administration, surgical incision, and pain

Expected outcome

The patient will develop minimal sequelae from inactivity and will progressively increase activity.

Interventions

1. Note the type of anesthetic administered intrapartally and the recovery time; reposition the patient after the prescribed period of bed rest.

2. Demonstrate or review pulmonary hygiene measures. Assist the patient with deep breathing and coughing every 2 to 4 hours, after administering analgesics if possible. Place the bed in semi-Fowler's to high Fowler's position. Splint the incision with a pillow or intertwined fingers.

3. While the patient is on bed rest, instruct her in leg exercises (paddling or modified knee bends, for example); schedule time for exercises and offer encouragement.

4. Assist the patient with progressive ambulation. Begin by having the patient dangle her legs over the side of the bed, then progress to her sitting at bedside and taking accompanied walks over designated lengths.

5. Additional individualized interventions: _____

Rationales

1. General anesthesia recovery times vary. Position changes and turning usually take place every 2 hours during the first 24 hours of prescribed bed rest. Spinal anesthesia recovery requires lying flat in bed in the supine or side-lying position for 8 to 12 hours.

2. Pulmonary hygiene measures help clear accumulated lung secretions. Premedication fosters compliance by decreasing pain and anxiety.

3. Blood stasis in peripheral vessels predisposes the patient to thrombophlebitis.

4. Hypotension and resulting vertigo commonly accompany early ambulation. Actual or anticipated pain and interference from I.V. lines and urinary catheter may frighten or confuse the patient and result in reluctance to move.

5. Rationales: _____

COLLABORATIVE PROBLEM

Altered nutrition: less than body requirements related to fasting status imposed by anesthesia and surgery and by physiologic response to abdominal surgery

Expected outcome

The patient will maintain fluid requirements and progress to a regular diet.

Interventions

1. Administer a balanced electrolyte and glucose I.V. solution at a rate of about 100 to 125 ml/hour; continue until the patient can tolerate solid food.

2. Assess the patient's abdomen, noting size, tension, and bowel sounds. Ask if flatus has been expelled.

Rationales

1. I.V. feedings supply fluid but not the caloric or nutritional requirements of postpartum course.

2. Peristalsis usually returns within 24 hours and is characterized by a soft, nondistended abdomen with active bowel sounds. Bowel sounds (normoactive, greater than 5 per minute) may occur during the recovery period.

3. Offer water and surgical (clear) liquid, and progress the diet, as tolerated. Note the patient's ability to retain food and express hunger. Keep the I.V. line in place until the patient can successfully retain liquids.

4. Assist the patient with menu selection, encouraging foods high in protein, vitamin C, and iron.

5. Additional individualized interventions: _____

3. The patient should return to a regular diet as tolerated, based on what she wants. Ascertaining her ability to retain liquids before removing the I.V. line obviates the need to restart the I.V. line if dyspepsia, nausea, or emesis should occur.

4. Protein and vitamin C promote wound healing, and iron helps correct anemia.

5. Rationales: _____

NURSING DIAGNOSIS

Knowledge deficit related to postpartum course and implications for subsequent pregnancies

Expected outcome

The patient will express an understanding of the normal postpartum course and implications for subsequent pregnancies.

Interventions

1. Decide when the patient is most ready to learn, based on her freedom from discomfort and distraction and her willingness to ask questions or express her concerns or doubts. Provide privacy. Actively listen, allowing time for questions.

2. Provide information on postpartum course, including:
• hygiene: Sutures or clips are usually removed on the 5th day and may be removed after discharge. Showering is frequently allowed by the next day if the patient is ambulating without difficulty.
• exercise: Heavy work, including lifting of heavy objects, is not permitted until the postpartum visit with the practitioner, usually in 2 weeks. Driving is prohibited for 4 to 6 weeks.
• coitus: Sexual relations may safely be resumed after the postpartum examination, usually in 3 to 6 weeks. Contraception alternatives are given as part of discharge planning and during the return visit to the doctor at 3 to 6 weeks.
• activities: The patient should concern herself predominantly with caring for herself and her infant.

3. Provide information, as appropriate, on vaginal birth after cesarean section and repeat elective cesarean section births. Using general guidelines, suggest that vaginal birth after cesarean section may be accomplished if the underlying condition has been corrected or does not recur. "Once a section, always a section" no longer holds true.

4. Additional individualized interventions: _____

Rationales

1. The patient will more readily receive and retain information if she is ready to learn.

2. Information gives the patient an active role in her own care and allows time to make adaptations in the home. The patient should know that heavy bleeding may occur after marked exertion. Maternal injury or pregnancy may result if sexual relations are resumed before postpartum examination. The stressors of a new infant and major surgery may easily lead to fatigue and depression; help from family members may be beneficial.

3. Certain conditions preclude vaginal birth. A trial labor may be encouraged in the absence of diagnosed maternal or fetal dysfunction. Criteria for trial labor include pelvic adequacy, preferably one prior low cervical transverse unextended uterine incision, informed consent, and immediate professional and logistical support for a cesarean section delivery if the trial should fail.

4. Rationales: _____

Intrapartum

Documentation checklist

During the hospital stay, document:

❏ patient status and assessment findings, including a history of previous pregnancies and their outcomes
❏ changes in patient status
❏ pertinent laboratory and diagnostic findings
❏ fundal height and tone
❏ pain — quality, location, frequency, and intensity
❏ the patient's response to surgery
❏ the patient's and family's reaction to the surgery
❏ patient and family teaching guidelines
❏ discharge planning guidelines.

Associated plans and appendices

❏ Abruptio placentae
❏ Hemorrhage
❏ Normal antepartum
❏ Placenta previa
❏ Pregnancy complicated by diabetes mellitus
❏ Pregnancy-induced hypertension
❏ Prolapsed umbilical cord
❏ Puerperal infection
❏ Puerperium
❏ Sexually transmitted diseases
❏ Thromboembolic disease
❏ Aspects of psychological care — maternal (appendix D)
❏ Preparing for nonemergency surgery (appendix E)
❏ Selected methods of family planning (appendix F)

Associated nursing diagnoses

❏ Constipation related to anticipatory abdominal pain
❏ Risk for altered parenting related to postponed bonding secondary to inability to touch, hold, or care for infant because of effects of anesthesia, pain, or infant condition
❏ Self-esteem disturbance related to perceived inability to give birth "naturally"

Labor and vaginal birth

Definition
Labor is a physiologic process in which the fetus, after an approximate 282-day habitus in utero, is expelled. There are four stages of labor. The first stage can be further divided into the latent, active, and transition phases. Prelabor is an amorphous stage that occurs several weeks before true labor and results in increased uterine activity, which serves to ready the cervix for its eventual effacement and dilation.
• First-stage labor is characterized by cervical effacement and dilation, readying for the passage of the fetal head.
• Second-stage labor results in expulsion of the fetus.
• Third-stage labor results in placental separation and expulsion.
• Fourth-stage labor is the 1 to 4 hours after placental delivery in which the contracting uterus controls bleeding. During this period, the mother is at risk for hemorrhage and complications associated with uterine atony, anesthesia induction, and metabolic disorders.

Delivery in the occiput or vertex presentation accounts for 95% to 97% of all labors, and this fetal presentation is assumed in this plan. The positional changes necessary to accommodate the fetal head to the maternal pelvis include engagement, descent, flexion, internal rotation, extension, external rotation, and expulsion. Anywhere from 5 to 30 minutes after expulsion, placental separation usually occurs, and placental delivery is enacted either spontaneously or manually.

Management of the labor process aims to maintain optimal maternal and fetal well-being, identify and ameliorate distress, and prevent or minimize complications.

Etiology and precipitating factors
• Etiology: The labor process is hypothesized to result from oxytocin release by the neurohypophysis; estrogen stimulation; progesterone withdrawal; increased maternal prostaglandin and fetal cortisol levels; increased uterine size; calcium release from the sarcoplasmic reticulum; pressure of the presenting part on the cervix and lower uterine segment; or placental aging.
• Signs of impending labor include:
– lightening — a decrease in fundal height, reshaping and enlarging of the lower abdomen, flattening of the costal region, and a subjective maternal feeling of fetal "dropping" that occur with the descent of the fetus to or through the pelvic inlet and lower uterine development. This phenomenon occurs several weeks before true labor and is more pronounced in primigravid patients.
– false labor — brief, irregular uterine contractions of the lower abdomen and groin that do not progress and do not result in cervical dilation. These contractions, more common in patients of high parity and late in pregnancy, should be considered harbingers of true labor and be monitored closely.
– bloody show — the vaginal discharge of blood-tinged mucus that indicates the approach of labor; it may occur hours to days before actual labor. This mucous plug of the cervical canal should be differentiated from frank bleeding.

Physical findings
Stage 1: Latent phase
• Cervical dilation: 0 to 3 cm
• Cervical effacement in primiparous patient usually complete before dilation; occurs with dilation in multiparous patient
• Duration of latent phase: 8 to 10 hours
• Uterine contractions: mild, 5 to 30 minutes apart, and last 10 to 30 seconds
• Membranes ruptured or intact
• Scant brown or pink vaginal discharge or mucous plug
• Station: primiparous patient — usually 0; multiparous patient — 0 to –2
• Fetal heart tones (FHT): clearest at level of or below umbilicus, depending on fetal position

Stage 1: Active phase
• Cervical dilation: 4 to 7 cm
• Duration of active phase: about 6 hours
• Uterine contractions: moderate, 3 to 5 minutes apart, and last 30 to 45 seconds
• Scant to moderate bloody mucus
• Station: 0 to +1
• FHT: heard slightly below umbilicus or lower abdomen

Stage 1: Transition phase
• Cervical dilation: 8 to 10 cm (cervical dilation is complete at 10 cm at the end of stage 1)
• Duration of transition phase: 1 to 2 hours
• Uterine contractions: strong, 2 to 3 minutes apart, and last 45 to 60 seconds
• Copious bloody mucus
• Station: +2 to +3
• FHT: clearest directly above symphysis pubis

Stage 2: Expulsion of fetus
• Cervical effacement 100%
• Duration of stage 2: 20 to 50 minutes
• Uterine contractions: strong, 2 to 3 minutes apart, and last 60 to 90 seconds; fetal bradycardia during contraction may occur
• Membranes may rupture
• Copious bloody mucus
• Station: fetal descent continues at a rate of 1 cm/hour in primiparous patient and 2 cm or more in multiparous patient until perineal floor is reached
• Urge to push begins
• Perineum bulges, flattens
• Crowning occurs
• Infant is born

Stage 3: Expulsion of placenta
• Usually occurs within 5 to 30 minutes of delivery
• Uterine shape globular, usually firmer; fundus rises
• Dark vaginal bleeding — gush or trickle
• Umbilical cord protrudes further from introitus
• Placenta intact: shiny presentation of fetal side of placental separation occurs from inner to outer margins (Schultze mechanism); rough presentation of maternal side of placental separation occurs from outer margins inward (Duncan mechanism)

• Placenta, membranes, and umbilical cord intact and free of anomaly

Stage 4
• Fundus firm or becomes firm when massaged, midline at level of umbilicus
• Moderate lochia rubra
• Episiotomy and laceration repair clean without ecchymosis or discharge, minimal edema; tenderness commensurate with analgesia, usually mild; edges well approximated
• Possibly extrusion of hemorrhoids

Diagnostic studies
• Diagnosis is based on physical findings. Little testing is done unless maternal or fetal disorder or disease is suspected.
• Fern test identifies integrity of membranes; crystalline frond-like or fern pattern (arborization) indicates amniotic fluid; neither urine, blood, nor vaginal secretions elicit this configuration.
(See *Clinical pathway: Vaginal delivery,* pages 110 and 111.)

COLLABORATIVE PROBLEM
Onset of true labor related to hormonal and physical changes

Expected outcome
The patient will exhibit signs of true labor as evidenced by regular contractions increasing in frequency and intensity, progressive cervical dilation, and pain not relieved by walking.

Interventions
1. Assess contractions for location, regularity, frequency (from the start of one contraction to the start of the next one), intensity (determined by palpation or intrauterine pressure monitoring), duration, and relief from analgesics. Assess degree of effacement, station, position, and texture or consistency of cervix.

Rationales
1. True labor is characterized by regular contractions of increasing intensity and frequency. The patient experiences pain in her back and abdomen that is not stopped by analgesics. Cervical dilation is progressive. Early in labor, the cervix is posterior; as labor progresses, the cervix moves anteriorly. Before term begins, the cervix is firm (green), but as the patient approaches term, the cervix ripens and softens.

2. On the patient's admission to the obstetric unit, review the patient profile for:
• last menstrual period (LMP) and estimated date of confinement (EDC)
• pelvic adequacy — pelvic size is identified by the doctor and includes diagonal conjugate (distance of sacral promontory to lower margin of symphysis pubis), ischial spines, pelvic walls, and sacrum
• obstetric, gynecologic, and outstanding medical histories
• age
• height and weight
• blood type and Rh of patient and baby's father
• medications being taken
• allergies
• streptococcus B screening results
• prenatal care and progress
• prenatal preparation for childbirth
• patient concerns and perceptions about pregnancy and labor
• support systems.

3. If there is no gross or frank bleeding, use strict aseptic technique to perform a vaginal examination, assessing the following:
• status of membranes and presence of amniotic fluid

• cervical dilation, effacement, position, and texture or consistency

• identification of presenting part

• station.

4. Take vital signs, including temperature, pulse and respiratory rates, and blood pressure; compare with prepregnancy and prenatal measurements. Assess for peripheral edema and reflexes; note any abnormalities. Integrate findings with history and physical examination.

2. The patient profile establishes a database and helps prevent or identify patient problems.

3. Bleeding may indicate previa or premature separation, and manipulation may further compromise patient status.
• Nitrazine paper test or the more reliable fern test confirms rupture of membranes. Pale, straw-colored fluid with a pH of 6.5 to 7.5 is normal.
• Softness and degrees of dilation and effacement assist in staging labor. Cervical location in relation to the vagina and presenting part may identify preterm labor by its posterior position. *Note:* Dilation reflects the average diameter of the cervical opening; a diameter of 10 cm is considered complete or fully dilated and should allow passage of a full-term fetus. Effacement reflects cervical thinning and shortening that occurs late in pregnancy or during labor; complete effacement obliterates the cervical canal and transforms the 2-cm cervical length to a paper-thin, circular orifice.
• Identification of presenting part is essential to safe labor management. Position, which is changeable, may also be identified by Leopold's maneuvers.
• Station relates the level of the presenting fetal part to an imaginary line between the maternal ischial spines.

4. This information establishes a database, identifies the high-risk patient, and aids in early recognition and management of complications.

(Text continues on page 132.)

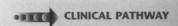

CLINICAL PATHWAY

Vaginal delivery

Patient problem	Active labor	Birth to 2 hours
Fluid balance	• No active bleeding • Temperature < 100.4° F (38° C) • No palpable bladder	• Minimal to moderate lochia flow • Firm fundus, no palpable bladder • Postanesthesia care unit and postanesthesia recovery score ≥ 8
Education	• Teach patient about activity level (based on anesthesia or analgesia administered).	• Patient states understanding of safety limits.
Pain and discomfort	• Patient used comfort options and alternative pain-control methods during progression of labor	• Patient states she is comfortable.
Family integration	• Patient's stated preferences for birth experience are discussed. • Patient's identified support systems or significant others are available.	• Patient begins breast-feeding 60 to 90 minutes after delivery (for breast-feeding). • Patient and significant others exhibit bonding behaviors (eye contact, touching, holding). • Patient's identified support systems are available.
Assessment	• Assess fetal heart rate and uterine activity every 30 minutes, then every 15 minutes in second stage of active labor. Assess intake and output (I & O) every shift and determine 24-hour total. Assess bladder every 2 hours. • Take vital signs (VS) every hour and temperature every 4 hours; if membranes rupture, take temperature every 2 hours. • Review prenatal course.	• Assess lochia, fundus, and VS every 15 minutes x 4. • Check voiding every 2 hours.
Teaching	• Support mother in birth plan. • Review clinical pathway. • Discuss comfort options. • Teach patient how to use 0 to 10 pain scale.	• Initiate parent-infant contact. • Have mother breast-feed (for breast-feeding). • Initiate self-care and begin self-care teaching. • Teach safety measures.
Discharge planning		
Tests	• Hepatitis surface antigen (if no prenatal test done) • Complete blood count (CBC) • Cervical examination (when necessary) • Doctor notified of any missing prenatal tests	
Interventions	• Insert straight catheter (if necessary). • Begin fetal monitoring. • Start I.V. line (if applicable).	• Apply ice to perineum as necessary. • Use straight catheter as necessary.
Consults	• Anesthesia • Social services (SS), if needed	
Medications	• Provide analgesia. • Maintain epidural (if applicable). • Maintain I.V. line (if applicable).	• Administer analgesia. • Discontinue I.V. line.
Nutrition	• Ice chips or fluids by mouth (optional)	• Diet as tolerated
Activity and safety	• Activity as tolerated • Ambulation encouraged early in labor	• Up with assistance, then activity as tolerated

2 to 6 hours after delivery	6 to 24 hours after delivery	Discharge
• Minimal to moderate lochia flow • Firm fundus • No orthostatic hypotension • Spontaneous voiding	• Minimal to moderate lochia flow • Firm fundus • Temperature < 100.4° F (38° C) • Spontaneous voiding	• Temperature ≤ 101° F (38.3° C) • Spontaneous voiding
• Patient identifies learning needs regarding herself and infant. • Patient demonstrates self-medication.	• Patient initiates care for herself and infant. • Patient demonstrates safe use of medication.	• Patient states understanding of discharge instructions and has questions answered. • Patient states understanding of information about follow-up care and concerns (nurse, doctor, lactation consultant, and community resources provide information).
• Patient states understanding of 0 to 10 pain scale.	• Patient states comfort measures are effective.	• Patient states comfort measures are effective.
• Patient expresses positive birth experience. • Milk production is stimulated (for breast-feeding).	• Family or significant others provide support (make positive comments, assist in providing care). • Patient achieves latch score ≥ 7.	• Patient states readiness for discharge (is emotionally ready, has assistance at home, has infant car seat).
• Assess lochia and fundus. • Check voiding. • Take VS on admission to postpartum unit at 2 hours, then every 6 hours x 4.	• Assess VS, lochia, and fundus every 6 hours x 4, then every shift if patient is stable.	• Assess VS, lochia, and fundus every shift if patient is stable and at time of discharge.
• Reinforce self-care and infant care teaching. • Reinforce teaching about breast-feeding and nipple integrity (for breast-feeding). • Teach self-medication program.	• Teach infant feeding. • Review discharge plan.	• Encourage patient to increase fiber and fluid intake. • Complete discharge instructions.
• Refer patient to discharge class or provide discharge video.	• Prepare patient for discharge.	• Review discharge instructions and follow-up appointments, and coordinate home care and follow-up phone calls.
• Rh$_o$(D) immune globulin (RhoGAM) workup for Rh-negative mother (obtain results as soon as possible)		
• Provide perineal hygiene. • Use straight catheter as necessary. • Obtain signature on circumcision permission form. • Provide breast pump as necessary. • Apply ice to perineum.	• Discontinue ice to perineum. • Provide sitz baths.	• Give sitz bath. • Encourage self-care.
• Home health and SS (if needed) • Lactation (for breast-feeding)	• SS (if needed) • Consider community resources (if applicable)	
• Administer analgesia. • Administer Rh$_o$(D) immune globulin (if necessary).	• Administer Rh$_o$(D) immune globulin (if indicated).	• Administer rubella vaccine (if necessary).
• Regular diet	• Regular diet	• Regular diet
• Activity as tolerated	• Up as tolerated	• Up as tolerated

Adapted with permission from TriHealth Health System, Cincinnati, Ohio.

Intrapartum

5. Apply an external fetal monitor; note fetal heart rate (FHR).

5. These interventions allow you to establish fetal status and a fetal database (see *Fetal heart activity*, page XXX). External (indirect) electronic fetal monitoring typically is used for patients with low-risk pregnancies. Transducers applied to the abdomen measure fetal heart activity as well as the frequency and duration of uterine contractions. External monitoring is noninvasive, easily applied, and independent of cervical dilation, membrane rupture, or fetal head engagement. Related nursing responsibilities include assessing, monitoring, and documenting fetal heart and uterine activity; performing appropriate and timely independent nursing actions; and reporting nonreassuring and ominous fetal heart rate patterns to the doctor.

6. Draw blood for:
• hemoglobin (Hb) level and hematocrit (HCT)

• serology (if needed: usually performed prenatally but may be repeated)
• type and crossmatch if patient is at greater risk for bleeding.

6. Profile of blood analysis establishes a database.
• Hb level and HCT assess the blood's oxygen-carrying capacity and identify anemia and possible blood loss.
• Serology determines exposure to sexually transmitted disease.
• A sample is needed to confirm blood type and Rh and to hold blood for emergency use.

7. If the patient's signs and symptoms indicate the need, obtain a clean-catch urine sample to determine protein and glucose levels and the presence of bacteria.

7. Small amounts of urine glucose (1+) are normal and attributed to an increased glomerular filtration rate and impaired tubular reabsorption; some proteinuria (1+) may be seen in vigorous labor as a result of protein catabolism. Bacteriuria may indicate infection. Aberrations warrant further analysis and remediation.

8. Additional individualized interventions: _____

8. Rationales: _____

NURSING DIAGNOSIS

Risk for ascending genital tract infection related to vaginal insult secondary to multiple vaginal examinations, proximity to rectum, normal nonsterile environment of pudenda, and access provided by rupture of membranes before labor

Expected outcome

The patient will exhibit no signs of infection as evidenced by stable vital signs, including temperature within normal limits, and no foul-smelling amniotic fluid.

Interventions

1. Perform all vaginal assessments using strict aseptic technique.

2. Administer a disposable cleansing enema of sodium phosphate (seldom done).

3. Change the underpad regularly and whenever it becomes wet or soiled.

Rationales

1. This minimizes the potential for pathogenic bacterial invasion through the dilating cervix.

2. Protocol varies among hospitals. If the patient has not had recent diarrhea, an enema may be given to minimize the fecal contamination that occurs when maternal pushing ensues. Stimulation of the bowel may stimulate the uterus.

3. This removes contaminants and minimizes vaginal exposure to pathogens.

Fetal heart activity

Evaluation of fetal heart activity provides valuable information for fetal assessment. This chart describes baseline fetal heart rate (FHR) and variations of fetal heart activity. FHR patterns that restore confidence about fetal status are called *reassuring*; those that fail to remove doubt about fetal status are called *nonreassuring*.

Term	Description	Implications
Baseline FHR	Mean FHR, measured between contractions or during intervals between periodic changes. Ranges from 120 to 160 beats per minute (bpm) in normal term fetus. May fluctuate 5 to 15 bpm normally.	• Decreased FHR suggests fetal sleep. • Increased FHR suggests fetal movement.
Tachycardia	Persistent (≥ 10 minutes) FHR above 160 bpm. Generally associated with loss of variability. Mild tachycardia: FHR 161 to 180 bpm; severe tachycardia: FHR > 180 bpm.	• May indicate maternal fever, amnionitis, maternal use of parasympatholytic agents (such as atropine) or beta sympathomimetic agents (such as terbutaline [Brethine]), maternal hyperthyroidism, early fetal hypoxia, fetal anemia, fetal infection, fetal tachyarrhythmias, or fetal heart failure. • Indicates fetal compromise when associated with decelerations or absence of variability; less serious when periodic changes are absent.
Bradycardia	Persistent (≥ 10 minutes) FHR below 110 bpm. Mild bradycardia: FHR 80 to 100 bpm; severe bradycardia: FHR < 80 bpm.	• May indicate fetal head compression from occiput posterior or occiput transverse fetal position, especially during second stage of labor. • May indicate fetal hypoxia, maternal use of beta blockers (such as propranolol [Inderal]), maternal connective tissue disease, maternal hypothermia, congenital or acquired fetal heart block, or postterm pregnancy. • May signal fetal compromise if associated with loss of variability and decelerations. • Reassuring if associated with good variability because fetus responds appropriately to stress.
Variability	Normal cyclic irregularity in cardiac rhythm. Short-term variability: beat-to-beat (R wave–to–R wave) change of consecutive cardiac cycles, generally 3 to 8 bpm. Long-term variability: cyclic fluctuations or "waviness," generally 3 to 5 cycles per minute. Short-term variability single most reliable predictor (among FHR characteristics) of fetal status.	• Baseline variability is associated with fetal wakefulness. • Increased variability is associated with mild and early fetal hypoxia, fetal activity or stimulation, and uterine manipulation. • Decreased variability is associated with fetal sleep, hypoxia or acidosis, extreme prematurity, maternal use of central nervous system (CNS) depressants (such as analgesics, narcotics, barbiturates, and tranquilizers) or parasympatholytics (such as atropine), general anesthesia, congenital anomalies of cardiovascular system and CNS, and fetal tachycardias. When preceded by late decelerations, decreased variability indicates fetal compromise.
Acceleration	Transient increase in FHR baseline (generally above 15 bpm) lasting 15 seconds.	• May indicate partial umbilical cord occlusion, uterine contractions, fetal movement, or fetal stimulation during pelvic examination. • Reassuring, signaling fetal well-being, when associated with fetal movement and normal variability.
Early deceleration	Transient decrease in FHR below baseline. (FHR seldom falls below 100 or 110 bpm, or 20 to 30 bpm below baseline.) Concurrent with uterine contractions; uniformly shaped; associated with average variability.	• May indicate fetal head compression, associated with active phase of labor and cervical dilation of 4 to 7 cm. • Reassuring; not associated with tachycardia, hypoxia, or loss of variability.

Fetal heart activity *(continued)*

Term	Description	Implication
Late deceleration	Transient repetitive FHR decrease below baseline. Occurs late in contraction phase; nadir of deceleration occurs after acme of uterine contraction. Most important, with late decelerations, return to baseline occurs *after* contraction is over. Return and descent typically are smooth and gradual. Commonly associated with loss of variability and increasing baseline FHR. Seldom precedes or follows acceleration.	• May indicate uteroplacental insufficiency resulting from maternal hypotension, uterine hypertonicity, hyperactivity (such as from oxytocin augmentation or labor induction), epidural or spinal anesthesia, hypertensive disorders, abruptio placentae, placenta previa, amnionitis, diabetes mellitus, collagen vascular disease, intrauterine growth restriction, postmaturity, or fetal hypoxia. • Nonreassuring; indicates fetal compromise when persistent or associated with elevated baseline FHR and loss of short-term variability.
Variable deceleration	Abrupt, transient decrease in FHR. Variable in duration, intensity, and timing relative to uterine contraction. Often preceded or followed by small, transient acceleration. Return to baseline is variable. Significant when lasting more than 60 seconds with FHR below 70 bpm.	• May indicate oligohydramnios and umbilical cord compression from short, knotted, or prolapsed cord; cord wrapped around fetal body part; or cord between fetus and maternal pelvis. • Reassuring if baseline FHR and short-term variability are normal. • Indicates fetal hypoxia and acidosis if pattern becomes progressively more severe and prolonged or sustained. Seen late in labor with fetal descent and maternal pushing.

4. Monitor vital signs. Note early rupture of membranes; presence of meconium; and odor, color, and consistency of amniotic discharge. Correlate findings with white blood cell count. Assess FHR with electronic fetal monitoring. For a low-risk patient, auscultate every 30 minutes during active stage 1 labor and every 15 minutes during stage 2. For a high-risk patient, auscultate every 15 minutes during active stage 1 labor, then every 5 minutes during stage 2. After the patient's membranes rupture, take her temperature every 2 hours until delivery.

5. Additional individualized interventions: _____
_____

4. Indications of infection include a temperature greater than 100.4° F (38° C); thick, yellow, and foul-smelling amniotic fluid; and a history of early membrane rupture. Meconium-stained fluid may indicate a compromised fetus. Leukocytosis is a normal occurrence during labor, and its presence does not necessarily indicate infection.

5. Rationales: _____
_____

COLLABORATIVE PROBLEM

Increased myometrial activity and cervical changes associated with stage 1 labor

Expected outcome

The patient will progress from the latent to the transition stage.

Interventions

1. Using palpation or external monitoring, assess uterine contractions for location, intensity, duration, and frequency. Assess hourly; as labor progresses, assess every 30 minutes, 15 minutes, and after every contraction. If fetal monitor is unavailable, assess FHT after every contraction when patient is completely dilated.

Rationales

1. The relation among factors assists in monitoring the progression of labor.

2. Assess cervical dilation and effacement and fetal station. Use the Friedman graph to correlate cervical dilation, fetal descent, and duration of labor. Include significant activities and occurrences (for example, amount, type, and dosage of medications; artificial or spontaneous rupture of membranes; color and amount of amniotic fluid; and marked change in fetal status). Note FHR and variability.

3. Assess bloody show and passage of the mucous plug. Concurrently evaluate for cord prolapse.

4. Assess amniotic fluid for color, amount, and odor. Assist the doctor with amniotomy.

5. Monitor vital signs hourly and temperature every 4 hours if the patient's membranes have not ruptured; otherwise, every 1 to 2 hours. If blood pressure is elevated or analgesia has been administered, monitoring every 10 to 15 minutes may be warranted. Perform monitoring between contractions. Integrate findings with medical history and significant physical findings. Check FHT every 15 minutes.

6. Transfer the patient to the delivery suite or set up the birthing room when the patient exhibits perineal bulging, when contractions result in display of occiput: +1 to +2, or when the multiparous patient has advanced to 0 to +1 station.

7. Additional individualized interventions: _____

2. Cervical dilation and fetal descent are more reliable measures of labor progression. The Friedman graph serves as an objective tool for monitoring labor as well as a medicolegal chronology.

3. Early in labor, the cervical mucous plug may be passed. As labor progresses, the bloody show becomes more copious. Bright red bleeding in any amount or umbilical cord protrusion warrants immediate evaluation and intervention.

4. Rupture of the membranes usually occurs spontaneously during labor. The decision to rupture the membranes is a medical one. The ensuing benefits of a more rapidly progressing labor and availability of amniotic fluid to monitor fetal well-being must be weighed against the potential for ascending genital tract infection and prolapsed umbilical cord.

5. The findings help evaluate maternal and fetal responses to labor and increased risks posed by actual or incipient hypertensive and cardiac disorders.

6. These signs indicate that delivery is imminent.

7. Rationales: _____

NURSING DIAGNOSIS

Anxiety related to unknown surroundings and hospital procedures, absent or minimal childbirth preparation, and fatigue or excitement

Expected outcome

The patient will express less anxiety.

Interventions

1. Introduce yourself as a primary caregiver to the patient and significant others. Give factual information. Explain the hospital's admission policies and procedures; listen to concerns and allow time for questions.

Rationales

1. Identifying the caregiver and establishing rapport decrease anxiety. Factual information minimizes fear of the unknown.

Intrapartum

2. Ascertain the patient's level of childbirth preparation, then review, reinforce, or teach, as appropriate. Have the patient give a brief demonstration of breathing and relaxation techniques.

3. Ascertain the patient's age, marital status or presence of significant other, previous childbearing experiences, ethnicity and degree of acculturation, use of personal space, and response to teaching. Be nonjudgmental.

4. Ensure privacy during the examination; drape the patient and minimize exposure.

5. Allow for cultural or religious rituals or practices when medically possible.

6. Assess the patient's support systems.

7. Additional individualized interventions: _____

2. Activities give the patient and partner a sense of control.

3. Information provides a database for psychosocial needs.

4. These interventions demonstrate respect for the patient.

5. Incorporation of symbolic practices may be a source of comfort and strength and may enhance the patient's ability to cope with labor and delivery.

6. Support systems can help decrease anxiety.

7. Rationales: _____

NURSING DIAGNOSIS

Decreased cardiac output related to uterine contractions with diversion of blood from uterine artery, to position, and to use of Valsalva's maneuver

Expected outcome

The patient will experience minimal sequelae secondary to labor-induced alterations in cardiac output.

Interventions

1. Monitor the patient's maternal vital signs every hour and FHR every 15 minutes as her condition warrants.

2. Assist, teach, or reinforce measures that allow the patient to relax between contractions.

3. Monitor the patient for supine hypotensive syndrome (vena cava syndrome), including hypotension and tachycardia. Encourage the right lateral or semi-Fowler position; use a tilted position instead of the supine position.

4. Additional individualized interventions: _____

Rationales

1. Evaluation of levels assists in determining maternal and fetal status.

2. Uteroplacental blood flow is reestablished between contractions.

3. Compression of the ascending vena cava results in decreased cardiac output and, ultimately, decreased placental perfusion. The lateral recumbent position increases uterine perfusion.

4. Rationales: _____

COLLABORATIVE PROBLEM

Risk for fluid volume deficit related to decreased gastric motility, subsequent medical limitation of oral intake, and diaphoresis associated with the work of labor

Expected outcome

The patient will exhibit no signs of fluid volume deficit as evidenced by good skin turgor, moist mucous membranes, good urine output, and urine specific gravity within normal limits.

Interventions

1. Monitor the patient's hydration status, including the condition of her skin, mucous membranes, and eyes and subjective sensation of thirst.

2. Continue to restrict oral intake; ice chips, ice pops, and hard candy may be allowed.

3. Monitor fluid intake and output. Note amount of diaphoresis.

4. Administer an I.V. infusion of balanced salt solution with glucose to a fasting patient in advanced labor.

5. Additional individualized interventions: _____
_____

Rationales

1. A well-hydrated state is characterized by smooth, supple skin; moist mucous membranes; and absence of thirst.

2. Prolonged gastric emptying occurs during labor. Vomiting may result in aspiration, a significant source of obstetric morbidity.

3. This allow evaluation of renal function; minimal satisfactory output is 30 to 50 ml/hour.

4. I.V. fluid administration prevents dehydration and acidosis; provides a vehicle for glucose and insulin administration in a diabetic patient; and allows prophylactic oxytocin administration.

5. Rationales: _____
_____

NURSING DIAGNOSIS

Altered urinary elimination related to pressure of the presenting fetal part and to regional anesthesia

Expected outcome

The patient will regain and maintain normal bladder function.

Interventions

1. Assess for a filling bladder by palpating above the symphysis pubis.

2. Assist the patient to the toilet every 2 to 4 hours. Perform nursing measures to promote voiding (for example, running water and putting the patient's hands in water).

3. Catheterize, if necessary, between contractions with a small, well-lubricated catheter. Alternatively, insert an indwelling urinary (Foley) catheter after the epidural catheter is in place; remove the catheter at delivery.

4. Additional individualized interventions: _____

Rationales

1. The urge to void may be absent. The symphysis pubis acts as an anatomic landmark to locate the bladder.

2. Bladder distention may interfere with fetal descent and contribute to postpartum uterine atony. Decreased bladder tone, urine retention, and infection may result.

3. Using such a catheter minimizes trauma from catheter insertion. An indwelling urinary catheter also decompresses the bladder, allowing fetal descent.

4. Rationales: _____
_____

COLLABORATIVE PROBLEM

Pain related to uterine hypoxia, pressure of presenting part, and cervical dilation

Expected outcome

The patient will express pain appropriate to progressive labor.

Interventions

1. Monitor contractions for frequency, intensity, and duration; correlate with cervical dilation, effacement, and station.

Rationales

1. Monitoring tracks the progression of labor.

Intrapartum

2. Keep the patient informed of her progress. Allow her to listen to FHR.

3. Encourage ambulation if the patient:
• is in latent or active stage 1 labor
• has received only a light narcotic (walking epidural)
• has intact membranes (ruptured membranes if the head is well engaged)
• has no vaginal bleeding
• shows no signs of fetal distress.

4. When the patient is confined to bed, minimize discomfort in the following ways:
• Allow her to find a comfortable position.
• Tell her to avoid the supine position.
• If she lies in the supine position, place a wedge under her left hip.
• Encourage her to assume the lateral or semi-Fowler position.

5. Encourage talking, watching TV, reading, and playing board games, and encourage the patient to focus on past experiences or on an object in a room away from her.

6. Promote comfort measures; encourage the patient to use pelvic rocking, administer back rubs and effleurage, apply cold or warm compresses to the back, and apply hot socks (warmed in a microwave) to the back and underbelly.

7. Cluster nursing activities so the patient can rest. Keep the room quiet and free of distractions.

8. Coach the patient through controlled-breathing techniques, progressing through the following levels as stage 1 progresses:
• level 1 — slow, deliberate inhalations through the nose; exhalation through the nose or mouth
• level 2 — shallow, rapid inhalations through the nose, slowing as each contraction wanes; exhalation through the mouth
• level 3 — increasingly rapid and shallow respirations; inhalation and exhalation through the mouth; molding the mouth during exhalation to a hee-hoo configuration.

9. Administer analgesics (if the patient desires), which can vary in strength and range from butorphanol (Stadol) to meperidine (Demerol). Butorphanol is given I.V. at 1 to 2 mg every 2 hours when active labor has been established and the cervix is dilated 4 cm or more.

10. Assist the practitioner with single injection or indwelling catheter insertion for nalbuphine (Nubain) or butorphanol or epidural block. Continue frequent monitoring of maternal vital signs and electronic monitoring of FHR.

2. These interventions include the patient in the health care team and involve her in her own care.

3. Ambulation provides diversion and offers psychological comfort.

4. The lateral recumbent position increases uterine perfusion and, ultimately, the progression of labor.

5. These distraction techniques help prevent contractions from becoming the focus of the patient's attention.

6. These activities reduce abdominal and back discomfort.

7. Fatigue diminishes the patient's ability to cope.

8. Controlled breathing increases relaxation, distraction, and coping abilities.

9. Once contractions become intense, analgesics may be given to control pain and allow the patient to rest between contractions. Analgesics should not be given too early because they may slow the labor process or within 1 hour of delivery because of their depressant effect on the fetus.

10. No drug has a single action; adverse reactions may affect the mother or fetus.

11. Help the practitioner with placement of the epidural or intrathecal catheter. If the patient has a walking or narcotic epidural, she will receive narcotics at a rate of 2 ml/hour instead of the more traditional rate of 5 to 7 ml /hour.

12. Additional individualized interventions: _____
_____

11. As its name implies, a walking epidural allows the patient to walk without prolonging labor. As she approaches transition, she can receive a stronger dose of narcotics.

12. Rationales: _____
_____

NURSING DIAGNOSIS

Risk for fetal injury related to uteroplacental insufficiency

Expected outcome

The fetus will experience minimal, if any, injury as evidenced by normal FHR and no signs of fetal distress.

Interventions

1. Review prenatal record for date of LMP and EDC. Note results and dates of sonography.

2. Assess fetal position and presentation by abdominal and vaginal palpation (Leopold's maneuver). Auscultate FHR to confirm findings.

3. Establish baseline FHR. Assess FHR on admission; after rupture of membranes, assess every 15 minutes for 45 minutes and as the patient's condition warrants (every 15 minutes through the first stage, every 5 minutes or after each contraction during the second stage). Auscultate FHR for 30 seconds or more after a contraction; electronically monitor for 15 minutes.

4. While monitoring FHR, note these factors: bradycardia (less than 110 beats/minute), tachycardia (more than 160 beats/minute), late decelerations, variable decelerations, and absent short-term (less than or equal to 2 beats/minute) variability.

5. Assist the doctor with fetal scalp sampling when acid-base balance must be ascertained.

6. Additional individualized interventions: _____

Rationales

1. This intervention establishes gestational maturity. The earlier ultrasonography is performed, the more accurate it is.

2. Indications for cesarean section delivery include transverse lie and most breech presentations.

3. Assessment evaluates fetal well-being in response to labor. Normal findings include an FHR of 120 to 160 beats/minute, transient decelerations or accelerations associated with contractions or fetal movement, early decelerations, and average variability.

4. These levels indicate fetal distress and warrant interventions to increase uteroplacental functioning, including:
• continual monitoring for FHR change
• administering oxygen to the patient and placing her in the recumbent position
• rehydration
• decreasing or discontinuing oxytocin infusion
• emergency treatment of prolapsed umbilical cord
• control of pyrexia.

5. Fetal blood pH levels of 7.25 or higher are considered normal during labor; levels between 7.20 and 7.24 are considered preacidotic. Serial fetal blood pH determinations in tandem with a complete clinical profile are better determinants of fetal acidosis.

6. Rationales: _____
_____

Intrapartum

NURSING DIAGNOSIS

Risk for maternal injury and infection related to the second stage of labor

Expected outcome

The patient will experience minimal, if any, injury or infection and will successfully expel the fetus.

Interventions

1. Increase the frequency of maternal and fetal assessments. Prepare for delivery, using the physiologic guidelines listed in intervention 6 on page 115.

2. Convert the birthing bed for delivery, elevating the head of the bed 30 to 60 degrees. Help the patient assume the lithotomy position, taking care to avoid pressure in the popliteal area.

3. Assist the scrubbed and gowned doctor or nurse-midwife with patient preparation, including perineal scrubbing and sterile draping. The practitioner may choose to wear double gloves.

4. Coach the patient through expulsive and bearing-down efforts and with controlled breathing during contractions. Repeat instructions frequently. Allow the patient to rest between contractions. Keep her appraised of her progress as the infant's head, shoulder, and body are delivered. If the patient has an epidural catheter in place, she may not feel contractions and will need direction to know when to push.

5. Assist with clamping of the umbilical cord. Note fundal height and consistency. Keep a hand on the patient's abdomen. Do not massage.

6. Monitor the patient for globular configuration of uterus, rise of uterus in abdomen, and gush of blood from vagina and protrusion of umbilical cord.

7. Additional individualized interventions: _____

Rationales

1. Greater physiologic stress on the mother and fetus warrants evaluation of their well-being. Infection-control procedures require wearing a scrub suit, mask, goggles, and cap.

2. Elevation makes it easier for the patient to use abdominal muscles for pushing. Pressure on the popliteal area may compromise peripheral circulation.

3. A sterile environment must be maintained. The practitioner may wear double gloves if the patient is at high risk for acquired immunodeficiency syndrome (see appendix K, Overview of isolation precautions).

4. Pushing is involuntary and assists in expulsion. Recovery time is needed between contractions to reestablish uteroplacental circulation.

5. A firm, contracted uterus will not bleed. The examiner's hand allows for immediate assessment of atony.

6. These signs indicate placental separation. Spontaneous delivery of the placenta usually occurs in 5 to 30 minutes. Evaluation of the integrity of the placenta minimizes the potential for retained fragments.

7. Rationales: _____

NURSING DIAGNOSIS

Risk for altered parenting related to delayed bonding

Expected outcome

The patient and her child will develop early bonding.

Interventions

1. Allow the mother to see her infant immediately after delivery. After the cord is clamped, place the infant on the mother's abdomen or put it to her breast, if she is breast-feeding.

2. Determine the infant's Apgar score while the mother holds the infant.

3. Additional individualized interventions: _____

_____

Rationales

1. While the episiotomy is being repaired, the mother should have ample time to become acquainted with her infant. Greeting, touching, caressing, and examining the newborn infant are common behaviors that enhance bonding.

2. Allowing the mother to hold the infant while its Apgar score is determined promotes bonding.

3. Rationales: _____

_____

Documentation checklist
During the hospital stay, document:
- ❏ patient status and assessment findings, including a history of previous pregnancies and their outcomes
- ❏ changes in patient status
- ❏ pertinent laboratory and diagnostic findings
- ❏ pain — quality, location, frequency, and intensity
- ❏ any signs of pending infection, alteration in voiding, or dehydration
- ❏ the patient's interaction with her infant
- ❏ patient and family teaching guidelines
- ❏ discharge planning guidelines.

Associated plans and appendices
- ❏ Normal antepartum
- ❏ Puerperium
- ❏ Aspects of psychological care — maternal (appendix D)

Additional nursing diagnoses
- ❏ Ineffective individual coping related to fatigue
- ❏ Knowledge deficit related to lack of childbirth preparation
- ❏ Sleep pattern disturbance related to regular, intense uterine contraction

Oxytocin-induced or oxytocin-augmented labor

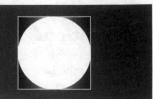

Definition

Oxytocin infusion functions exactly as the naturally occurring endogenous hormone oxytocin produced by the posterior pituitary gland: It stimulates uterine contractions. This oxytocic effect is greatest at term. Its ability to induce or stimulate labor and to augment a labor characterized by inadequate uterine contractions is addressed here. Management is directed at stimulating a labor as close to normal as possible, ensuring maternal and fetal well-being, and preventing complications associated with oxytocin induction.

Etiology and precipitating factors

- Etiology: not applicable.
- Inductions usually take place from 38 weeks on.
- Conditions that warrant labor augmentation include hypotonic uterine dysfunction during the active phase of the first stage of labor or during the second stage.
- Conditions that warrant labor stimulation include gestational age greater than 42 weeks as well as medical conditions that necessitate early delivery, such as maternal history of precipitate labor in a multigravid patient, polyhydramnios or hydramnios, Rh isoimmunization, severe preeclampsia near or at term, prolonged premature rupture of membranes, diabetes, abruptio placentae, incomplete or inevitable abortion, and fetal death.

Physical findings

Genitourinary

- Uterine dysfunction: prolonged phase or stage of labor beyond expected norms, lack of progress in dilation or effacement, or lack of descent of presenting fetal part
- Uterine contractions infrequent and of short duration and mild intensity

Subjective

- Maternal exhaustion

Diagnostic studies

- Fetal sonography evaluates fetal size and position.
- Radiologic pelvimetry, although seldom performed, may be used to evaluate fetal size and position and to rule out cephalopelvic disproportion.
- Fern test confirms rupture of membranes.
- Blood glucose level provides database for glucose and insulin management of diabetic patient.

COLLABORATIVE PROBLEM

Risk for maternal injury related to necessity for medically indicated oxytocin induction (three expected outcomes)

Expected outcome 1

The patient requiring oxytocin induction will be identified.

Interventions

1. Review the patient's history, including estimated date of confinement, gynecologic and obstetric histories, and electronic fetal and uterine contraction record.

2. Assess whether the patient is a candidate for oxytocin use. Note the following:
- parity fewer than 5
- no uterine overdistention or previous scarring (in some instances, such as vaginal births after cesarean section [VBACs], oxytocin will be used)
- no mechanical obstruction or cephalopelvic disproportion
- active labor that has progressed to 50% effacement and 2- to 3-cm dilation
- near-term fetus, vertex presentation, fetal heart rate (FHR) within normal range.

Rationales

1. Augmentation is considered only after a trial of labor has failed to progress. The patient's history provides a database for care planning and early identification of problems.

2. The potency of oxytocin precludes its use in various conditions. The profile enhances the scenario for a normal vaginal birth and good maternal and fetal outcomes.

3. Assess the status of the fetus and determine if dystocia (failure to progress) is occurring.

4. Additional individualized interventions: _____

3. If the patient has no signs of progression (such as increasing effacement or cervical dilation) or if there are signs of fetal compromise, a cesarean section may be necessary to prevent fetal or maternal injury.

4. Rationales: _____

Expected outcome 2

The patient will experience minimal or no injury while undergoing stimulated or augmented uterine contractions as evidenced by positive FHR or no signs of fetal distress.

Interventions

1. Before induction, reassess uterine contractions. Assess the patient's blood pressure and pulse rate. Monitor FHR with a minimum tracing of 30 minutes.

2. Start a primary I.V. line of physiologic electrolyte solution. Use an infusion pump, and piggyback oxytocin with secondary I.V. set.

3. On initiation of oxytocin induction, FHR and uterine contractions must be electronically monitored continuously and charted every 15 minutes and at each increase in dose.

4. Administer oxytocin per order and protocol, using the following guidelines:

• 1 ml (10 units) of oxytocin/1,000 ml diluent
• infuse at a rate of 1 to 2 mU/minute; slowly increase the infusion by 1 to 2 mU/minute every 30 to 60 minutes until a contraction pattern similar to normal labor is established.

5. Additional individualized interventions: _____

Rationales

1. This information establishes a baseline.

2. Electrolyte solution minimizes oxytocin's antidiuretic effect. Hemodynamic changes associated with the drug demand a controlled flow rate to minimize the potential for overdose. Piggybacking allows for emergency discontinuance of the drug in cases of drug-induced tetany or hypersensitivity without compromising venous access.

3. Oxytocin acts rapidly and has a half-life of about 3 minutes when administered I.V. Fetal distress or uterine hyperactivity warrants immediately decreasing or discontinuing the drug infusion.

4. One syringe (Tubex) contains 10 units/ml, the pharmacologic equivalent of 10 USP posterior pituitary units.
• The infusion will contain 10 mU of oxytocin/ml.
• These findings indicate that the pattern of normal labor has been established. Response time is variable. If progressive cervical changes have not occurred and delivery is imminent with the prescribed parameters, labor induction has failed and surgical delivery may be appropriate.

5. Rationales: _____

Expected outcome 3

The patient will exhibit no signs of oxytocin-induced uterine hyperactivity as evidenced by contractions less than every 90 seconds or shorter than 75 to 90 seconds in length or a resting uterine tone less than 15 to 20 mm H_2O.

Interventions

1. Continue assessments of maternal vital signs as well as the frequency, intensity, and duration of contractions and the resting tone. Note all significant patient activities and procedures on tracing strip.

Rationales

1. Assessment assists in monitoring drug response and labor progression.

Intrapartum

2. Monitor for signs of hyperstimulation, including:
• contraction frequency greater than every 90 seconds
• sustained or prolonged contractions greater than 75 seconds
• resting uterine tone of 15 mm H_2O or more between contractions
• resting uterine tone of ^{3}25 mm Hg or more between contractions (measured with a fluid-filled intrauterine pressure catheter [IUPC]) or ^{3}35 mm Hg (measured with a sensor-tipped IUPC).

3. Immediately decrease or stop the oxytocin drip and infuse the primary I.V.

4. Have 0.25 mg subcutaneous terbutaline (Brethine) available.

5. Additional individualized interventions: _____

2. Hyperstimulation may result from overdose or uterine hypersensitivity to oxytocin given in therapeutic amounts. Regardless of the cause, hyperstimulation, with its strong or protracted contractions, may cause abruptio placentae, uterine rupture, cervical and vaginal lacerations, impaired uteroplacental blood flow with resulting fetal hypoxia, postpartum hemorrhage, or death.

3. Plasma concentrations of short-lived oxytocin quickly drop once the drug is stopped.

4. Although management of hyperstimulation is usually palliative, terbutaline may be given to relieve uterine tetany.

5. Rationales: _____

COLLABORATIVE PROBLEM

Risk for fetal injury related to uteroplacental insufficiency (two expected outcomes)

Expected outcome 1

The patient at risk for uteroplacental insufficiency will be identified.

Interventions

1. Electronically monitor FHR 30 minutes before induction and before increasing oxytocin dosage. Monitor for insufficiency, following these guidelines:
• FHR less than 110 or more than 160 beats/minute (bradycardia or tachycardia, respectively)
• repetitive late or variable decelerations
• absent or short-term variability (less than or equal to 2 beats/minute)
• meconium staining of amniotic fluid.

2. Monitor maternal vital signs, especially blood pressure.

3. Additional individualized interventions: _____

Rationales

1. Hypertonic or tetanic contractions impair uteroplacental blood flow. Fetal hypoxia and distress follow.

2. Epidural anesthesia may cause hypotension, resulting in decreased blood flow to the placenta and subsequent fetal hypoxia.

3. Rationales: _____

Expected outcome 2

The fetus will experience no injury as evidenced by no signs of fetal distress and appropriate interventions to support maternal circulation and oxygenation.

Interventions

1. Decrease or stop the oxytocin drip and infuse the primary I.V. if uteroplacental insufficiency should occur. Notify the doctor.

2. Position the patient in recumbent position, and administer oxygen by mask at 8 to 10 L/minute.

3. Additional individualized interventions: _____

Rationales

1. If the effects of oxytocin are not quickly reversed, emergency surgical delivery of a compromised infant may be necessary.

2. This position increases uterine perfusion. Supplemental oxygen enhances alveolocapillary perfusion.

3. Rationales: _____

NURSING DIAGNOSIS

Pain related to oxytocic effect

Expected outcome

The patient will experience minimal pain.

Interventions

1. Establish rapport with the patient and significant other.

2. Before induction, explain the procedure, rapidity of onset, and anticipated progression of labor. Encourage questions. Review breathing and relaxation techniques.

3. Assess pain and its characteristics, including quality, frequency, location, and intensity. Keep the patient informed of her progress.

4. Perform comfort measures, including position changes, relaxation techniques, massage and effleurage, music, hydrotherapy, and application of heat (from socks filled with rice and heated inside a microwave) or cold (from a cold soda can); provide pharmacologic analgesia.

5. Additional individualized interventions: _____

Rationales

1. A positive relationship increases trust and decreases anxiety.

2. Fear of the unknown increases the patient's perception of pain. Oxytocin's rapid and pronounced onset and course of action may leave the patient little time to garner her resources.

3. A pain profile monitors, in part, how labor is progressing.

4. Increased tissue perfusion plus the stimulation of the afferent fibers decreases the sensation of pain. Analgesics may be given after active labor has been clearly established; if given earlier, their depressive characteristics may compromise fetal status. The patient may have a walking (narcotic) epidural early on (when she is dilated 2 cm), which can be converted to a standard (caine) epidural after she dilates 4 cm and approaches transition.

5. Rationales: _____

Documentation checklist

During the hospital stay, document:
❏ patient status and assessment findings, including a history of previous pregnancies and their outcomes
❏ changes in patient status
❏ pertinent laboratory and diagnostic findings
❏ fundal height and tone
❏ appearance of any perinatal or genital lacerations or suture lines

❏ pain — quality, location, frequency, and intensity
❏ the patient's response to treatment
❏ the patient's and family's reaction to the need for induction therapy
❏ patient and family teaching guidelines
❏ discharge planning guidelines.

Intrapartum

Associated plans and appendices
❏ Abortion
❏ Abruptio placentae
❏ Cesarean section birth
❏ Labor and vaginal birth
❏ Pregnancy complicated by diabetes mellitus
❏ Pregnancy-induced hypertension
❏ Premature rupture of membranes
❏ Rh isoimmunization
❏ Aspects of psychological care — maternal (appendix D)

Additional nursing diagnoses
❏ Risk for ascending genital tract infection related to premature rupture of membranes
❏ Risk for fluid volume deficit related to hemorrhage secondary to uterine abruption
❏ Risk for fluid volume excess related to potent antidiuretic effect of oxytocin

Part 3

Postpartum

Puerperium

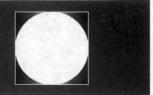

Definition
The puerperium usually extends from after the third stage of labor to 6 weeks after delivery. During this period, the anatomic and functional changes of pregnancy reverse. Management is directed at monitoring these changes, minimizing the discomfort associated with them, and preventing conditions that can result in maternal morbidity and mortality, such as hemorrhage, thromboembolic disease, and infection.

Etiology and precipitating factors
Not applicable.

Physical findings
See *Normal postpartum findings*.

Diagnostic studies
In the absence of pathology, trauma, or complications, few tests are conducted.

Normal postpartum findings

When assessing the postpartum patient, the acronym BUBBLE-HE can help you to remember assessments specific to the postpartum period — *B*reasts, *U*terus, *B*owel, *B*ladder, *L*ochia, *E*pisiotomy, *H*omans' sign and hemorrhoids, and *E*motion. You will also need to assess the patient's temperature, pulse, blood pressure, and weight.

- **Breasts:** Initially soft, nontender, and without erythema or discharge; colostrum secretion begins by 2nd day postpartum, with subsequent tenderness and engorgement that persist for approximately 3 days
- **Uterus:** Firm and nontender; fundus midline located midway between the symphysis pubis and umbilicus after third-stage labor; at or 1 cm (1 fingerbreadth) above umbilicus within 12 hours, persisting for 48 hours; then regressing at a rate of 1 cm/day; prepregnancy size attained within about 4 weeks. During assessment of the uterus, abdomen may appear soft and somewhat flabby, with red or purple striae prominent; possible distasis recti abdominis (separation of abdominal recti muscles) may occur
- **Bowel:** Patient may experience discomfort secondary to episiotomy or hemorrhoids; may require stool softener
- **Bladder:** Proteinuria for up to 3 days; lactosuria persisting for several weeks
- **Lochia:** Musky, fleshy, or earthy aroma; rubra for several days; progresses to serosa after 3 or 4 days, to alba after 10 days; combined volume equals about 100 ml
- **Episiotomy:** Area and sutured lacerations clean, dry, and odorless; edges well approximated, with minimal edema and some tenderness
- **Homans' sign and hemorrhoids:** Positive sign may indicate lower-extremity thrombophlebitis: hemorrhoids may extrude from the rectum as a result of pregnancy and labor
- **Emotion:** Patient may initially appear passive and preoccupied with her needs; increasing participation in self-care and interest in infant follow; mood swings may range from laughing and crying to talking incessantly about infant.
- **Temperature:** May increase to 100.4° F (38° C) during the first 24 hours
- **Pulse:** Bradycardia of 50 to 70 beats/minute lasting up to 1 week
- **Blood pressure:** Essentially unaffected and congruent with previous readings
- **Weight:** Immediate loss of 10 to 12 lb (4.5 to 5.4 kg); additional 5-lb (2.3-kg) loss during 1st week

COLLABORATIVE PROBLEM
Altered genitourinary (GU) function related to completion of pregnancy process and to delivery

Expected outcome
The patient will experience normal alterations associated with puerperium.

Interventions

1. Assess delivery data, including:
- vital signs
- medical and obstetric histories; blood type and Rh factor
- maternal age, parity, and delivery outcome
- course of labor and delivery
- anesthetic, drugs, and parenteral fluids administered
- time of delivery
- GU and abdominal assessments
- urine output.

2. Assess vital signs every 15 minutes for 1 hour, every 30 minutes for 1 hour, every hour for 4 hours, and then every 4 hours for the remainder of hospital stay or as the patient's condition warrants. Perform a physical examination concurrently.

3. Assess the patient's uterus every 15 minutes for 1 hour, every 30 to 60 minutes for the next 4 hours, and then every 4 hours for the remainder of the hospital stay or as the patient's condition requires. Have the patient empty her bladder before the examination. Monitor fundal height, position, and tone.

4. Assess vaginal discharge, noting frank bleeding and passage of clots as well as the color, amount, consistency, and odor of lochia.

5. Assess the episiotomy and perineum for *redness, edema, ecchymosis, drainage,* and well *approximated* suture edges (the REEDA parameters), and pain.

6. Assess fluid intake and output, including time, amount, and color of each voiding for 24 hours, as well as bladder distention.

7. Assess the patient's breasts for size, temperature, tenderness, discharge, and fissures.

8. Assess the patient's calves bilaterally for color, size, temperature, pulses, pain, Homans' sign, paresthesias, and paralysis.

Rationales

1. The course of the puerperium may be altered or affected by various physiologic and psychological factors.

2. Besides the physiologic adaptations noted in *Normal postpartum findings,* only mild fluctuations should occur. An elevation in temperature may indicate infection (in most cases, GU infection or thrombophlebitis). An increased pulse rate may result from blood loss. A rise in blood pressure may indicate pregnancy-induced hypertension or a chronic hypertensive state.

3. A firm, contracted uterus that continues to regress is undergoing normal involutional changes. A distended bladder may distort findings by displacing the uterus upward.

4. Frank bleeding requires immediate intervention. Occasional small clots result from pooled vaginal blood associated with the recumbent position; large or multiple clots, especially in conjunction with frank bleeding, require immediate intervention. Lochial discharge normally contains red blood cells, decidual shreds, epithelial cells, multiple microorganisms and, later, white blood cells. An alteration in predesignated flow from rubra to alba may indicate placental subinvolution, retained placental fragments, or infection.

5. Minimal edema, tenderness, and occasional ecchymosis are expected. Pronounced pain accompanied by ecchymosis and edema may indicate perineal hematoma or trauma. Drainage or tension along the episiotomy line may signal infection.

6. Diuresis of the extracellular fluid associated with normal pregnancy should result in the patient's voiding large amounts of urine for about 24 hours. Assessment of each voiding determines the degree of bladder emptying.

7. Assessment provides the framework for managing the patient, whether she chooses to breast-feed or bottle-feed.

8. Assessment establishes a baseline and allows for early diagnosis of thromboembolic dysfunction related to position, immobility, and increased coagulation factors associated with pregnancy.

Postpartum

9. Assess prepregnancy, actual, and desired weights. Note the type and amount of foods consumed and cultural preferences.

10. Additional individualized interventions: _____

9. Appetite is usually excellent and intake greater than usual for several days. Observations provide a framework for diet teaching.

10. Rationales: _____

Nursing diagnosis

Risk for fluid volume deficit related to blood loss secondary to uterine atony or retained placental fragments

Expected outcome

The patient will not develop uterine atony and will have improved uterine tone.

Interventions

1. Gently massage the boggy uterus at the fundus while supporting the lower uterine segment.

2. Assist the patient with bladder training every 3 hours if she cannot urinate spontaneously and completely empty her bladder.

3. Put the suckling infant to the patient's breast.

4. Have on hand oxytocin, methylergonovine (Methergine), and carboprost tromethamine (Hemabate).

5. Administer analgesics for afterbirth pains.

6. Additional individualized interventions: _____

Rationales

1. Gentle massage stimulates uterine contraction, helps expel any retained placental fragments, and restores positive uterine tone. Aggressive manipulation may tire the myometrium and result in further atony. Support minimizes the risk of uterine inversion.

2. The uterus that is displaced by a distended bladder may become atonic.

3. Suckling stimulates the release of oxytocin, which increases myometrial contractions.

4. Pharmacologic agents may be used to stimulate uterine contraction, but unless the patient has excessive bleeding or subinvolution, their use is questionable because they do not decrease bleeding or enhance involution.

5. Contractions cause discomfort. Greater pain is associated with increased parity, marked intrapartum abdominal distention, retained placental fragments, and oxytocin stimulation.

6. Rationales: _____

Collaborative problem

Risk for injury or trauma related to hematoma formation secondary to blood vessel injury during delivery

Expected outcome

The patient will experience no complications associated with hematoma formation.

Interventions

1. Assess the perineum for signs of hematoma, including tense vaginal growth, ecchymosis, and severe pain. Also note possible inability to void, increased pulse and respiratory rates, and decreased blood pressure, hemoglobin level, and hematocrit.

2. Prepare for incision and drainage of hematomas, possible blood replacement, and antibiotic therapy.

3. Additional individualized interventions: _____
_____

Rationales

1. These signs and symptoms result from the pressure of entrapped blood in confined vaginal or vulvar spaces. Vital signs and lowered blood values assist in quantifying the amount of blood loss.

2. Large and enlarging hematomas require surgical intervention, replacement for blood lost, and antimicrobial prophylaxis or treatment. Peritoneal and retroperitoneal hematomas may require laparotomy for evacuation.

3. Rationales: _____
_____

NURSING DIAGNOSIS

Risk for ascending genital tract infection related to vaginal tears or lacerations, surgical episiotomy, and endometrial exfoliation

Expected outcome

The patient develops no or minimal infection.

Interventions

1. Note trends in temperature; correlate your findings with the patient's antepartum status and presenting symptoms.

2. Instruct the patient to wash her perineum with mild soap and water daily and to use a peri bottle after each elimination.

3. Instruct the patient to wipe her perineum from front to back and to apply perineal pads front to back.

4. Replace sterile perineal pads after each elimination and at least once every 4 hours, regardless of lochia flow.

5. Instruct the patient to wash her hands before and after touching her genitals.

6. Additional individualized interventions: _____
_____

Rationales

1. Persistent low-grade fever for more than 24 hours postpartum or actual pyrexia suggests infection.

2. Washing removes secretions and contaminants.

3. These interventions reduce the risk of fecal contamination.

4. A warm, moist pad contaminated with organisms from the external genitalia and skin provides a good medium for bacterial growth.

5. Soiled hands act as vectors.

6. Rationales: _____
_____

COLLABORATIVE PROBLEM

Altered immune system response related to Rh isoimmunization and lack of rubella antibodies

Expected outcome

The patient will not become sensitized and will begin to produce rubella antibodies.

Postpartum

Interventions

1. Administer 300 mcg of Rh$_o$ (D) immune globulin (RhoGAM) within 72 hours of delivery to the Rh$_o$ (D)-negative nonsensitized patient who has an Rh-positive spouse, an Rh$_o$ (D)-positive neonate, and a negative direct Coombs' test of umbilical cord blood.

2. Administer live rubella vaccine to the patient who:
• has no allergies to eggs or neomycin
• has hemagglutination inhibition titers of less than 1:18
• plans to delay her next pregnancy for at least 3 months.

3. Additional individualized interventions: _____
_____

Rationales

1. Rh$_o$ (D) immune globulin suppresses maternal antibody formation and protects a subsequent pregnancy from circulatory fetomaternal incompatibility.

2. Allergy to eggs or neomycin strongly predisposes the patient to vaccine allergy. Low titers indicate a lack of immunity. The vaccine renders lifelong immunity against rubella. The virus is teratogenic and can be transmitted to the fetus during the first trimester. Because blood products (including Rh$_o$ (D) immune globulin) can interfere with the rubella vaccine, the patient should have her rubella titer checked about 6 weeks' postpartum.

3. Rationales: _____

COLLABORATIVE PROBLEM

Pain related to episiotomy repair and to afterbirth pains of the contracting uterus

Expected outcome

The patient experiences minimal or no perineal or pelvic pain.

Interventions

1. Assess the perineum.

2. Apply an ice pack to the perineum immediately after delivery.

3. Assist with heat treatments beginning 12 hours postpartum, including:
• moist heat or sitz baths for 20 minutes three times daily with a water temperature of 100° to 110° F (37.8° to 43.3° C)
• dry heat or heat lamp to exposed perineum for 20 minutes twice daily with the heat source 18″ to 24″ (46 to 61 cm) from the perineum
• whirlpool bath, alone or with a heat lamp.

4. Teach the patient to sit with less discomfort by contracting her buttocks before sitting.

5. Apply a local anesthetic to the affected area after every perineal cleaning and pad change.

6. Offer analgesia to the patient who complains of afterbirth pains or gives nonverbal indications of pain. If the patient is receiving I.V. oxytocin, check the flow rate.

Rationales

1. This assessment validates the expected response and eliminates other causes, such as hematoma and infection.

2. Cold minimizes edema and provides local anesthesia.

3. Heat soothes and promotes tissue healing by increasing blood and lymph flow to the area; moist heat also cleans the area, decreasing the risk of infection.

4. This maneuver supports underlying structures.

5. Local anesthetic sprays and ointments have an immediate, numbing effect.

6. A normal postpartum occurrence, uterine contractions cause discomfort that may require analgesia. If I.V. oxytocin is infusing too rapidly, it may increase contractions.

COLLABORATIVE PROBLEM

Rectal pain related to anorectal varices

Expected outcome

The patient experiences minimal or no rectal pain.

Interventions	Rationales
1. Assess the anorectal area, and integrate physical findings with the patient's prepregnancy history.	**1.** Assessment identifies problems and may indicate which established treatments the patient needs.
2. Apply a covered ice pack or cold witch hazel compresses directly to the hemorrhoids for 20 minutes every 4 hours for 24 hours immediately postpartum.	**2.** Cold minimizes edema and provides local anesthesia.
3. Tell the patient to take a warm, 20-minute sitz bath of 100° to 110° F (37.8° to 43.3° C) 20 minutes after defecating.	**3.** Heat reduces discomfort and increases blood flow, which improves healing.
4. Advise the patient to lie on her side and avoid protracted sitting and standing.	**4.** These actions minimize rectal pressure.
5. Demonstrate how to digitally replace externally protruding hemorrhoids.	**5.** This maneuver reduces the pressure caused by the hemorrhoids.
6. Teach the patient diet and bowel hygiene measures that will help her establish regular bowel habits. Include information on drinking an adequate amount of fluids and eating high-fiber foods.	**6.** Anticipation of or actual passage of a hardened stool may result in holding back, which further aggravates the condition.
7. Administer pharmacologic agents, as indicated, including creams, ointments, stool softeners, laxatives, and analgesics.	**7.** Local anesthetics produce an immediate numbing effect. Stool softeners and laxatives promote painless passage of soft stools. Analgesia decreases perineal discom-
8. Additional individualized interventions: _____	**8.** Rationales: _____

COLLABORATIVE PROBLEM

Altered urinary elimination related to pregnancy-induced hypervolemia, birth-induced trauma, overdistention, and the effects of anesthesia

Expected outcome

The patient maintains or returns to normal urinary tract function.

Interventions	Rationales
1. Monitor fluid intake and output for 24 to 48 hours.	**1.** Fluid output reflects renal function.
2. Note time, amount, and color of each elimination.	**2.** Optimally, the patient should void every 3 to 4 hours. Symptoms of incomplete emptying and retention with overflow (voiding small amounts frequently) imply poor bladder tone and predispose the patient to GU infection and uterine atony.

3. Help the patient to void spontaneously by:
• encouraging the patient to void whenever she feels the urge.
• providing medication every 3 to 4 hours as necessary for pain before ambulation.
• suggesting that the patient run tap water while in the bathroom and pour clean water over her perineum while voiding.
• encouraging voiding during a sitz bath or shower if elimination is difficult.

4. Assess for urinary urgency and frequency, dysuria, hematuria (differentiate from urine contaminated with vaginal discharge) and, possibly, pyrexia.

5. Catheterize the patient only if necessary — for instance, when the patient cannot void every 6 to 8 hours or has persistent urine retention with overflow. Use an indwelling urinary (Foley) catheter to measure residual urine; if there is more than 50 ml of urine, keep the catheter in place. Continue perineal care while the catheter is in place.

6. Teach the patient Kegel exercises as soon as the anesthetic has worn off and the patient is receptive. Instruct her to mimic holding back urine for 10 seconds and then release; have her perform 10 exercises consecutively four times daily.

7. Additional individualized interventions: _____
_____

3. These measures act as a physical and occasional psychological impetus to void.

4. These are indications of urinary tract infection, which warrants antimicrobial therapy.

5. Catheterization further predisposes the patient to a GU infection. The GU system is compromised by a traumatized, edematous, and hyperemic bladder; neural impairment associated especially with the size of a gravid uterus; conduction anesthesia; and use of morphine sulfate (Duramorph).

6. Kegel exercises strengthen the pubococcygeal muscles and prevent or ameliorate pelvic floor relaxation and urinary stress incontinence.

7. Rationales: _____
_____

COLLABORATIVE PROBLEM

Breast engorgement in the nonnursing patient related to milk production secondary to prolactin secretion

Expected outcome

The patient develops minimal or no breast engorgement or milk production.

Interventions

1. Assess the patient's breasts immediately postpartum and every 8 hours, noting colostrum secretion for 2 to 3 days; initial diffuse breast nodularity followed by tense, warm, engorged, and painful breasts; and low-grade fever.

2. Provide breast support with a firm, well-fitted bra or breast binder.

3. Teach the patient to avoid self-breast stimulation and stimulation from the infant or sexual partner, from a breast pump or manual expression of milk, and from hot showers or baths.

4. Institute pain-relief measures, including applying an ice bag to the patient's breasts and providing oral analgesics (most commonly codeine and aspirin).

Rationales

1. Colostrum is the first lacteal secretion to appear. Engorgement and resulting symptoms are the product of venous and lymphatic stasis.

2. These measures provide support until mechanical suppression of lactation, which usually is accomplished in 2 to 3 days.

3. Avoiding breast stimulation decreases milk production.

4. These measures control local and central pain.

5. Additional individualized interventions: _____
_____

5. Rationales: _____
_____

COLLABORATIVE PROBLEM

Breast engorgement in the lactating patient related to milk production secondary to prolactin secretion

Expected outcome

The patient develops minimal engorgement and begins producing milk

Interventions	Rationales
1. Assess the patient's breasts as you would those of the nonnursing patient.	**1.** The physiologic course, uninterrupted by mechanical suppression, is the same for either patient. Engorgement is the natural harbinger of lactation.
2. Provide pain-relief measures, including breast support, cold soaks, and analgesics.	**2.** The patient may need pain-relief measures that do not inhibit milk secretion until her symptoms subside.
3. Massage the breasts; the patient should then express milk, either manually or with a breast pump.	**3.** The patient may need to express milk mechanically until symptoms abate.
4. Put the infant to the breast as soon as comfortable and have the patient empty her breasts regularly.	**4.** These actions minimize further engorgement and enhance prolactin secretion.
5. Additional individualized interventions: _____	**5.** Rationales: _____

NURSING DIAGNOSIS

Knowledge deficit related to postpartum sexual activity

Expected outcome

The patient is informed about about postpartum sexual activity.

Interventions	Rationales
1. Assess the patient's knowledge base. Allow her to ask questions. Anticipate and prepare a scenario for teaching. Teach the patient in a quiet area when she is rested, relaxed, and free of pain.	**1.** An appropriate setting enhances rapport and learning.
2. Provide factual information on resuming sexual activities, including the following: • Episiotomy usually heals by the 3rd postpartum week. The patient should not resume intercourse until her doctor has examined her, usually 4 to 6 weeks postpartum. • Menses usually resume in the nonnursing patient in 6 to 8 weeks.	**2.** Involution of the placental site is probably not complete until the 6th postpartum week. Intercourse before healing may lead to infection or pregnancy.
3. Additional individualized interventions: _____	**3.** Rationales: _____

Documentation checklist

During the hospital stay, document:

❏ patient status and assessment findings, including fluid intake and output, cardiovascular status, Rh and rubella status, signs of dehydration, alterations in voiding patterns, presence of hemorrhoids or perineal tears or hematomas, appearance of episiotomy (if present), and appearance of lochia
❏ changes in patient status
❏ pertinent laboratory and diagnostic findings
❏ pain — quality, location, frequency, and intensity
❏ the patient's response to treatment
❏ the patient's and family's reaction to the birth
❏ the patient's and family's reaction to possible thromboembolic disease.
❏ fundal height and tone
❏ appearance of perinatal or genital lacerations or suture lines
❏ appearance of the breasts, including signs of engorgement
❏ patient's and family's interaction with the infant
❏ patient and family teaching guidelines, including breast-feeding support if applicable, sexuality activities, and normal maternal care needs
❏ discharge planning guidelines.

Associated plans and appendices

❏ Selected daily dietary allowances — maternal (appendix B)
❏ Aspects of psychological care — maternal (appendix D)
❏ Selected methods of family planning (appendix F)
❏ Parent teaching guides (appendix J)

Additional nursing diagnoses

• Fear related to perceived inability to care for infant
• Ineffective individual coping related to hormonal processes and fatigue
• Ineffective thermoregulation related to postpartum chill secondary to postdelivery vasomotor response

Hemorrhage

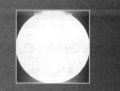

Definition
Hemorrhage is blood loss of 500 ml or more after delivery. Excessive loss most commonly occurs early in the puerperium, usually within the first 24 hours, although hemorrhage may occur from 4 to 6 weeks postpartum.

Ideally, management is prophylactic and includes recognizing and controlling predisposing conditions and scrupulously managing labor and delivery. Recognizing and correcting hypovolemia is essential.

Etiology and precipitating factors
• Early hemorrhage can result from uterine overdistention and atony, lacerations (with or without hematoma formation), retained placental fragments, and hypofibrinogenemia. Late hemorrhage can result from subinvolution, the retained products of conception, myomas, and infection.
• Patients at risk include those with a history of postpartum uterine atony or hemorrhage, an overdistended uterus from hydramnios, multiple gestation or an infant large for gestational age, high parity, placenta previa, abruptio placentae, or a medically complicated pregnancy; those who undergo protracted or precipitate labor and delivery or oxytocin augmentation or induction; those who receive relaxant anesthesia; and those who retain a dead fetus for a prolonged period after intrauterine death.

Physical findings
Cardiovascular
• hypotension
• tachycardia
• tachypnea
• pallor, cyanosis, and cold and clammy skin
Genitourinary
• Uterine atony
 – soft, boggy uterus that will not stay contracted
 – bright red vaginal bleeding; amount varying from continual trickle to profuse
 – passage or expression of multiple or large clots
 – distended bladder
• Laceration
 – continued bright red vaginal bleeding despite a well-contracted uterus, with no clots passed
 – possibly visible tear of the cervix, external genitalia, or anus

• Hematoma
 – perineal, vaginal, urethral, bladder, or rectal pressure
 – tense, severely painful vaginal protrusion
 – ecchymotic perineum; purple cast to vaginal mucosa
 – possibly inability to void
• Hypofibrinogenemia
 – multisite bleeding from any orifice or invasive site
 – frank vaginal bleeding without clotting
• Retained placenta
 – uterine tone ranging from firm and contracted to somewhat boggy, depending on amount of retention
 – fragmented or missing cotyledons or membranes immediately after delivery
• Subinvolution (late hemorrhage, most commonly 4 to 6 weeks postpartum)
 – fundal height greater than postpartum stage would warrant; poor uterine tone
 – persistent or recurrent lochia; persistent lochial flow
 – possibly leukorrhea
Subjective
• Pain with lacerations and hematoma
• Apprehension, restlessness, and anxiety with hypovolemia

Diagnostic studies
• Accurate and complete history and physical examination may furnish enough data for a definitive diagnosis of hypovolemia and may make diagnostic studies unnecessary.
• Ultrasonography may identify larger retained placental fragments.
• Hemoglobin level and hematocrit decrease.
• Coagulation factors — fibrinogen decreases and activated partial thromboplastin time increases.

COLLABORATIVE PROBLEM

Fluid volume deficit related to blood loss secondary to uterine atony or to retained placental fragments or lacerations (two expected outcomes)

Expected outcome 1

The patient exhibiting signs of early uterine atony and hemorrhage will be identified.

Interventions

1. Ascertain from delivery personnel:
- outstanding medical and obstetric histories
- length and characteristics of labor
- type of delivery
- course and outcome of placental delivery
- postdelivery assessment, including estimated blood loss.

2. Perform a postpartum assessment every 30 minutes for 1 hour, then every 4 hours and as the patient's condition warrants. Note the following:
- fundal height and tone
- amount and characteristics of vaginal discharge and bleeding
- signs of hematoma on perineum
- presence and number of clots
- presence of bladder distention
- number and weight of pads used.

3. At the same time, monitor the patient's capillary refill time (it should be less than 3 seconds) and vital signs, and integrate the findings with your physical examination.

4. Note trends in hemoglobin level and hematocrit, compare them with prenatal and intrapartum values, and integrate them with estimated blood loss.

5. Monitor the patient's fluid intake and output every 8 hours; if the patient has overt bleeding and constitutional signs of deterioration, monitor hourly.

6. Additional individualized interventions: _____

Rationales

1. This information helps identify the high-risk patient. The expected blood loss from vaginal birth is 300 to 500 ml; from cesarean section birth, 900 to 1,100 ml.

2. Postpartum assessment provides a database and promotes early detection of any aberrations. A distended bladder prevents effective uterine contraction. Noting the number and weight of pads used helps estimate blood loss and replacement needs. (*Note:* One milliliter of blood weighs 1 g.)

3. Increased capillary refill time and restlessness indicate early shock. Extensive blood loss may occur before the classic signs of hemorrhage (hypotension, tachycardia, tachypnea, and pallor) occur.

4. A 500-ml blood loss is usually mirrored by a decrease of 4 percentage points in hematocrit.

5. Fluid output reflects renal function; minimal levels should range from 30 to 50 ml/hour.

6. Rationales: _____

Expected outcome 2

The patient has minimal further dysfunctional bleeding and returns to normovolemia.

Interventions

1. Evaluate the bladder for distention; catheterize if distended.

Rationales

1. A distended bladder displaces the uterus upward and prevents uterine contraction.

2. Gently massage the boggy uterus at the fundus while supporting the lower uterine segment.

2. Gentle massage stimulates uterine contraction, helps expel retained placental fragments, and restores uterine tone. Aggressive or forceful manipulation may tire the myometrium and result in further atony. Support minimizes the risk of uterine inversion.

3. Start an I.V. infusion of a balanced solution using a large-bore needle. Type and crossmatch for blood products.

3. The I.V. line provides venous access and an immediate infusion site for replacement blood products before peripheral vasoconstriction associated with shock occurs.

4. If a normotensive patient develops atony and hemorrhage, administer 0.2 mg of methylergonovine (Methergine) I.M., 10 to 40 units of oxytocin I.V. in 1,000 ml of a physiologic electrolyte solution, or 250 μg/L of carboprost tromethamine (Hemabate) I.M. Note the patient's uterine tone and monitor blood pressure carefully.

4. Oxytocic agents stimulate uterine contractions and, therefore, control postpartum bleeding. Uterine hyperactivity may result with overdose.

5. After initial I.V. or I.M. doses, administer one of the following oral oxytocic agents to the normotensive patient:
• ergonovine (Ergotrate), 0.2 to 0.4 mg two to four times daily for 2 days
• methylergonovine, 0.2 mg two or four times daily for up to 7 days.

5. Oxytocic agents control atony and hemorrhage; if the patient was hypertensive during pregnancy, these drugs may be contraindicated.

6. Administer whole blood, plasma, or platelets.

6. Whole blood replaces actual losses and helps restore normovolemia. Plasma contains fibrinogen, which corrects defects associated with disseminated intravascular coagulation. Platelets assist in coagulation to treat coagulopathies.

7. Prepare the patient for surgery for diagnosed lacerations, hematoma, or retained placenta.

7. Lacerations require surgical ligation; larger hematomas require evacuation. Nonadherent, retained placenta may require dilatation and curettage. Adherent, retained placenta accreta associated with profound blood loss may warrant hysterectomy.

8. Additional individualized interventions: _____

8. Rationales: _____

COLLABORATIVE PROBLEM

Risk for genital infection related to bacterial contamination secondary to trauma and hemorrhage

Expected outcome

The patient exhibiting early signs of infection will be identified and will receive the appropriate nursing interventions.

Interventions

1. Monitor for signs of infection, including:
• tender uterus
• chills and pyrexia
• change in lochial flow, purulent drainage, or odorous discharge
• pelvic or perineal discomfort disproportionate to the type and course of delivery.
Correlate findings with intrapartum and immediate postpartum surveys.

Rationales

1. Assessment helps identify the high-risk patient and the origin of the infection.

Postpartum

2. Obtain a specimen of lochia or any discharge for culture and sensitivity testing, and initiate antibiotic therapy.

2. Culture and sensitivity testing identifies the causative organism and its sensitivity to various antibiotics. Culture specimens should be obtained before therapy is initiated because antibiotics may mask infection.

3. Additional individualized interventions: _____

_____

3. Rationales: _____

_____

Documentation checklist

During the hospital stay, document:
- ❏ patient status and assessment findings
- ❏ changes in patient status
- ❏ pertinent laboratory and diagnostic findings
- ❏ fundal height and tone
- ❏ appearance of perinatal or genital lacerations or suture lines
- ❏ amount of blood loss
- ❏ fluid status—intake and output
- ❏ signs of infection
- ❏ pain—quality, location, frequency, and intensity
- ❏ patient's response to treatment
- ❏ patient's and family's reaction to hemorrhage
- ❏ patient and family teaching guidelines
- ❏ discharge planning guidelines.

Associated plans and appendices

- ❏ Abruptio placentae
- ❏ Inappropriate size or weight: large for gestational age
- ❏ Multiple gestation
- ❏ Placenta previa
- ❏ Pregnancy complicated by diabetes mellitus
- ❏ Puerperal infection
- ❏ Puerperium
- ❏ Aspects of psychological care—maternal (appendix D)

Additional nursing diagnoses

- ❏ Altered peripheral tissue perfusion related to hypoxia secondary to blood loss
- ❏ Fear related to blood loss
- ❏ Impaired tissue integrity related to perineal or genital lacerations

Puerperal infection

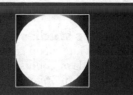

Definition

Puerperal infection is postpartum infection of the genital tract. Although it may occur at any time in the puerperium, it usually occurs within 10 days of delivery. The infection may be local and involve the breasts as well as structures of delivery, including the external genitalia, vagina, uterus, and parametria; or it may progress by way of the circulatory or lymphatic systems to pelvic cellulitis, septic thrombophlebitis, peritonitis, or bacterial shock. Aseptic technique and advances in technology have decreased the incidence, but infection is still a leading cause of maternal morbidity. Ideally, management is prophylactic and directed at early recognition of infection and prompt, aggressive antibiotic therapy. The differential diagnosis of pyrexia as well as careful assessment and physical examination are critical in ruling out other sources of infection, such as decreased respiratory function, pyelonephritis, thrombophlebitis, and wounds.

Etiology and precipitating factors

• Infection results from polymicrobial invasion by one or more of the following organisms: anaerobic bacteria, including *Bacteroides, Peptostreptococcus, Peptococcus,* and *Clostridium,* and aerobic bacteria, including *Escherichia coli,* beta-hemolytic streptococci, *Klebsiella, Proteus mirabilis, Pseudomonas, Staphylococcus aureus,* and *Neisseria gonorrhoeae.*
• The risk increases with anemia and malnutrition; antenatal coitus when or after membranes have ruptured; intrapartum invasive techniques, breaks in aseptic technique, and improper perineal care; prolonged labor, especially with ruptured membranes; prolonged rupture of membranes; hemorrhage, especially if blood loss is greater than 1,000 ml; operative delivery; manipulation; and trauma.

Physical findings

• Localized infection of external genitalia (sutured laceration or episiotomy; infected trauma of perineum, vulva, vagina, cervix, or abdominal surgical wound)
 – low-grade fever (temperature less than 101° F [38.3° C]); possibly chills and rapid onset of pyrexia
 – localized pain; wound pain disproportionate to extent of repair
 – edema, erythema, necrosis of wound edges; edges no longer approximated; sanguinopurulent or purulent discharge
 – dysuria, with or without urine retention
• Mastitis

 – severe breast engorgement
 – chills, rapid temperature elevation to 101° F (38.3° C) and higher; constitutional symptoms
 – hard, red, painful breast; possibly purulent discharge from nipple
• Endometritis or metritis
 – irregular fever, with temperature varying from 101° to 103° F (38.3° C to 39.4° C); proportionate tachycardia
 – soft, tender uterus larger than involutional stage would warrant; protracted afterbirth pains
 – profuse, foul-smelling, bloody, occasionally frothy lochia; scant, odorless lochia in beta-hemolytic streptococcal infection
• Salpingitis or oophoritis
 – pyrexia of 103° to 104° F (39.4° to 40° C)
 – unilateral or bilateral lower abdominal pain
• Parametritis or pelvic cellulitis
 – persistent pyrexia (102° to 104° F [38.8° to 40° C]), chills, and constitutional symptoms
 – frequent unilateral or bilateral abdominal tenderness; pain on pelvic examination associated with uterine movement, possibly preceded by signs and symptoms of endometritis
 – possibly uterine fixation and pelvic mass on vaginal examination
 – possibly abscess formation that may be palpated vaginally, rectally, or abdominally, depending on location; inguinal focal point under skin may cause edema, erythema, tenderness
• Thrombophlebitis
 – pyrexia 4 to 10 days postpartum
 – pain, erythema, and edema of affected leg
 – pelvic, lower abdominal, or flank pain; chills and spiking fever in pelvic thrombophlebitis; fever may spike to 105° F (40.5° C) and then fall precipitously
 – decreased ventilatory function if small pulmonary emboli ensue
• Peritonitis
 – commonly preceded by signs and symptoms of endometritis
 – marked pyrexia, tachycardia, rapid and shallow respirations; constitutional symptoms
 – severe abdominal pain with rigidity
 – abdominal distention with decreased bowel sounds; nausea, vomiting (often projectile and eventually containing feces), and diarrhea
 – excessive thirst or brown tongue and foul breath
 – anxious expression and restlessness

Diagnostic studies

• Elevated white blood cell (WBC) count (a patern of upward trends or counts of 15,000 to 30,000/mm³) usually occurs in 36 to 48 hours.

• Culture of blood, urine, or intrauterine material, revealing the causative agent, confirms diagnosis.
• Ultrasound may reveal signs of pelvic or femoral thrombophlebitis.

COLLABORATIVE PROBLEM

Risk for postpartum infection related to the trauma of labor, delivery, and self-inoculation as well as the iatrogenic introduction of pathogens (two expected outcomes)

Expected outcome 1

The patient develops minimal or no infection.

Interventions

1. Ascertain from delivery personnel:
• outstanding medical and obstetric histories
• course of labor and delivery and recovery time
• estimated blood loss
• anesthetic, drugs, and parenteral fluids administered.

2. Inspect the perineum, using a good source of light. Note the color and integrity of the perineum, and assess the episiotomy for pain, *r*edness, *e*dema, *e*cchymosis, *d*rainage, and *a*pproximation of suture edges (the REEDA parameters).

3. Assess fundal height and tone. Massage the boggy uterus.

4. Assess lochia for type, amount, odor, and characteristics. Correlate your findings with postpartum data.

5. Assess the patient's breasts for erythema, pain, engorgement, and nipple discharge. Correlate your findings with normal postpartum changes, and note whether the patient is breast-feeding.

6. Monitor the patient's vital signs, especially temperature, every 4 hours and as her condition warrants. Note pyrexia trends (temperatures in excess of 100.4° F [38° C] on any 2 of the first 10 days postpartum, exclusive of the first 24 hours, to be taken orally by a standard technique at least four times daily [Joint Committee on Maternal Welfare]).

7. Note the white blood cell count, and integrate the data into a complete clinical profile.

8. Perform perineal care and hygienic measures. Make sure caregivers and the patient wash their hands. Clean the perineum and frequently change pads, provide sitz baths, and apply antibiotic creams.

Rationales

1. Assessment identifies the high-risk patient. All puerperal patients are at risk for infection because of their denuded placental attachment sites and thin, highly vascular decidua.

2. Careful inspection provides a database and assists in the early identification of a hematoma or inflammation and infection.

3. Assessment confirms the normal involutional process. Massage stimulates contractility and expulsion of placental fragments. Infection is commonly associated with subinvolution.

4. Assessment confirms the normal involutional process and helps identify signs of infection.

5. Assessment helps differentiate normal postpartum changes from signs of breast infection.

6. In conjunction with a physical examination, trends can help in formulating a medical diagnosis.

7. Leukocytosis accompanies inflammation. However, normal postpartum levels are increased (15,000 to 30,000/mm³), and diagnosis depends on integrating all pertinent suspect data.

8. These measures limit exposure to contaminants and promote healing.

9. Monitor the patient's fluid intake and output, and encourage a fluid intake of eight to ten 8-oz glasses per day.

10. Help the patient select a balanced diet; encourage intake of protein, vitamin C, and iron.

11. Assess breath sounds, respiratory rate, and effort. Assist the patient with pulmonary hygiene, including coughing and deep breathing every 4 hours.

12. Assess the patient's calves bilaterally for color, size, temperature, Homans' sign, pain, pulses, and paresthesias. Assist with progressive ambulation. Encourage frequent position change in bed.

13. Encourage rest and uninterrupted sleep. Coordinate assessments and procedures to promote rest.

14. Teach the patient proper hand-washing technique to prevent infection as well as the signs and symptoms of infection and when to call the doctor.

15. Additional individualized interventions: _____

9. Temperature increases may result from dehydration; fluid output reflects renal function.

10. Protein and vitamin C promote healing. Iron, whether from food or supplements, can help correct anemia.

11. Pulmonary exercises improve oxygenation and prevent pooling or accumulation of secretions, minimizing the risk of atelectasis and pneumonia.

12. Assessment provides a database that can help identify thrombophlebitis.

13. Rest decreases the metabolic rate, increasing the physiologic and emotional resources needed for healing.

14. A patient who is discharged early may be at home when infection develops.

15. Rationales: _____

Expected outcome 2

The patient manifesting early signs of infection will be identified and will receive appropriate interventions.

Interventions

1. Note temperature trends. Monitor for infection (see discussion of physical findings on page 141).

2. Administer the following medications as indicated after specimens have been taken for culture and sensitivity tests:
• antibiotics such as penicillin, gentamicin (Gentacidin), clindamycin (Cleocin), tetracycline (Sumycin), cefoxitin (Cefoxin, Mefoxin), chloramphenicol (Chloromycetin), or metronidazole (Flagyl)
• oxytocic agents, such as ergonovine (Ergotrate) and methylergonovine (Methergine).

3. Check with the lactation consultant about discontinuing breast-feeding in the patient with a diagnosis of suppurative mastitis.

4. Closely monitor fluid intake and output; administer I.V. fluids with electrolytes; withhold food and fluids if the patient has persistent vomiting or paralytic ileus.

5. Insert a nasogastric tube, monitor continuous nasogastric suction, and assess bowel sounds.

6. Additional individualized interventions: _____

Rationales

1. Compilation of data assists in early identification and treatment of infection.

2. Various antibiotic drugs are used either alone or in combination to combat and resolve infection; oxytocic agents help stimulate uterine contractions and the expulsion of retained placental fragments.

3. In suppurative mastitis, breast milk becomes infected. The suckling infant's nose and throat usually harbor the organism — most commonly *S. aureus* — that causes the infection and, possibly, reinfection.

4. Dehydration secondary to pyrexia, vomiting, and diarrhea as well as fluid retention associated with peritonitis depletes the patient's fluid and electrolytes.

5. Paralytic ileus associated with peritonitis warrants mechanical decompression. Restoration of bowel function is gauged by the cessation of symptoms and the patient's ability to expel flatus.

6. Rationales: _____

Postpartum

NURSING DIAGNOSIS

Pain related to inflammatory processes and exudate entrapment

Expected outcome

The patient experiences minimal pain.

Interventions

1. Establish rapport with the patient and significant others. Call her by her preferred name.

2. Assess the characteristics of any pain, including quality, frequency, location, and intensity.

3. Minimize distracting environmental stimuli.

4. Perform comfort measures, including encouraging and assisting with position changes, implementing relaxation techniques and massage, and provide pharmacologic analgesia.

5. Additional individualized interventions: _____

Rationales

1. A positive relationship increases trust and decreases anxiety. This in turn may decrease regressive behaviors, anger, resistance, and noncompliance.

2. A pain profile may assist in formulating a medical diagnosis.

3. External stimuli may increase the perception of pain. Unwarranted interruptions of rest periods sap the patient's emotional reserve.

4. Increased tissue perfusion and stimulation of afferent fibers decrease the perception of pain. Pharmacologic analgesia provides central pain control.

5. Rationales: _____

Documentation checklist

During the hospital stay, document:
❏ patient status and assessment findings
❏ changes in patient status
❏ pertinent laboratory and diagnostic findings
❏ fundal height and tone
❏ appearance of perinatal or genital lacerations or suture lines
❏ pain — quality, location, frequency, and intensity
❏ patient's response to treatment
❏ patient's and family's reaction to infection
❏ patient and family teaching guidelines
❏ discharge planning guidelines.

Associated plans and appendices

❏ Cesarean section birth
❏ Hemorrhage
❏ Normal antepartum
❏ Premature rupture of membranes
❏ Puerperium
❏ Aspects of psychological care — maternal (appendix D)

Additional nursing diagnoses

❏ Fluid volume deficit related to dehydration secondary to pyrexia, decreased fluid intake, and emesis
❏ Knowledge deficit related to source of infection, its course and outcome, and implications for the infant
❏ Risk for altered body temperature related to bacterial contamination and pathogenic invasion of genital tract

Thromboembolic disease

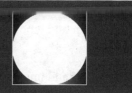

Definition

Thromboembolic disease is a complication of the puerperium that includes thrombophlebitis and phlebothrombosis, forms of deep vein thrombosis (DVT). Thrombophlebitis is the formation of a thrombus or clot after vein inflammation. The inflammatory process may cause the thrombus to attach more firmly to the vein, minimizing the opportunity for dislodgment and embolism. Phlebothrombosis is the formation of a clot in the absence of inflammation, possibly resulting in a greater risk of dislodgment and, subsequently, pulmonary embolism. All thrombi have the potential to dislodge and result in embolism.

Venous stasis is a major factor in the development of thrombosis. Predominant sites of thrombus formation include the legs, thighs, and pelvis. Management aims to prevent or recognize early symptoms of the disease, prevent further complications, and provide pain relief.

Etiology and precipitating factors

• Risk factors include a history of oral contraceptive use and venous thrombosis, obesity, and prolonged inactivity or sitting during pregnancy.

Physical findings

Cardiovascular

• DVT
  – initial low-grade fever followed by pyrexia and chills; tachycardia
  – marked pain and edema of affected extremity, more frequently the left leg; abrupt in onset
  – possibly increased warmth of extremity or positive Homans' sign
• Superficial thrombophlebitis
  – slight temperature elevation; possibly normal temperature
  – slight increase in pulse rate
  – warmth, redness, and tenderness at affected site

Subjective

• Calf pain

Diagnostic studies

• Accurate and complete history and physical examination may furnish enough data for a definitive diagnosis, possibly rendering diagnostic studies unnecessary.
• Doppler ultrasonography detects reduced or obstructed venous blood flow.
• Impedance plethysmography identifies amount of blood passing through the affected vessel.
• Phlebography confirms thrombus and impeded venous flow.

COLLABORATIVE PROBLEM

Altered peripheral tissue perfusion related to venous stasis (two expected outcomes)

Expected outcome 1

The patient experiencing early signs of peripheral dysfunction will be identified.

Interventions	Rationales
1. Ascertain from delivery personnel the patient's outstanding medical and obstetric histories, type and time of delivery, length of labor, anesthetic or analgesic administered, and postdelivery complications.	**1.** Information helps identify high-risk patients: those with a history of varices or thromboses, prolonged immobility associated with surgical delivery or the lithotomy position, and postdelivery complications.
2. Assess the calves and thighs bilaterally for size, color, temperature, peripheral pulses, pain, paresthesia, paralysis, and Homans' sign.	**2.** Assessment provides a database and promotes early recognition of dysfunction.
3. Monitor vital signs, especially temperature.	**3.** Persistent low-grade fever may indicate inflammation.

4. Monitor for and report signs of superficial venous thrombosis.

5. Monitor for and immediately report signs of DVT, including:
• sudden onset of severe leg or thigh pain accompanied by edema
• possibly positive Homans' sign
• increases in temperature and pulse rate and chills.

6. Additional individualized interventions: _____

4. Although superficial venous thrombosis is considered less serious because the risk of embolism is low, indications still need to be reported.

5. Phlegmasia alba dolens, or "milk leg," is a serious postpartum complication that usually involves the deep venous system from groin to foot and has the potential to generate life-threatening emboli.

6. Rationales: _____

Expected outcome 2

The patient demonstrates good peripheral circulation.

Interventions

1. Maintain the patient on bed rest. Fully elevate the affected leg on a pillow. Avoid compressing the popliteal space.

2. Do not position the patient with her knees flexed or legs up.

3. Apply warm packs to the affected leg; remove them for 10 minutes every hour.

4. Administer broad-spectrum antibiotics if the patient has a fever.

5. Administer 5,000 to 7,500 units of heparin subcutaneously every 4 to 6 hours or by continuous I.V. drip at a rate of 1 unit/ml of estimated blood volume. The dosage depends on activated partial thromboplastin time (APTT).

6. After acute inflammation has subsided, help the patient ambulate progressively. Apply fitted elastic support hose or pneumatic compression stockings.

7. Additional individualized interventions: _____

Rationales

1. Bed rest minimizes pressure on the peripheral venous system. Elevation improves blood return to the heart.

2. These positions may impede peripheral flow or cause pelvic pooling, thus compromising an already weakened system.

3. Warm packs cause vasodilation, which improves blood flow and decreases pain, although the patient may still need analgesics.

4. Fever indicates inflammation or infection.

5. An anticoagulant, heparin prevents further thrombus formation. An APTT that is 1½ to 2½ times the control in seconds indicates effective anticoagulant therapy.

6. Support hose or stockings compress superficial veins and promote deep venous flow.

7. Rationales: _____

Nursing diagnosis

Altered cardiopulmonary tissue perfusion related to pulmonary embolism secondary to dislodgment of deep vein thrombus

Expected outcome

The patient shows no signs of cardiopulmonary dysfunction.

Interventions

1. Monitor and report immediately signs of impaired cardiopulmonary status, including:
• any nonspecific alteration after an uncomplicated postpartum course, such as vague chest pain, anxiety, or apprehension
• a respiratory rate greater than 20 breaths/minute
• chest pain, shortness of breath, tachypnea, restlessness, pallor, or diaphoresis
• possibly crackles, friction rub, or increased jugular pressure.

2. Additional individualized interventions: _____

Rationales

1. Anticoagulant pharmacotherapy is indicated in suspected or confirmed embolism to minimize the risk of further and possibly fatal thrombus formation. The classic symptoms of pleuritic pain, hemoptysis, and dyspnea do not frequently occur; an increased respiratory rate is the most common and telling sign of embolism.

2. Rationales: _____

NURSING DIAGNOSIS

Risk for fluid volume deficit related to blood loss secondary to overheparinization

Expected outcome

The patient experiencing bleeding will be identified and treated accordingly.

Interventions

1. Monitor APTT and hematocrit (HCT).

2. Monitor for signs of bleeding, including epistaxis, hematemesis, dark and tarry stools, hematuria, ecchymosis, petechiae, prolonged bleeding from sites of invasive procedures, and oozing or bleeding from any orifice.

3. Have protamine sulfate 1% on hand.

4. Additional individualized interventions: _____

Rationales

1. APTT is the most accurate indicator of effective heparinization. Decreasing HCT is consistent with blood loss.

2. Such signs of bleeding usually precede frank bleeding.

3. Protamine sulfate inactivates heparin.

4. Rationales: _____

Documentation checklist

During the hospital stay, document:
❏ patient status and assessment findings, including fluid intake and output and cardiovascular status
❏ changes in patient status
❏ pertinent laboratory and diagnostic findings
❏ pain — quality, location, frequency, and intensity
❏ patient's response to treatment
❏ patient's and family's reaction to thromboembolic disease
❏ patient and family teaching guidelines
❏ discharge planning guidelines.

Associated plans and appendices

❏ Normal antepartum
❏ Puerperium

❏ Aspects of psychological care — maternal (appendix D)

Additional nursing diagnoses

❏ Impaired gas exchange related to obstructed pulmonary tree secondary to emboli
❏ Ineffective individual coping related to sudden onset of a complication affecting the patient's health and activities
❏ Knowledge deficit related to heparin or warfarin use, indications, adverse effects, and interactions
❏ Pain related to edema and compromised peripheral vascular circulation
❏ Risk for trauma related to prolonged standing and sitting secondary to compromised peripheral vasculature

Postpartum

Part 4

Newborn infant assessment guides

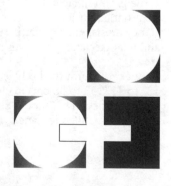

Newborn infant nursery assessment

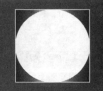

Assessment determines the infant's initial condition, establishes a baseline for subsequent care, and identifies potential and existing problems. The initial assessment takes place immediately after birth (see *Newborn infant postdelivery assessment*, page 152).The more complete physical assessment usually is finished within the infant's first 24 hours. (See *Ballard gestational-age assessment tool*, page 153.)

Physical assessment

Conduct the assessment in a well-lighted, warm, draft-free room. For the general survey and measuring and weighing, undress the infant completely, but leave a diaper over the infant's genital area to avoid soiling. (Remove the diaper to weigh the infant and to assess the hips, lower spine, genitals, and rectum.) Although any organized, consistent, and complete assessment method is satisfactory, the most common way to proceed is from head to toe (cephalocaudal), assessing vital signs; auscultating the heart, lungs, and abdomen; and then palpating the abdomen. These assessments are performed when the infant is quiet. Continue the general survey by assessing the infant's color, size, proportion, symmetry, nutritional status, posture, positioning, activity, reflexes (see *Major neonatal reflexes,* page 154), and behavior. Note gross abnormalities and disproportionate sizes. Assess hip abduction last because it frequently evokes infant crying. The features described below are common findings for the full-term normal neonate.

Skin

The skin appears soft, smooth, nearly transparent, elastic, and ruddy to pale pink, with desquamation by the 2nd or 3rd day. The nail beds and scrotum are more deeply pigmented in black infants, with possible mongolian spots in darker-skinned infants. Physiologic jaundice commonly appears after the first 24 hours. The neonate has lanugo, especially over the shoulders and back, and vernix caseosa, especially under the fingernails and in labial folds. The skin may show transient harlequin-like color changes, mottling with stress, acrocyanosis, milia, miliaria rubra, erythema toxicum, and telangiectatic nevi. Nails are formed and firm.

Head

About one-fourth the body length, the head measures 13″ to 15″ (33 to 38 cm) in circumference. It is flexed onto the chest. The smooth skull, with flat, soft, nonbulging or sunken fontanels, may be asymmetrical from uterine position, molding during birth, or positional compression. The anterior diamond-shaped fontanel measures 1″ to 2½″ (2.5 to 6 cm) at its widest diameter; the smaller posterior diamond-shaped fontanel measures ½″ to 1″ (1 to 2.5 cm). Skull sutures feel like ridges. A ¾″ (2-cm) illumination ring is apparent during transillumination of the frontoparietal skull, ½″ (1 cm) over the occiput.

Neck

The infant's neck is short, supple, and mobile, with tonic neck, neck righting, and otolith righting reflexes. The prone infant can hold its neck in line with its back and turn its head from side to side. The infant in a sitting position shows momentary ability to hold its head erect.

Eyes

Usually tightly closed, the infant's eyes are slate gray, dark blue-gray, or brown. Frequently, there is edema of the eyelids. The infant's cry is tearless. Transient strabismus may be evident. The pupils, usually equal, are round, with direct and consensual constriction in response to light. Reflexes include the red reflex and the optical blink reflex. Doll's eye fixation is also evident.

Ears

The ear canal is patent. The tops of the firm, elastic pinna parallel the eye's inner and outer canthi. Earlobes may have preauricular tags. The infant responds to loud sound with the startle (acoustic blink) reflex.

Nose and throat

Broad and patent, the nostrils may contain a mucous discharge. The infant is an obligate nasal breather and can sneeze and cry lustily. The tongue lies midline in the mouth; the palate is intact. The infant is edentulous with minimal salivation. Rooting, sucking, swallowing, yawn, and gag reflexes are present. White, glistening areas, called Epstein's pearls, may appear on the hard palate.

Chest and lungs

The circumference of the rounded chest measures 12″ to 13″ (30.5 to 33 cm). Anteroposterior and lateral diameters are equal. The xiphoid tip protrudes anteriorly at the apex of the costal angle. The infant has chiefly abdominal respirations (40 to 60 breaths/minute), intermittently slow and shallow or deep and rapid, with apneic episodes lasting 6 to 15 seconds. Breath sounds are bilaterally clear, loud, bronchovesicular, and hyperresonant. They commonly are diminished on the chest side opposite the head's direction, and fine crackles may be heard at the end of inspiration. Possibly enlarged, the breasts may secrete milky fluid.

Heart
Following respiratory trends, the heartbeat (110 to 160 beats/minute) sounds clear and regular and frequently is labile. The point of maximal intensity may be seen at the fourth intercostal space left of the midclavicular line. S_1 is louder than S_2 at the apex, and S_2 is louder than in the pulmonic area. S_2 splitting is common; innocent systolic murmurs may be evident.

Abdomen
Soft, cylindrical, and protruding, the abdomen may show a superficial venous pattern. The umbilical stump is drying and darkening. The following can be palpated; the liver (soft with a smooth edge) 1 to 2 cm below the right costal margin; the spleen tip along the lateral aspect of the left upper quadrant; kidneys, on deep palpation, with lower poles 1 to 2 cm above the umbilicus. Urine, if apparent, is clear; bowel sounds are present; and regurgitation may accompany feedings. Femoral pulses are equal. The crawling reflex is present.

Male genitalia
The penis is straight. The foreskin covers and adheres to the glans penis, which has a midline urethral opening at the tip. Testes in the edematous scrotum (or in the inguinal canal from which they can be milked) measure about 1 cm.

Female genitalia
The labia majora cover the labia minora. The clitoris appears large. The infant may have a mucoid, occasionally blood-tinged vaginal discharge. The urethra is located anterior to the vaginal orifice.

Rectum
The infant has a patent anus. There is passage of a meconium plug or meconium. The anal reflex is evident. Perianal skin tags may be present.

Arms and legs
Arms and legs are straight and symmetrical in size, shape, and position. The body is flexed, and the hands are clenched. No simian crease appears in the palms. Plantar creases cover the soles. The hips are stable and do not dislocate. Ortolani's maneuver and Barlow's sign are negative. The infant has good muscle tone, especially with resistance to opposing flexion, and full range of motion in each major joint. Hands have 10 fingers; feet have 10 toes. Hands and feet may show some edema. Feet are flat with creased soles. Deep tendon and plantar reflexes are highly variable. Brachial and radial pulses are strong and equal bilaterally. Femoral pulses are strong, equal, and regular bilaterally.

Back
The spinal column is straight. The buttocks have a symmetrical midline crease.

Behavioral assessment
The neonate moves successively through behavioral states, or degrees of alertness. Behavioral assessment evaluates the neonate's ability to react to and integrate various stimuli during these states.

The most commonly used behavioral evaluation tool is the Brazelton neonatal behavioral assessment scale (BNBAS), developed by pediatrician T. Berry Brazelton in 1973. This tool evaluates the neonate's behavioral state and behavioral responses.

For best results, behavioral assessment should be conducted in a quiet, dimly lighted setting. Findings should be interpreted in light of the period of reactivity and the neonate's gestational age.

Behavioral states
During *deep sleep,* the neonate makes few or no spontaneous movements; any movements that occur are brief and jerky. Respirations are even and regular. No rapid eye movements (REMs) occur. The neonate can be aroused from this state only for a few moments at a time.

During *light sleep,* the neonate can easily be aroused and brought to wakefulness; REMs can be detected. The neonate may move the arms and legs occasionally; movements are smoother than during deep sleep. Breathing patterns vary as the neonate drifts from light sleep to drowsiness.

During the *drowsy state,* the neonate tries to become fully alert, moves more frequently and regularly, and opens the eyes periodically. Responses to auditory and tactile stimuli are sluggish.

During the *alert state,* the neonate seems to be transfixed by external stimuli.

During the *active state,* the neonate responds to external stimuli with regular eye and body movements.

During the *crying state,* the neonate responds to both internal and external stimuli, cries vigorously and without interruption, and makes thrusting movements.

Behavioral responses
The neonate's behavioral responses fall into six basic categories: habituation, orientation, motor maturity, variations, self-quieting ability, and social behaviors. See *Neonatal behavioral responses,* page 155, for a complete description of these responses.

Newborn infant assessment guides

Newborn infant postdelivery assessment

The Apgar scoring system, shown here, provides a way to immediately evaluate an infant's cardiopulmonary and neurologic status. The assessment is performed at 1 and 5 minutes after birth and repeated every 5 minutes until the infant stabilizes.

APGAR SCORING SYSTEM

Sign	0	1	2
Heart rate	Absent	Slow (< 100 beats/minute)	> 100 beats/minute
Respiratory effort	Absent	Slow or irregular	Good cry
Muscle tone	Flaccid; limp	Some flexion of arms and legs	Active motion with flexion
Reflex irritability: Response to catheter in nostril (tested before oropharynx is clear) or to slapping on soles	No response	Grimace; some motion	Cough, sneeze, or cry
Color	Blue or pale	Body pink; arms and legs pale or blue	Completely pink

Legend:
Totals indicate:
0 to 3 — Severe distress
4 to 6 — Moderate difficulty
7 to 10 — No difficulty

The initial assessment

Concomitantly, as you measure the Apgar score, make sure the infant has a patent airway and no obvious problems. Make the following assessments (which may vary from hospital to hospital). To prevent heat loss in the infant, perform the assessment with speed and accuracy.
• UMBILICAL CORD — Presence of two arteries and one vein on cut surface: the arteries are smaller-lumened, papular structures; the vein is larger with a thinner vessel wall. Note length and time of delivery and umbilical cord clamping.
GENERAL APPRAISAL — Total appearance, state of maturity, size and relation of body parts, presence of congenital anomalies or birth trauma, and spontaneity of movement.

• CRY — Quality
• SKIN — Color and condition
• TEMPERATURE — First, take rectal temperature to rule out imperforate anus; afterward, take axillary temperatures.
• LENGTH
• WEIGHT
• ABDOMEN — Palpate for masses. If necessary, pass gastric tube through mouth to rule out esophageal atresia. Aspirate stomach contents to rule out high intestinal obstruction.
• RESPIRATIONS — Observe whether infant can breathe with closed mouth to rule out choanal atresia.
• MOUTH — Palpate integrity of palate to rule out cleft palate.

Ballard gestational-age assessment tool

To use this tool, the examiner evaluates and scores the neuromuscular and physical maturity criteria, totals the scores, and then plots the sum in the maturity rating box to determine gestational age.

NEUROMUSCULAR MATURITY

NEUROMUSCULAR MATURITY SIGN	SCORE							RECORD SCORE HERE
	-1	0	1	2	3	4	5	
POSTURE	—						—	
SQUARE WINDOW (Wrist)	>90°	90°	60°	45°	30°	0°		
ARM RECOIL	—	180°	140° to 180°	110° to 140°	90° to 100°	<90°		
POPLITEAL ANGLE	180°	160°	140°	120°	100°	90°	<90°	
SCARF SIGN								
HEEL TO EAR						—		

TOTAL NEUROMUSCULAR MATURITY SCORE

PHYSICAL MATURITY

PHYSICAL MATURITY SIGN	SCORE							RECORD SCORE HERE
	-1	0	1	2	3	4	5	
SKIN	Sticky, friable, transparent	Gelatinous, red, translu-sent	Smooth, pink; visible vessels	Superficial peeling or rash; few visible vessels	Cracking; pale areas; rare visible vessels	Parchment-like; deep cracking; no visible vessels	Leathery, cracked, wrinkled	
LANUGO	None	Sparse	Abundant	Thinning	Bald areas	Mostly bald	—	
PLANTAR SURFACE	Heel-toe 40 to 50 mm: -1; <40 mm: -2	>50 mm; no crease	Faint red marks	Anterior transverse crease only	Creases over anterior two-thirds	Creases over entire sole	—	
BREAST	Imperceptible	Barely perceptible	Flat areola, no bud	Stippled areola; 1- to 2-mm bud	Raised areola; 3- to 4-mm bud	Full areola; 5- to 10-mm bud	—	
EYE AND EAR	Lids fused, loosely: -1; tightly: -2	Lids open; pinna flat, stays folded	Slightly curved pinna; soft, slow recoil	Well-curved pinna; soft but ready recoil	Formed and firm; instant recoil	Thick carti-lage; ear stiff	—	
GENITALIA, (Male)	Scrotum flat, smooth	Scrotum empty; faint rugae	Testes in upper canal; rare rugae	Testes descending; few rugae	Testes down; good rugae	Testes pendulous; deep rugae	—	
GENITALIA, (Female)	Clitoris prominent; labia flat	Prominent clitoris; small labia minora	Prominent clitoris; enlarging minora	Majora and minora equally prominent	Majora large; minora small	Majora cover clitoris and minora	—	

TOTAL PHYSICAL MATURITY SCORE

SCORE

Neuromuscular _____

Physical _____

Total _____

MATURITY RATING

TOTAL MATURITY SCORE	GESTATIONAL AGE (WEEKS)
-10	20
-5	22
0	24
5	26
10	28
15	30
20	32
25	34
30	36
35	38
40	40
45	42
50	44

GESTATIONAL AGE (Weeks)

By dates _____

By ultrasound _____

By score _____

Newborn infant assessment guides

Adapted with permission from Ballard, J.L., Khoury, J.C., Wedig, K., et al. (1991). New Ballard Score, expanded to include extremely premature infants. *Journal of Pediatrics*, 119(3), 417-423. Used with permission from Mosby, Inc.

Major neonatal reflexes

This chart summarizes the neonatal reflexes that exist at birth or shortly thereafter. Some reflexes, such as the pupillary and blink reflexes, persist throughout life. Others, including Babinski's, doll's eye, grasp, Moro's, sucking, tonic neck, and trunk incurvation reflexes, disappear within a few weeks or months of birth.

Reflex	How to elicit	Normal response
Babinski's	Lightly stroke one side of neonate's foot upward from heel and across ball of foot.	Toes fan; great toe dorsiflexes.
Blink (corneal)	Momentarily shine bright light directly into neonate's eyes.	Neonate blinks.
Crossed extension	With neonate in a supine position, extend one leg and stimulate sole with light pin prick or finger flick.	Neonate swiftly flexes and extends opposite leg as if trying to push stimulus away from other foot.
Doll's eye	With neonate in a supine position, slowly turn neonate's head to left or right.	Eyes remain stationary.
Grasp • Palmar • Plantar	Press finger against neonate's palm. Press object against ball of neonate's foot.	Fingers momentarily close around object. Toes curl downward and around object.
Moro's (startle)	Make loud noise or suddenly disturb neonate's equilibrium.	Neonate stiffens and then briskly abducts and extends arm with hands open and fingers extended in "C" shape. Legs flex and abduct, and arms return to embracing posture. Crying is usual.
Placing	Hold neonate so that top of foot or anterior portion of lower leg lightly touches underside of flat surface.	Hips and knees flex; foot rises onto surface.
Pupillary	Darken room and shine penlight directly into each eye for several seconds.	Pupils constrict equally bilaterally.
Rooting	Touch finger to neonate's cheek or to corner of mouth.	Neonate turns head toward stimulus, opens mouth, and searches for stimulus.
Stepping	Hold neonate so that sole touches flat surface. (Test this reflex when testing placing reflex.)	Neonate makes walking or stepping motion.
Sucking	Place finger (or nipple) in neonate's mouth.	Neonate sucks on finger (or nipple) forcefully and rhythmically.
Tonic neck (fencing)	With neonate in a supine position, turn head over shoulder to one side.	Arm and leg partially or completely extend on side to which head is turned; opposite arm and leg flex.
Trunk incurvation (Galant)	With neonate in a prone position, stroke one side of spine about (½") 1 cm from midline.	Trunk curves to stimulated side; shoulders and pelvis move in same direction.

Initial size and vital signs

Size includes length and weight. Vital signs include temperature, heart rate, and respiratory rate. Average ranges follow:

Length: crown to rump: 12" to 14" (31 to 35 cm); head to heel: 19" to 21" (48 to 53 cm)

Weight: 2,500 to 4,000 g (5 lb, 5 oz to 8 lb, 13 oz)

Temperature: axillary (skin): 97.7° to 98.6° F (36.5° to 37° C); rectal (core): 96° to 99.5° F (35.5° to 37.5° C)

Heart rate: 110 to 160 beats/minute

Respiratory rate: 40 to 60 breaths/minute

Neonatal behavioral responses

Behavioral response	Description	When to assess
Habituation	Process of becoming accustomed to environmental stimuli, such as light and noise	During deep sleep, light sleep, or drowsy state
Orientation	Responsiveness to visual and auditory stimuli. Normally, neonate moves both head and eyes when orienting to visual or auditory stimulus. Nystagmus and gaze aversion after direct eye contact are normal. Neonate typically stops activity in response to auditory stimulus; sudden or loud stimulus usually causes crying.	During alert or active state
Motor maturity	Posture, muscle tone, muscle coordination, and movements. These should all be within normal parameters; arm and leg movements should be smooth, symmetrical, and equal. However, motor responses may vary greatly during first 24 hours after birth.	During alert state
Variations	Frequency of changes in activity level, behavioral state, and skin color	During each behavioral state
Self-quieting ability	Promptness and effectiveness with which neonate self-quiets when crying. Self-quieting behaviors include moving hands toward mouth, sucking on fist, changing position, and responding to auditory or visual stimuli when crying.	During crying state
Social behaviors	Reflexive cuddling, smiling, and other behaviors, such as crying to be fed followed by stopping sucking after hunger has been sated.	During alert or active state

Newborn developmental care

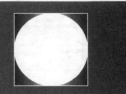

Definition

Developmental care is an approach to care giving that considers both a newborn's developmental stage and the effects of the environment on the newborn. The approach takes into account that the senses develop at different stages during gestation, with touch and taste developing early in gestation and vision and hearing developing later, and seeks to modify the newborn's environment appropriately. Developmental care also uses cue-based care — responding to the signals the infant gives off that it is stable or under stress — to modify care to reduce the infant's stress. It is particularly useful in caring for the premature or sick newborn.

In a typical hospital nursery, a newborn receives a great deal of visual and auditory stimuli. In a typical neonatal intensive care unit (NICU), the sick or premature infant is bombarded with such stimuli at a point in its development when it can least handle such stress. The effects of such stimuli can have life-long effects. For instance, the average sound level in a NICU is in the 50- to 90-decibel range — much higher than the typical home or office. Incubator fans can reach 80 decibels, a level that can cause hearing loss in an adult. Bright lights and loud intercom systems further interfere with the newborn's attempts to sleep. Such effects can result in poor weight gain, increased episodes of apnea and bradycardia, hypoxic spells, and poor feeding tolerance.

To combat these effects, the National Committee for NICU Design standards recommends decreasing ambient light to between 1 and 60 foot-candles at the bedside and keeping noise levels below 50 decibels on average, with transient sounds not to exceed 70 decibels and noise from equipment not to exceed 40 decibels. Other developmental care interventions include clustering care and cycling lights to provide longer stretches of uninterrupted sleep. By providing the infant with cue-based care in a less stressful environment, developmental care can help decrease the complications of prematurity and shorten the infant's length of stay in the NICU.

Physical findings
Stability signals*
- Regular color — even, without mottling or cyanosis
- Respiratory effort — easy, with no evidence of distress, apnea, or tachypnea
- Regular heart rate without bradycardia or tachycardia
- Minimal tremors of extremities
- Good muscle tone; good posture
- Smooth movements of extremities
- Hand-to-mouth movements
- Hand grasping
- Sucking and rooting reflex — strong
- Hand holding
- Tucking of body parts
- State regulation, steady sleep-wake patterns
- Self-consoling efforts
- Focused, alert look
- "Ooh" face
- Cooing
- Smiling

Stress signals
- Frequent color changes — mottling, cyanosis
- Irregular respiratory rate and labored breathing; periodic apnea or tachypnea
- Irregular heart rate and periodic bradycardia or tachycardia
- Noticeable tremors of the extremities
- Seizure activity
- Yawning
- Gagging
- Hiccuping
- Straining
- Sneezing, coughing, choking
- Sighing
- Poor muscle tone
- Poor posture
- Flaccid trunk or extremities
- Hypertonia or hypotonia
- Finger splaying
- Facial grimace
- Hand over face
- Fetal tuck
- Irritability
- Uncoordinated movements
- Irregular sleep-wake patterns
- Gaze aversion
- Staring
- Panicked look
- Inability to regulate state

* Must be considered along with gestational age; however, even the most immature infant will exhibit some stability signals given the right environment

Diagnostic studies

Although none are specific to developmental care, different assessment tools can be used to measure gestational age (see *Ballard gestational-age assessment tool,* page 153) and determine the development of behavioral and neurologic systems. The most commonly used tool for the premature infant is the Assessment of Preterm Infant Behavior (APIB) developed by Dr. T. Berry Brazelton. Using the Neonatal Individual Developmental Care and Assessment Program (NIDCAP) requires extensive training.

NURSING DIAGNOSIS

Sensory/perceptual alteration: visual, auditory, kinesthetic, gustatory, tactile, and olfactory related to excessive stimulation of the intensive care environment

Expected outcome

The infant will exhibit no stress signals.

Interventions

1. Assess the intensive care environment for:
• sources of loud sounds
• sources of excessive light
• cycling of lights, if any
• location of infant's bed in relation to equipment and traffic of unit.

2. Reduce sound levels by:
• limiting conversation at bedside
• speaking in a quiet voice
• not placing objects on top of the Plexiglas incubator top
• limiting use of overhead intercom systems
• switching monitor alarms to lights only when possible or decreasing sound level of first signal
• keeping radios off or on very low volume near bedside
• padding the inside of trash can lids to muffle sound
• placing strips of felt or other insulating material inside bedside cabinet or table drawers to muffle sound
• periodically using sound-proof incubator covers to protect the infant
• requesting acoustical tiles in the ceiling over bedside to absorb sound
• requesting carpeting or carpet strips on the floor
• instituting one quiet hour per day to sensitize staff members and parents to the need for quiet.

3. Reduce light levels by:
• dimming lights when possible
• cycling lights
• using window shades
• using procedural or bedside lights instead of overhead lights
• having individual controls for lights at each bedside
• using an incubator cover throughout the day during sleep periods.

Rationales

1. Assessment suggests types of adjustments that can improve the unit's environment.

2. Such measures reduce sound, which can reduce infant stress.

3. These techniques reduce light levels in the unit, which can reduce infant stress.

Newborn infant assessment guides

4. Assess the infant's ability to respond to stimuli. Observe for:
- stress signals
- stability signals
- neurologic deficits
- alertness or inattention
- inappropriate response to noise, eye contact, or feeding and absent normal reflexes
- effects of medications on behavior.

4. Assessment results suggest the types and amounts of sensory stimulation to provide or reduce.

5. Provide appropriate visual stimulation by:
- dimming bright lights
- suspending a black-and-white mobile with geometric shapes 7″ to 9″ (18 to 23 cm) from the infant's eyes (if the infant is in an incubator, tape a picture to one side of the incubator)
- holding the infant at eye level for eye contact and, if possible, holding the infant upright on shoulder.

5. The infant should be able to look at and respond to an object (stability signals); too much visual stimulation may cause the infant to look away or sigh or cause respiratory or cardiac changes (stress signals). A mobile may be too stimulating for a very immature infant.

6. Provide appropriate auditory stimulation by:
- talking to the infant in a low tone, using quiet, soft voice inflections
- calling the infant by name and speaking to it while giving care
- singing, playing tapes, or periodically turning on a radio to a very low volume
- avoiding excessive noises and conversations around the infant
- reducing monitor noises if possible.

6. The infant should display appropriate auditory responses, such as turning its head toward sounds (stability signal); overstimulation may cause apnea, bradycardia, or minimal body response (stress signals).

7. Provide appropriate tactile stimulation by:
- stroking the infant gently from head to toe with warmed hands and fingers
- holding and caressing the infant (if appropriate)
- giving the infant a pacifier for nonnutritive sucking satisfaction
- touching the infant with articles of different textures, such as cotton balls or smooth and napped cloth, or placing the infant on sheepskin or lambs wool
- changing the infant's position every 2 hours (if appropriate)
- providing boundaries for the infant (especially the premature infant) by placing blanket rolls behind the infant's back while it lies on its side or by swaddling the infant so that the soles of its feet touch a boundary and the infant maintains a flexed position and good body alignment
- carrying the infant in a strap-on carrier (if appropriate).

7. Tactile responses, such as motor activity, should be appropriate to the infant's condition and the stability or stress signals given. Overstimulation may cause hyperactivity or hypoactivity; tactile deficiency may cause inappropriate crying spells or responses only during procedures. Providing boundaries helps keep the infant's body in alignment, with hips flexed, and gives the infant a sense of stability with boundaries that feel like the boundaries of the uterus.

8. Provide gustatory stimulation by offering a pacifier for nonnutritive sucking; if the infant is receiving enteral feedings, give the infant breast milk or formula as indicated.

8. The infant should display gustatory responses, such as hand-to-mouth activity, feeding, and nonnutritive sucking.

9. Provide uninterrupted rest and sleep periods and cluster care. Base your care on the infant's stability and stress signals.

9. Rest periods and clustering care help prevent overstimulation. Stress signals indicate that care must stop, even if it must be started again in a few minutes.

10. Additional individualized interventions: _____

10. Rationales: _____

NURSING DIAGNOSIS

Knowledge deficit related to developmental care for sick infant

Expected outcome

The parents verbalize appropriate understanding of their infant's developmental care needs.

Interventions

1. Teach the parents about:
• the developmental level of their infant
• disease process
• care procedures
• stability and stress signals
• their role in the infant's care.

2. Teach the parents about such care-giving techniques as:
• clustering care based on stability and stress signals
• kangaroo care (skin-to-skin contact)
• nesting and containment techniques
• controlling auditory and visual stimuli in the NICU.

3. Have the parents and family give return demonstrations of developmental care techniques.

4. Encourage the parents and family to participate in the infant's care.

5. Teach the parents and family how to balance the infant's activities with rest and how to evaluate its tolerance for activities. Provide written materials at the appropriate reading level for the parents' reference at home.

6. Additional individualized interventions: _____

Rationales

1. Learning about the infant's developmental level in relationship to the infant's condition and care procedures relieves anxiety and allows parents to prepare for the infant's discharge. Giving them a role in their infant's care allows them a sense of control.

2. Such teaching promotes family compliance and helps dispel fears about equipment and procedures. Kangaroo care promotes bonding with the infant and is linked with increased weight gain as well as temperature and cardiopulmonary stability.

3. Return demonstrations boost family members' feelings of adequacy and independence and may alert the nurse to the need for more instruction.

4. Participation helps alleviate feelings of inadequacy and prepares family members to care for the infant at home.

5. The stimulation of activity is crucial for normal infant growth and development, which may be delayed by prolonged hospitalization. Activity tolerance varies from infant to infant. Once they are home, parents can use written materials to remember what they were taught.

6. Rationales: _____

Documentation checklist

During the hospital stay, document:
❏ infant status and assessment findings, especially neurobehavioral assessment data such as stress and stability signals
❏ changes in infant status
❏ pertinent laboratory and diagnostic findings
❏ the infant's response to treatment, specifically developmental care interventions
❏ the family's reaction to the infant's diagnosis
❏ parent-infant interaction

❏ family teaching guidelines, with special emphasis on stability and stress signals and developmental care techniques
❏ discharge planning guidelines.

Associated plans

All infant care plans have applications relevant to developmental care. See the plan appropriate to the individual infant.

Additional nursing diagnoses

❐ Altered family processes related to birth of high-risk infant
❐ Altered growth and development related to functional immaturity and prolonged environmental stress
❐ Altered parenting related to infant's need for intensive care nursery
❐ Altered nutrition: less than body requirements related to excessive stimulation of intensive care environment
❐ Anxiety (parental) related to vulnerability of small infant to illnesses
❐ Caregiver role strain related to infant status and need for intensive care
❐ Ineffective infant feeding pattern related to overstimulation of the intensive care environment
❐ Powerlessness (parental) related to health care environment and limited infant interaction
❐ Risk for injury (visual and auditory) related to excessive, long-term stimulation of the intensive care environment

Part 5

Infant

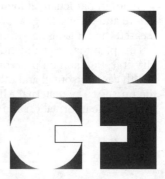

Acquired immunodeficiency syndrome — infant

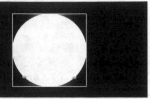

Definition

Acquired immunodeficiency syndrome (AIDS) represents end-stage infection with the human immunodeficiency virus (HIV). It is characterized by T-cell–mediated immunodeficiency that is unexplained by congenital conditions or drug suppression. Because of profound immunosuppression, people with AIDS develop opportunistic infections from bacteria, fungi, protozoa, and viruses. Consult the 1993 Centers for Disease Control and Prevention (CDC) Revised Classification System for HIV Infection/AIDS Surveillance Case Definition for a diagnostic composite and the inclusive surveillance case definition for AIDS.

No other definition of AIDS has been developed for infants and children, and the classification system and surveillance definition may not apply. For this reason, two definitions have emerged: one for infants and children up to age 15 months who have been exposed to their infected mothers perinatally and the other for older children with perinatal infection and for infants and children who have acquired the virus through other means. AIDS in infants and children younger than 15 months who have perinatal infection and who were exposed to infected mothers in the perinatal period is defined by one or more of the following criteria:
• identification of HIV in the blood or tissues
• presence of HIV antibody (confirmed by repeatedly reactive screening test plus a positive Western blot analysis) and evidence of both cellular and humoral immunodeficiency and a symptomatic infection
• signs and symptoms coinciding with those contained in the revised classification system.

The CDC reports that the incidence of vertical transmission of HIV from mother to infant has declined 27%. Factors leading to the sharp decline include better awareness of the dangers of HIV, the use of precautions such as condoms during sexual intercourse, voluntary testing, and better treatment methods for HIV-positive women. In particular, zidovudine (Retrovir) treatment before and during pregnancy and during labor has decreased the transmission from mother to infant.

This plan focuses on identifying infants at risk for HIV infection and on preventing HIV transmission to health care personnel and others who care for infants in the nursery. The maternal AIDS plan (see page 30) has prerequisite information and should be used with this plan.

Data included in the definition and plan are adapted from the CDC, "1993 Revised Classification System for HIV Infection and Expanded Case Definition for AIDS Among Adolescents and Adults," *Morbidity and Mortality Weekly Report,* December 18, 1992.

Etiology and precipitating factors
• Presence of HIV, a retrovirus
• Infant born to an HIV-seropositive mother (by perinatal transmission)
• Infant receiving HIV-seropositive blood transfusion

Physical findings
Maternal history
• Drug abuse or needle sharing
• Sexual partner or partners with a positive HIV antibody test or AIDS-positive HIV, enzyme-linked immunosorbent assay (ELISA), and Western blot test as confirmation
Infant status at birth
• No obvious disease signs (HIV testing is not routinely performed unless the mother's blood is known to be seropositive)
• Highly variable findings and symptoms, depending on the type of infection

Behavioral findings
• Loss of developmental milestones already achieved as immune system worsens and neurologic impairment progresses

Diagnostic studies
• ELISA — reveals HIV antibody, although seroconversion may take up to 6 months; in the neonate, HIV antibodies may appear from maternal infection, reflecting the placental transfer of maternal antibody
• Western blot test — confirms positive ELISA
• Immunoglobulin (Ig) level (antibody [IgM, IgA] detection) — identifies antibodies that do not readily cross the placenta
• p24 HIV antigen testing — identifies the presence of antigen
• CD4 count — helps quantify the progression of HIV infection
• Blood and tissue cultures — identifies HIV

COLLABORATIVE PROBLEM

Risk for infection related to perinatal transmission of HIV and immunosuppression (three expected outcomes)

Expected outcome 1

The infant at risk for HIV infection will be identified.

Interventions

1. Assess the infant's potential for developing HIV infection, including:

• maternal history of drug abuse, needle sharing, sexual partners with AIDS, positive HIV antibody test, or two positive ELISA tests on the same sample
• HIV antibody in the infant's blood or tissues

• tissue and blood cultures to identify infection with or without symptoms as well as abnormal Ig levels, CD4 and CD4:CD8 ratio, p24 antigen levels, and absolute cell count.

2. Discourage breast-feeding in HIV-positive mothers.

3. Give the infant 2 mg/kg of zidovudine by mouth every 6 hours for the first 6 weeks of life.

4. Additional individualized interventions: _____

Rationales

1. Assessment helps identify the high-risk population and the infant's potential exposure and plan appropriate measures.
• A mother with this history is at high risk for developing AIDS and could transmit the disease to the infant.

• Early testing of the infant may reflect placental transfer of maternal antibody or infection, with the HIV antibody persisting for as long as 15 months.
• Testing reveals humoral and cellular immunodeficiency.

2. Breast milk may transmit the HIV virus.

3. Zidovudine can effectively decrease the vertical transmission of HIV

4. Rationales: _____

Expected outcome 2

The infant exposed to HIV or who tested HIV-positive and who is experiencing HIV-related illness will be identified.

Interventions

1. Assess the infant for signs that may indicate HIV infection, including:
• failure to thrive
• weight loss more than 10% at the time symptoms appear
• elevated temperature
• diarrheal episodes (more than three times daily)
• lymph nodes measuring about ¼" (0.5 cm) at two or more sites
• hepatomegaly and splenomegaly
• rash.

Rationales

1. Infants may have signs and symptoms that persist for more than 1 month before a definitive AIDS diagnosis is made. In infants, signs and symptoms usually involve multiple organ systems and seldom occur alone.

2. Assess the infant for:
- cytomegalovirus disease
- herpes simplex virus infection with ulcer lasting longer than 1 month
- lymphoid interstitial pneumonia
- toxoplasmosis of the brain
- HIV dementia
- HIV wasting syndrome
- bacterial sepsis
- coccidioidomycosis and histoplasmosis (disseminated)
- lymphoma
- other viral, fungal, or protozoal infections.

3. Assess the infant for signs of opportunistic infection.

4. Additional individualized interventions: _____

2. Opportunistic infections occur because the infant's immune system is compromised and suppressed.

3. Zidovudine therapy suppresses bone marrow, making the infant vulnerable to opportunistic infections.

4. Rationales: _____

Expected outcome 3

The infant displays minimal effects of the infectious process.

Interventions

1. Provide supportive care and treatment of potential and existing infections by preparing and administering anti-infective therapy.

2. Screen visitors for viral or other infections.

3. Follow CDC recommendations for minimizing the risk of HIV transmission.

4. Additional individualized interventions: _____

Rationales

1. Anti-infective therapy treats opportunistic infections. Drugs of choice include penicillin G (Wycillin), ampicillin (Omnipen), methicillin (Staphcillin), carbenicillin (Geopen), cephalothin (Keflin), kanamycin (Kantrex), gentamicin (Garamycin), amikacin (Amikin), streptomycin, neomycin (Mycifradin), tobramycin (Nebcin), and amphotericin B (Fungizone).

2. Because of immunosuppression, the infant is predisposed to infection from others.

3. CDC studies show that these measures help reduce HIV transmission.

4. Rationales: _____

NURSING DIAGNOSIS

Risk for injury related to transmission of HIV to personnel and other infants in the nursery

Expected outcome

Caregivers and infants in the nursery who were previously HIV-negative do not become infected with HIV.

Interventions

1. Wear gloves when examining or handling all unbathed infants, when drawing blood, and before potential contact with body fluids, rashes, or skin breaks (for example, at I.V., catheter, dressing, or other exposure sites).

Rationales

1. Gloves prevent the infant's body fluids from coming in contact with skin breaks, which may permit transmission of the virus. *Note:* Neonates still have amniotic fluid and materials from the amniotic sac on their skin.

2. Wash hands with antiseptic solution before entering the nursery, before and after caring for the infant, and before and after touching contaminated articles.

3. Exclude the infant from the nursery, depending on whether the infant has enteritis, draining wounds, congenital syphilis, or a viral infection, such as cytomegalovirus, herpes, or rubella. (Do not exclude the infant solely on the basis of HIV infection.)

4. Wear a scrub or cover gown per hospital policy; change to a new gown for each infant.

5. Provide for proper disposal, decontamination, and sterilization of all equipment, supplies, and articles that come in contact with the infant (treat as hazardous waste), as follows:
• Use disposable products if possible.
• Dispose of used gowns, catheters, and other materials in clearly marked containers, according to local, state, and federal regulations.
• Follow standard sterilization, disinfection, cleaning, and housekeeping procedures, according to hospital policy.
• Double-bag nondisposable infectious material, using a water-soluble plastic inner liner, and color-code the bags.
• Disinfect spills with a 1:10% solution of 5.25% sodium hypochlorite (household bleach) or approved chemical germicides.
• Clearly label laboratory specimens and secure them in a plastic bag. Then notify the laboratory.

6. Follow the protocol in appendix K, Overview of isolation precautions.

7. Additional individualized interventions: _____

2. Hands are considered contaminated unless washed properly.

3. Isolation of the infant with a positive culture for any infection helps prevent transmission to other infants.

4. A scrub gown permits easy hand washing. A new gown prevents cross-contamination.

5. Sequestering, disinfecting, and sterilizing infectious material isolate and destroy the virus, helping to avoid self-inoculation as well as contamination of others and the environment.

6. These guidelines describe ways to prevent HIV transmission.

7. Rationales: _____

Nursing diagnosis

Fear (parental) related to infant's future death as a result of HIV infection

Expected outcome

The parents express less fear.

Interventions

1. Assess the level and cause of fear by:
• listening to expressions of fear
• determining what the parents know about AIDS
• observing nonverbal expressions of fear.

Rationales

1. The parents' fear level may increase with lack of information and distorted perceptions.

2. Provide information about AIDS based on what is known, including:
• cause of disease
• presence of HIV in infant
• possible implications of testing positive for HIV
• possible additional information and treatment as research efforts progress
• potential for positive future because disease may take 6 months or more to develop or may never develop
• importance of maintaining hope.

2. Increased knowledge reduces anxiety and fear and gives some reassurance that the disease may not develop. Although AIDS currently results in death, research to develop effective identification, prevention, and treatment intensifies daily.

3. Maintain a calm, positive attitude when interacting with the parents.

3. A calm, positive attitude conveys caring and concern.

4. Encourage the parents to use a support network, such as clergy, family, or others.

4. A support system can help the parents cope with a potentially critically ill child.

5. If the mother has AIDS or is positive for HIV, support her decision to seek counseling related to birth control and future pregnancies.

5. Abortion is an option for some pregnant women who test positive for HIV or who have AIDS. Prevention of pregnancy is critical for females who are HIV-positive and for those with AIDS.

6. Refer the parents to community resources and home health care services.

6. These referrals provide the parents and family with continued support before and after discharge.

7. Additional individualized interventions: _____

7. Rationales: _____

Documentation checklist

During the hospital stay, document:
❏ patient status and assessment findings, including signs of infection
❏ mother's current status
❏ changes in patient status
❏ pertinent laboratory and diagnostic findings
❏ patient's response to treatment
❏ parent-infant interaction
❏ the family's reaction to the infant's HIV status
❏ family teaching guidelines
❏ discharge planning guidelines.

Associated plans and appendices

❏ Acquired immunodeficiency syndrome — maternal
❏ Drug addiction and withdrawal
❏ Inappropriate size or weight for gestational age: small for gestational age
❏ Sepsis neonatorum and infectious disorders
❏ Overview of isolation precautions (appendix K)

Additional nursing diagnoses

❏ Altered nutrition: less than body requirements related to immunosuppression and infectious processes
❏ Anticipatory grieving (parental) related to potential loss of infant
❏ Anxiety (parental) related to interpersonal disease transmission and contagion and threat of future death of infant

❏ Ineffective individual coping related to situational crisis, inadequate support system, or unrealistic perceptions
❏ Risk for altered parenting related to reaction to HIV diagnosis
❏ Risk for caregiver role strain related to impact of HIV diagnosis and care
❏ Risk for infection related to immunosuppression

Anemia

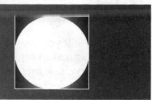

Definition

Anemia is characterized by a decreased number of erythrocytes and lower-than-normal hemoglobin (Hb) levels. At birth, the average red blood cell (RBC) count is 5,000,000/mm³. Levels fall to 3,000,000 to 4,000,000/mm³ during the next 8 weeks because new RBCs are not produced for replacement. Hb levels, normally between 16 and 20 g/dl (cord blood) at birth, fall to 10 to 11 g/dl during the next 8 weeks and between 7 to 9 g/dl in preterm infants. Physiologic anemia results from decreased Hb and RBC production, a 90-day survival rate for RBCs, increased blood volume, and hemodilution because of rapid growth. Preterm infants develop anemia earlier and with greater severity than full-term infants.

Blood volume at birth is normally about 90 ml/kg, with an average of 300 ml in a full-term infant. Optimal blood volume is transferred to the infant at birth if the cord is clamped 30 seconds after delivery and if the infant is placed below the level of the placenta to allow gravity to enhance blood transfer.

This plan focuses on care of the infant at risk for or with acute or chronic anemia.

Etiology and precipitating factors

• Hemolysis of RBCs in hemolytic disease (ABO and Rh erythroblastosis or other genetic conditions)
• Lag in hematopoiesis while growth occurs
• Defects in clotting mechanisms from vitamin K deficiency, causing deficiencies in coagulation factors
• Platelet abnormality from infections
• Iron deficiency from lack of iron intake and low iron stores
• Blood loss before, during, or after parturition, as from the following situations:
  – trauma, rupture, or tear of cord
  – incision into placenta during cesarean delivery
  – disorders such as placenta previa and abruptio placentae
  – clamping of cord too soon with infant above level of placenta
  – fetofetal bleeding (chronic transfer of blood from one twin to the other) or fetomaternal hemorrhage
  – trauma during labor, causing intracranial hemorrhage or hemorrhage into liver, spleen, or kidneys
  – trauma after cardiac massage
  – multiple blood sampling

Physical findings

Maternal history
• Rh isoimmunization
• Obstetric accident, traumatic delivery, tear in cord
• Cesarean delivery
• Iron deficiency, poor nutrition
• Poor prenatal care
• Intrauterine or I.V. transfusion

Infant status at birth
• Premature or small for gestational age
• Twin or multiple birth
• Low blood volume from cord being clamped too soon with infant above level of placenta
• Low Apgar score, cyanotic skin

Cardiovascular
• Tachycardia (more than 160 beats/minute)
• Feeble or absent pulses
• Hypotension (30 to 50 mm Hg systolic)

Gastrointestinal
• Palpable enlarged liver
• Upper abdominal distention
• Failure to gain weight and poor feeding

Integumentary
• Pallor of skin and mucous membranes
• Cyanosis despite oxygen therapy
• Petechiae or ecchymoses with thrombocytopenia

Neurologic
• Weak cry
• Diminished activity or flaccidity
• Listlessness
• Temperature instability

Pulmonary
• Tachypnea and dyspnea
• Gasping and retractions
• Episodes of apnea or bradycardia

Behavioral findings
• Irritability
• Lethargy

Diagnostic studies
• Complete blood count (CBC) — reveals decreases in RBC count, Hb level (less than 14 g/dl for term infant and less than 13 g/dl for preterm infant), and hematocrit (HCT; less than 45%); reveals mean corpuscular volume with smaller newly formed RBCs and mean corpuscular hemoglobin with RBCs less filled with Hb

• Reticulocyte levels — increase in response to decreases in RBCs (attempts to replace RBCs)
• Bilirubin levels — increase as RBCs are destroyed
• Iron levels — decrease to less than 100 µg/dl

• Blood type and Rh factor of mother and infant — may be incompatible
• Stools — may reveal frank or occult blood

COLLABORATIVE PROBLEM

Fluid imbalance related to blood loss before, during, or after birth (two expected outcomes)

Expected outcome 1

The infant who is anemic or at risk for anemia will be identified and cared for accordingly.

Interventions

1. Assess the risk for anemia, taking into account:

• indications in maternal history

• prematurity or possibility of twins

• Apgar score

• traumatic birth

• blood type and Rh factor

• bilirubin level

• RBC count, HCT, and Hb level and decreased iron and serum-bound iron levels.

2. Assess for signs of anemia from blood loss, including:
• pallor
• tachypnea (more than 60 breaths/minute)
• tachycardia (more than 160 beats/minute)
• arterial hypotension (less than 30 mm Hg).

3. Assess for signs of anemia that indicate hemorrhage, including:
• abdominal distention
• periumbilical ecchymoses
• shifting dullness
• apnea
• seizure activity.

4. Assess for signs of anemia from hemolysis, including:
• jaundice
• lethargy or diminished activity
• poor feeding
• increased bilirubin level and decreased RBC count.

Rationales

1. If the risk is established, steps can be taken to offset the life-threatening condition.
• The mother's condition may predispose the infant to anemia.
• Anemia is more severe and occurs earlier in preterm infants.
• Apgar score indicates adequacy of circulation and oxygenation.
• Trauma that causes hematoma results in blood loss into tissue.
• Incompatibility may result in hemolytic disease and destruction of RBCs.
• An increased bilirubin level reveals the amount of RBC destruction.
• An HCT less than 45% (normal value at birth is 45% to 65%), a venous blood level of Hb less than 13 g/dl, a capillary blood level less than 14.5 g/dl (normal level at birth is 16 to 20 g/dl cord blood), and a serum-bound iron level less than 100 µg/dl indicate anemia. Decreases that are greater than normally expected after birth may indicate anemia.

2. These signs indicate hemorrhage caused by accident or great blood loss with possible shock and a decrease in the oxygen-carrying capacity of the blood.

3. These signs may indicate internal hemorrhage from trauma during labor or bleeding into the central nervous system.

4. These signs indicate hemolysis of RBCs.

5. Assess for signs of anemia from iron deficiency, including:
- pallor
- irritability
- decreased Hb levels, HCT, and iron levels.

6. Assess for signs of anemia from a platelet disorder, including:
- petechiae
- ecchymoses.

7. Assess for signs of anemia from a clotting disorder, including:
- pallor
- lethargy
- bleeding from umbilical cord
- bloody or black stools
- hematuria
- decreased Hb level, HCT, and platelet count.

8. Additional individualized interventions: _____

5. These signs indicate iron deficiency anemia.

6. These signs indicate anemia from thrombocytopenia.

7. These signs indicate anemia from poor response to vitamin K or from low levels of clotting factors (usually factors I and V).

8. Rationales: _____

Expected outcome 2

The infant shows no signs of anemia or its complications.

Interventions

1. Record Hb level and HCT initially and every 4 hours, as ordered.

2. If Hb level and HCT decrease below 40% and 13 g/dl, respectively, notify the doctor; check CBC and reticulocyte values, as ordered.

3. Calculate or measure blood volume according to hospital protocol, and closely monitor the amount of blood drawn.

4. Administer warmed and humidified oxygen, as needed.

5. Maintain a thermoneutral environment.

6. Monitor arterial blood pressure and central venous pressure by means of an umbilical artery catheter (UAC); measure other vital signs continuously.

7. Prepare for transfusion of packed RBCs; if the infant is symptomatic, give cytomegalovirus(CMV)-negative whole blood.

Rationales

1. Monitoring Hb level and HCT reveals changes that indicate improving or deteriorating status. Decreasing values may signal blood loss.

2. Decreased values indicate that the infant may need iron or an exchange transfusion if RBCs are not being produced.

3. Monitoring blood volume allows quick detection of imbalances. Blood volume may be calculated by using an average volume of 90 ml/kg and estimating the loss based on decreases in Hb level and HCT after birth (methods vary).

4. This treats tachypnea and dyspnea and prevents hypoxia from a decreased oxygen-carrying capacity of blood.

5. A thermoneutral environment reduces the metabolic demands for additional oxygen.

6. Monitoring provides an ongoing assessment of the infant's condition and the effects of treatment.

7. Transfusion may be needed to relieve hypoxia by increasing the RBC count and Hb level (see the "Hyperbilirubinemia" plan, page 228, for transfusion procedure). CMV-negative blood assures that the infant will not become infected with CMV by transfusion.

Infant

8. Carry out gavage feedings by gastric tube.

9. Prepare and administer vitamin K I.M. or I.V. if the infant is actively bleeding after birth.

10. If the infant is full term, prepare and administer oral liquid iron daily as a supplement; provide iron-fortified formula or vitamins with iron as alternatives. If the infant is premature, administer vitamin E before giving the iron; give oral iron supplements if the preterm infant is also receiving erythropoietin.

11. Additional individualized interventions: _____

_____

8. If the infant is feeding poorly, gavage feedings provide nutrition. Oral feedings are not given with a UAC in place.

9. Vitamin K protects against prolonged prothrombin time.

10. These measures treat iron deficiency and prevent anemia based on the reticulocyte level. If the situation is acute and the infant is bleeding, it will need blood. If the patient is a growing preterm infant, the infant will need vitamin E plus iron if it is receiving erythropoietin. Vitamin E is one of the major dietary factors affecting RBC production. Because vitamin E increases with gestational age, the premature infant is predisposed to anemia due to insufficiency. Likewise, serum ferritin levels decrease rapidly with initiation of erythropoietin; the premature infant requires iron supplementation to offset this deficiency.

11. Rationales: _____

_____

Nursing diagnosis

Knowledge deficit (parental) related to need for transfusion or medication administration after discharge

Expected outcome

The infant's parents receive appropriate information about treatment and continuing drug therapy.

Interventions

1. Inform the parents about:
• infant's condition
• reason for transfusion
• screen of blood products and selection of donors, according to blood bank standards
• their opportunity to select a donor if the donor fits blood bank guidelines
• infant's improved condition after the transfusion.

2. Teach the parents how to administer oral iron supplements, including:
• how to measure the correct amount in a dropper, and administer it
• time of day to give iron
• how to store iron
• what the iron does and its possible adverse effects. Explain that treatment may continue for 3 months or longer to maintain a normal iron level.

3. Instruct the parents in appropriate nutritional sources of iron, such as iron-fortified formulas and cereals.

4. Encourage questions and clarify information as requested. Allow for a return demonstration of preparing and giving the medication.

Rationales

1. Information helps relieve the parents' fears that the transfused blood may transmit acquired immunodeficiency syndrome, hepatitis, or other diseases to the infant.

2. Thorough instruction promotes compliance.

3. Adequate nutrition provides sufficient calories plus additional sources of iron to combat a deficiency.

4. Explanations and demonstrations reinforce understanding.

5. Refer the parents and family for possible community and home health care follow-up.

5. Referral to community and home health care services helps to support the parents and ensure compliance with the medical regimen.

6. Additional individualized interventions: _____

6. Rationales: _____

Documentation checklist
During the hospital stay, document:
❒ patient status and assessment findings, especially fluid status (intake and output)
❒ changes in patient status
❒ pertinent laboratory and diagnostic findings, especially HCT, CBC, and Hb and reticulocyte values
❒ patient's response to treatment, especially transfusions
❒ family's reaction to the need for transfusions
❒ parent-infant interaction
❒ family teaching guidelines
❒ discharge planning guidelines.

Associated plans and appendices
❒ Hyperbilirubinemia
❒ Intracranial hemorrhage
❒ Preterm infant
❒ Normal laboratory values for the newborn (appendix I)

Additional nursing diagnoses
❒ Altered family coping (parental) related to possible life-threatening illness of infant
❒ Altered individual coping (parental) related to possible life-threatening illness of infant
❒ Altered peripheral tissue perfusion related to decreased oxygen-carrying capacity of blood
❒ Anxiety (parental) related to possible life-threatening illness of infant
❒ Fear (parental) related to transmission of disease to infant by way of transfusion or to belief that allowing transfusion will violate religious convictions

Bowel obstruction

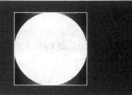

Definition

Bowel obstructions are congenital abnormalities of the GI system that occur in the intestinal tract. They may partially or completely obstruct the intestinal tract. Intestinal atresia of the duodenum, jejunum, or ileum is an interruption in the continuity of the bowel; it causes complete obstruction. Intestinal stenosis, which may affect any segment of the intestine, is a narrowing or constriction in the bowel; it causes an incomplete or partial obstruction. Single or multiple areas of stenosis or atresia may exist.

Another abnormality that causes obstruction is malrotation, in which the cecum fails to assume its correct anatomic position. The duodenum is pulled out of position, and duodenal bands maintain the abnormal position of the cecum. The loosely connected mesentery allows the small intestine to twist around it. This twisted loop of bowel (volvulus) causes obstruction and, possibly, strangulation of the superior mesenteric artery.

Such conditions as imperforate anus and strangulated inguinal hernia may also cause obstruction. Imperforate anus, an imperfect fusion of the anal area, may be a high or low type, depending on whether or not the rectum passes through the puborectalis muscle. It may be associated with a fistula leading to the vagina in girls or to the urethra in boys. In inguinal hernia, a portion of the intestine prolapses through the inguinal ring because of weakness or incomplete closure of the inguinal ring at 32 weeks' gestation or later. This prolapsed portion of the bowel may become incarcerated or strangulated, causing complete obstruction.

This plan focuses on the care of the infant who displays signs and symptoms of GI obstruction and on the prevention of complications before surgical intervention.

Etiology and precipitating factors

• Failure of the gut to recanalize in utero because of ischemic injury to the bowel below the duodenum or from abnormality in which the common bile duct and the pancreatic duct enter into the upper duodenum; either condition may cause atresia or stenosis

• Duplications of any length or segment of the GI tube, with or without continuity with the normal segment
• Functional obstructions caused by such conditions as achalasia, pyloric stenosis, megacolon, and meconium plug syndrome
• Incomplete closure of the inguinal ring, allowing the intestine to protrude through it

Physical findings

Maternal history
• Hydramnios or polyhydramnios
• Abnormal ultrasound results

Infant status at birth
• Usually appears normal at birth
• Closed anal area or only a small aperture, making the insertion of a rectal thermometer impossible; anal dimple possible (imperforate anus)

Gastrointestinal
• Bile-stained vomitus (early occurrence coincides with higher obstruction; later occurrence, with lower obstruction)
• Abdominal distention (intermittent with duodenal obstruction; persistent with jejunal or ileal obstructions and with imperforate anus or inguinal hernia strangulation)
• Diminished stools or failure to pass meconium
• Weight loss

Diagnostic studies

• X-ray studies of bowel and upper GI and small bowel series—may reveal pattern of double bubble from distended duodenum or dilated loops of bowel
• X-ray contrast studies of upper GI tract—may reveal malrotation; barium enema studies determine obstruction by inguinal hernia strangulation
• X-ray studies of infant in upside-down position—allows gas in colon to rise and outline blind rectal pouch and position in relation to anal opening (in imperforate anus)

COLLABORATIVE PROBLEM

Bowel obstruction related to congenital GI abnormality (two expected outcomes)

Expected outcome 1

The infant at risk for or with bowel obstruction is identified.

Interventions

1. Assess for signs and symptoms of partial or complete bowel obstruction, including:

• bile-stained vomitus (also noting amount of vomitus and time vomiting occurred)

• diminished or absent stools

• abdominal distention and tense abdomen

• abnormal results of upper and lower GI tract X-ray studies.

2. Assess for other congenital conditions, such as Down syndrome, herniation, and absence of an anus.

3. Additional individualized interventions: _____
_____

Rationales

1. Prompt recognition of GI abnormalities allows for immediate interventions to treat an acute condition and prevent complications.
• Greenish vomitus indicates bowel obstruction; earlier vomiting indicates that the obstruction is located higher in the GI tract.
• Diminished stools indicate partial or evolving obstruction; absent stools indicate complete obstruction.
• These signs indicate failure of the GI tract to rid itself of gas and secretions because of obstruction.
• Study results identify location and extent of obstruction.

2. These conditions commonly accompany GI anomalies.

3. Rationales: _____
_____

Expected outcome 2

The infant does not develop physical complications associated with bowel obstruction.

Interventions

1. Maintain fluid and electrolyte balance and caloric needs by:
• administering and monitoring I.V. solution (dextrose 10% in water administered at a rate calculated individually for the infant as ordered) with added electrolytes, if needed
• weighing the infant daily if its condition permits
• monitoring fluid intake and output hourly (with output including gastric drainage of at least 2 to 3 ml/kg/hour) and comparing output with I.V. intake.

2. Provide gastric decompression and monitor its effect by:
• measuring abdominal girth
• ensuring patency of gastric tubing by noting drainage and carefully aspirating it without exerting pressure
• noting vomiting
• auscultating bowel sounds.

3. Prevent pulmonary aspiration of vomitus by positioning the infant on its abdomen or side and administering oxygen if needed.

4. Maintain a neutral thermal environment by:

• monitoring the infant's axillary temperature every 2 hours
• placing the infant in an incubator or using a radiant warmer.

Rationales

1. Fluid and electrolyte balance and caloric needs must be maintained to prevent dehydration and hypoglycemia and their complications.

2. Gastric decompression prevents abdominal distention by removing contents.
• Increases in girth indicate distention.
• This action ensures properly functioning suction apparatus for decompression.
• Vomiting indicates ineffective decompression.
• Bowel sounds indicate that air and fluid are moving through the bowel.

3. Aspiration will compromise the infant's pulmonary system.

4. A neutral thermal environment prevents cold stress, which would further compromise the sick infant and increase its oxygen needs.
• Temperature readings reveal any decrease in body temperature.
• Thermoregulation can help maintain an optimal temperature (see the "Hypothermia and Hyperthermia" plan, page 247).

5. Prepare the infant for surgical intervention after a diagnosis has been made. Surgical removal or repair of the affected part corrects bowel obstruction (see the "Preoperative care" plan, page 284).

6. Additional individualized interventions: _____

5. Adequate physical and psychological preoperative preparation aids postoperative recovery.

6. Rationales: _____

Nursing diagnosis

Parental anxiety related to uncertain outcome of surgical intervention

Expected outcome

The parents express minimal anxiety through the crisis situation.

Interventions

1. Maintain a calm and accepting manner.

2. Encourage the parents to ask questions. Give honest and accurate answers or obtain information for them. For example, they may need to know that:
• small-bowel surgery involves resection and anastomosis of the intestinal segments
• malrotation involves releasing bands across the small bowel and releasing the cecum
• anal deformity involves removing the anal membrane; if the deformity is in a high position, a colostomy may be performed until the correction can be completed.
• inguinal hernia repair is needed if the mass cannot be reduced or the bowel becomes strangulated
• temporary gastrostomy may be performed or total parenteral nutrition administered after surgery.

3. Use pamphlets and drawings to reinforce and clarify information from the doctor about the surgical procedure, the prognosis, and postsurgical care.

4. Spend as much time as possible with the parents. Keep them informed of the infant's care and progress. Explain procedures and their rationales.

5. Additional individualized interventions: _____

Rationales

1. A calm, accepting manner allows the parents to feel comfortable expressing feelings and asking questions.

2. Encouragement promotes trust and decreases anxiety; information alleviates fear of the unknown.

3. Information may need to be repeated or reinforced because the parents may be too anxious to absorb it all at once; this action also provides for a better-informed consent before surgery.

4. These actions show your caring and supportive attitude.

5. Rationales: _____

NURSING DIAGNOSIS

Ineffective family coping: compromised related to emotional crisis of infant with a congenital defect and potential need for long-term care after surgery

Expected outcome

The parents are able to cope with parenting changes required to care for the sick infant needing surgery

Interventions

1. Help the parents appraise the crisis in terms of their needs and their infant's needs.

2. Involve the parents in care, as appropriate, encouraging as much contact with the infant as possible.

3. Help the parents express their feelings about loss of the "perfect child," the intensive care nursery, and changes in the infant's appearance if colostomy or gastrostomy must be performed as well as other feelings, such as their guilt during possible long-term treatment.

4. Reassure the parents of their ability to care for their infant after surgery.

5. Refer the parents to social services and community resources for additional help.

6. Additional individualized interventions: _____

Rationales

1. This will identify necessary changes and determine possible strategies to cope with the crisis.

2. Involving the parents encourages bonding with the infant.

3. By reassuring the parents that their feelings are normal, you show your acceptance of their concerns and fears.

4. Reassuring the parents creates self-confidence in their ability to care for their child.

5. Referral to other services ensures continuing support as the infant progresses and is ready to leave the hospital.

6. Rationales: _____

Documentation checklist

During the hospital stay, document:
❏ patient status and assessment findings, especially bowel sounds, feeding difficulties, abdominal distention, or family history of GI problems
❏ changes in patient status
❏ pertinent laboratory and diagnostic findings, especially pertinent X-ray studies and fluid and electrolyte levels
❏ patient's response to treatment
❏ family's reaction to the bowel obstruction
❏ parent-infant interaction
❏ family teaching guidelines
❏ discharge planning guidelines.

Associated plans
❏ Hypoglycemia
❏ Hypothermia and hyperthermia
❏ Postoperative care
❏ Preoperative care

Additional nursing diagnoses
❏ Altered family processes related to situational crisis
❏ Altered nutrition: less than body requirements related to feeding status and gastric decompression
❏ Fear (parental) related to possible loss of child as a result of surgery
❏ Knowledge deficit (parental) related to lack of exposure to information
❏ Pain related to abdominal distention or presence of gastric tubes
❏ Risk for altered body temperature related to extremes of age and weight, dehydration
❏ Risk for fluid volume deficit related to nutritional status and gastric decompression

Choanal atresia

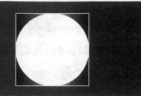

Definition

Choanal atresia is a congenital malformation of the respiratory tract in which the choanae (posterior nares opening into the nasopharynx) are obstructed by a membranous or bony structure covering the openings. One or both nares may be affected, with partial or complete obstruction.

Because the infant is an obligate nose breather, this malformation causes severe respiratory distress by preventing the inspiration of air.

This plan focuses on identifying the infant with choanal atresia and providing immediate care before surgical correction.

Etiology and precipitating factors
• Cause unknown

Physical findings
Infant status at birth
• Able to take first breath through mouth, with further attempts at breathing difficult or impossible
• Experiences severe retractions and cyanosis from air hunger when not crying; symptoms disappear when the infant cries because it can then breathe through the mouth
Integumentary
• Pink when crying, blue when not crying
Pulmonary
• Nose filled with thick mucus
• Catheter cannot be passed through the nose
• Suprasternal and substernal retractions
• Snorting respirations

Diagnostic studies
• X-ray of head or neck to determine abnormality

COLLABORATIVE PROBLEM

Ventilatory insufficiency related to obstruction from congenital defect

Expected outcome

The infant maintains airway patency and adequate respiratory efforts.

Interventions

1. Insert size 0 or 00 oral airway.

2. Perform endotracheal intubation if the oral airway cannot maintain a patent airway.

3. Assess respiratory efficiency, including:
• continued crying since delivery
• pink when crying and cyanotic when not crying
• accumulation of nasal secretions
• arching of head and neck when attempting to breathe
• retractions on inspiration.

4. Position the infant with the head of the bed elevated.

5. Prepare and assist with examination by otolaryngologist.

6. Prepare the infant for surgery to correct the defect.

Rationales

1. This immediate intervention allows for mouth breathing when the nares are obstructed.

2. Intubation accommodates breathing and prepares the infant for surgery.

3. Assessment allows differentiation of choanal atresia from other respiratory distress problems; the neonatal unit nurse may be the first to recognize choanal atresia in the infant.

4. Elevating the head of the bed improves air exchange in the infant.

5. In rare cases, examination may reveal that the obstruction is caused by a membrane only, which the otolaryngologist may puncture to allow breathing.

6. Surgery is necessary to achieve airway patency (see the "Preoperative care" plan, page 284).

7. Additional individualized interventions: _____

7. Rationales: _____

NURSING DIAGNOSIS

Ineffective family coping: compromised related to anxiety, guilt, and emotional conflict as a result of infant's defect

Expected outcome

The parents understand and adjust to their infant's condition and needs in the crisis situation.

Interventions

1. Allow and encourage the parents to express their feelings and fears about loss of the "perfect child."

2. Reinforce that in other ways the infant is normal and healthy and that surgery may correct the defect, leaving no visible effects.

3. Encourage the parents to hold and cuddle the infant and to give care as appropriate. Support their efforts to do so.

4. Provide accurate information about:
• condition of the infant and symptoms that must be watched for
• cause, prevalence, and nature of the defect
• equipment used and procedures performed on the infant
• rationales for care being given
• preparation for surgery and care after surgery, if anticipated.

5. Allow time for questions about and discussion of the prognosis and the infant's needs.

6. Additional individualized interventions: _____

Rationales

1. Expression of feelings helps promote trust and decrease the parents' anxiety.

2. Positive reinforcement helps reduce sadness and increase confidence in possible correction of the problem.

3. Involving parents in care promotes bonding and the development of the parent-child relationship.

4. Accurate information reduces the parents' anxiety and maximizes their understanding.

5. Open discussion reinforces information given and the parents' ability to cope with the crisis.

6. Rationales: _____

Documentation checklist

During the hospital stay, document:
❏ patient status and assessment findings, especially respiratory status
❏ changes in patient status
❏ pertinent laboratory and diagnostic findings, especially X-rays
❏ patient's response to treatment and surgery
❏ family's reaction to choanal atresia and surgery
❏ parent-infant interaction
❏ family teaching guidelines
❏ discharge planning guidelines.

Associated plans

❏ Postoperative care
❏ Preoperative care

Additional nursing diagnoses

❏ Altered nutrition: less than body requirements related to inability to ingest feedings while breathing through mouth
❏ Altered parenting related to interruption in bonding process
❏ Dysfunctional grieving (parental) related to loss of the "perfect child"
❏ Fear (parental) related to impending surgery and possible loss of child
❏ Knowledge deficit (parental) related to lack of information

Cleft lip and cleft palate

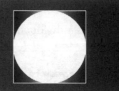

Definition

Cleft lip and cleft palate are the two most common forms of facial malformations. Cleft lip occurs in 1 of every 700 to 800 births and cleft palate, in 1 of every 2,500 births. Both malformations may accompany other birth defects, such as spina bifida, heart defects, extra fingers or toes, fusing together of fingers or toes, and talipes deformity. The abnormality may involve clefts of the lip and the palate, cleft of the lip only, cleft of the hard or soft palate only, or bilateral deformities.

Cleft lip with or without cleft palate — cosmetically the most distressing of the two abnormalities — develops when the maxillary prominence fails to fuse with the nasal elevations, causing failure of nostril and upper lip formation. Cleft lip develops during the 6th to 8th week of gestation and may be unilateral, involving only one nasal cavity, or bilateral, involving both. It may involve the lip only or extend to the nose.

Cleft palate occurs during formation of the fetal neck and jaws and develops when downward movement of the tongue is delayed, causing a failure of the palate to fuse above the tongue to form the roof of the mouth. Cleft palate develops during the 7th to 12th week of gestation and may be partial or complete. It may affect only the soft palate and uvula or extend to the hard palate. The malformation interferes with feeding and speech development.

Cleft lip with or without cleft palate is more common in boys; cleft palate is more common in girls. Treatment involves a team approach, including the nurse, pediatrician, orthodontist, speech therapist, plastic surgeon, and psychologist.

This plan focuses on care of the infant with one or both of these defects before surgical intervention. Surgical correction of cleft lip usually occurs from 6 weeks to 8 months after birth; sometimes it is performed immediately. Correction of cleft palate occurs between ages 1 and 2; the time of correction depends on the infant's condition, parental acceptance, and the surgeon's preference.

Etiology and precipitating factors

• Actual cause unknown; believed to be the result of inherited factors, mutant genes, or chromosomal abnormalities

• Environmental factors may include medications or teratogens ingested during a critical period of pregnancy or maternal exposure to radiation or infection

Physical findings

Family history

• Family member or relative with cleft lip or cleft palate

Infant status at birth

• Visible unilateral or bilateral cleft lip
• Mouth examination reveals visible cleft palate involving soft or hard palate with opening between the mouth and the nasal cavity

Gastrointestinal

• Difficulty sucking (with cleft lip and cleft palate)

NURSING DIAGNOSIS

Altered nutrition: less than body requirements related to inability to ingest food because of difficulty sucking (two expected outcomes)

Expected outcome 1

The infant experiencing early signs of inadequate nutrition will be recognized.

Interventions

1. Assess nutritional status and needs, including:

- sucking or swallowing ability

- daily caloric and fluid intake

- daily weight gain or loss.

2. Additional individualized interventions: _____
_____

Rationales

1. The infant's appetite is not affected by the defect, but the ability to suck properly is impaired, so intake may be reduced.
- The infant may be unable to form an adequate seal for sucking.
- Documented daily intake helps determine whether the infant is meeting nutritional needs or whether the feeding method needs to be changed, possibly to gastric gavage.
- Monitoring weight daily evaluates the success of the feeding pattern and reveals the optimal weight gain desired or the need for a change in feeding method to minimize weight loss.

2. Rationales: _____

Expected outcome 2

The patient exhibits good nutritional status.

Interventions

1. Based on assessment, calculate the minimum number of calories per kilogram per day and the number of milliliters per kilogram per day of feeding needed.

2. To help the breast-feeding mother, teach her to:

- massage her breasts and nipples before nursing

- apply pressure to the areola with her fingers, guide the nipple to side of the infant's mouth, and hold it there during feeding
- allow extra feeding time
- burp the infant frequently during feeding
- hold the infant in an upright or a sitting position while feeding

- pump her breasts and feed the infant with a bottle if the infant cannot breast-feed.

Rationales

1. This indicates the infant's nutritional requirements (see appendix G, Fluid and nutritional needs in infancy).

2. The infant with cleft palate may or may not be able to breast-feed; the infant with cleft lip may be able to breast-feed if the cleft doesn't affect sucking.
- Massaging breasts and nipples brings milk near the surface for ease in sucking and hardens breasts, helping the infant to hold the nipple in its mouth.
- Holding the nipple in the infant's mouth allows the infant to nurse with its gums rather than by sucking, if sucking is difficult.
- Feeding may take up to 1½ hours.
- The infant swallows more air during feedings.
- Holding the infant in an upright or a sitting position enhances swallowing and prevents milk from coming through the defect and out of the nose, thus decreasing the risk of aspiration.
- Pumping breast milk satisfies the mother's desire to breast-feed and provides an excellent source of nourishment.

Special feeding devices

Various devices, shown below, may be used to feed an infant with cleft lip or cleft palate.

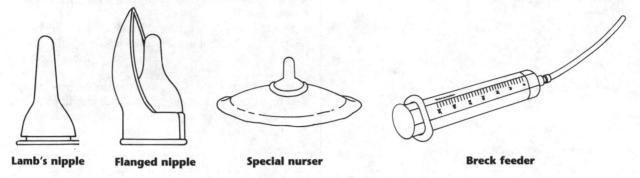

Lamb's nipple   **Flanged nipple**   **Special nurser**   **Breck feeder**

3. To help the bottle-feeding mother, teach her to:

• hold the infant in an upright or a near-sitting position during feeding

• select an appropriate nipple, such as one with a flange, a Lamb's nipple (big and soft with large holes), or a regular preterm nipple with a large hole, or use a Breck feeder (rubber-tipped Asepto syringe) or soft plastic bottle to squeeze formula into the infant's mouth (See *Special feeding devices.*)
• place the nipple at the side or back of the infant's tongue
• thicken milk with small amount of cereal

• feed the infant small amounts slowly, and burp the infant after each 10 to 15 ml of milk

• refrain from removing the nipple from the infant's mouth unless necessary
• give the infant some water after feeding
• gently wipe milk away from the infant's face and nose with a damp cloth and pat dry.

4. Additional individualized interventions: _____

3. Safe bottle-feeding maintains the infant's nutritional status.
• Holding the infant in an upright or a near-sitting position reduces the risk of aspiration and of swallowing air.
• The mother may have to experiment to find the nipple or device that is most suitable for the infant, depending on the defect.

• Placing the nipple at the side or back of the infant's tongue avoids the cleft and enhances swallowing.
• Thicker milk allows for easier swallowing because of increased gravity flow.
• Feeding slowly and burping regularly prevent regurgitation or vomiting by expelling the air the infant swallows during feeding.
• Removing the nipple may cause the infant to cry, making feeding more difficult.
• Water rinses milk away from the mouth and defect.
• Wiping removes milk that may have entered and drained from the nose.

4. Rationales: _____

NURSING DIAGNOSIS

Ineffective airway clearance related to possible aspiration of secretions or milk as a result of defect

Expected outcome

The infant maintains a clear airway.

Interventions

1. Assess the infant's respiratory status, noting:
- rate, depth, and effort
- dyspnea and cyanosis
- nasal flaring and chest retractions
- breath sounds
- skin color
- capillary refill.

2. Observe for abdominal distention.

3. Carefully suction the oropharynx and nasopharynx when needed.

4. Position the infant in an infant seat at a 30- to 45-degree angle.

5. Feed the infant in an upright position, and elevate the head of the crib 30 degrees after feedings.

6. Additional individualized interventions: _____

Rationales

1. Assessment provides data about respiratory status and function. Aspirating secretions or milk can cause tachypnea, abnormal breath sounds, bluish skin, or delayed capillary filling from decreased oxygenation.

2. Distention, resulting from swallowed air, compromises respirations.

3. Suctioning removes excess liquids and secretions in the hypopharynx.

4. Such positioning prevents the infant's tongue from falling back and obstructing the airway.

5. This position prevents aspiration of milk.

6. Rationales: _____

NURSING DIAGNOSIS

Altered oral mucous membrane related to defect and retention of formula in oral cavity

Expected outcome

The infant maintains good tissue integrity and intact oral mucus membranes.

Interventions

1. Assess for impairment by observing:
- reddened, tender areas on the lip or palate
- formula in the oral cavity or crust formation.

2. Clean cleft lip with a little water or half-normal saline solution and hydrogen peroxide after each feeding.

3. Apply a little cream or baby oil to the infant's lips.

4. Report persistent irritation for further treatment.

5. Additional individualized interventions: _____

Rationales

1. Impairment may cause irritation or inflammation of mucous membrane.

2. Cleaning rinses away milk after feeding. Hydrogen peroxide solution has bactericidal cleaning action.

3. Cream or oil prevents drying and cracking.

4. Persistent irritation may lead to infection if the mucosa breaks down.

5. Rationales: _____

NURSING DIAGNOSIS

Ineffective family coping: compromised related to anxiety, guilt, or emotional conflict as a result of infant's defect (two expected outcomes)

Expected outcome 1

The parents develop a trusting relationship with the caregivers and begin the adaptation process.

Interventions

1. Encourage and allow parental expression of feelings and fears about caring for the infant, what others might say, or loss of the "perfect child."

2. Allow the parents to see and hold the infant as soon after birth as possible, after the obstetrician has informed them of the defect.

3. Allow the parents to grieve the loss of the "perfect child."

4. Reinforce that the infant is in other ways normal and healthy.

5. Handle the infant in a caring manner, and encourage the parents to hold and cuddle the infant.

6. Allow for open visitation with the infant when desired, encouraging the parents' active role in giving care.

7. Encourage participation in a support group for parents of infants with congenital defects.

8. Additional individualized interventions: _____

Rationales

1. Society places great importance on physical appearance; impairment causes parental shock, guilt, and disappointment.

2. Delay in seeing the infant may heighten the parents' anxiety and sadness.

3. Grieving may help the parents accept the child with a defect.

4. Reinforcement helps reduce the parents' sadness and anger and helps them begin adapting to the crisis.

5. Such handling promotes bonding and the infant's normal social and emotional development.

6. Visits promote a flexible, secure environment for development of the parent-child relationship.

7. Such groups offer support and a positive view of the treatment outcome.

8. Rationales: _____

Expected outcome 2

The parents express their understanding of the infant's defect.

Interventions

1. Assess the parents' understanding of cleft lip and cleft palate.

2. Assure the parents in a calm, positive way that the defect can be repaired with surgery.

3. Provide information about:
• the infant's condition, its causes and prevalence, and the nature of the defect
• the infant's short-term needs, such as feeding
• the infant's long-term problems, such as impaired speech, dental problems, upper respiratory tract and ear infections, and possible need for surgery.

4. Allow the parents to ask as many questions as they want.

Rationales

1. Assessment reveals how much and what kind of information the parents need and what misinformation they may have.

2. This reassures the parents that the defect can be corrected and helps them in the grieving process.

3. Information increases the parents' understanding of the defect.
• Explaining the infant's condition helps resolve the parents' guilt feelings.
• This reduces anxiety about the most difficult problem in caring for the infant.
• This prepares the parents for long-term health needs. The palate is essential to speech formation, and changes in structure — even after surgery — may permanently affect speech. Mouth breathing may cause changes in the shape of the mouth and dental problems, with the need to straighten teeth and correct the shape of jaw. Middle ear infections from failure of the eustachian tube to drain may contribute to hearing loss. Upper respiratory tract infections are common. Depending on the deformity, the child may need subsequent surgeries for further correction.

4. The more questions the parents ask, the better able they will be to adapt.

5. Additional individualized interventions: _____

5. Rationales: _____

NURSING DIAGNOSIS

Knowledge deficit (parental) related to feeding of the infant and surgical procedure to correct defect

Expected outcome

The parents receive appropriate information about feeding and defect repair and express their understanding of the material.

Interventions

1. Inform the parents of the general timing of surgical repair and what to expect from the infant. Show them photographs of infants before and after surgical repair.

2. Instruct the parents in breast-feeding or bottle-feeding techniques, as appropriate.

3. Before surgery, teach the parents what care techniques they will need to use, including:
• feeding the infant without a nipple (with a syringe with 1″ to 2″ [2.5 to 5 cm] of latex tubing attached to a Breck feeder, for instance), unless specifically ordered to use a nipple by the plastic surgeon
• using restraints, such as jackets with pockets for tongue-depressor splints or a commercially available restraining device, to hold the infant's arms straight and away from its mouth until the suture line heals.
• periodically positioning the infant on its back (using an infant seat) so that the infant can be closely observed for excessive secretions.

4. Instruct the parents in postoperative care measures, including:
• incision care
• dietary modifications

• trying to prevent the infant from sucking and blowing

• not inserting silverware or straws into the infant's mouth
• rinsing the oral cavity with sterile water after feeding.

Rationales

1. If the infant's weight is optimal and it has no other neonatal anomalies, it may undergo surgery to repair a cleft lip shortly after birth; this can minimize the parents' shame or embarrassment. Surgery may also take place in 2 to 3 months or as late as 8 months to allow for bonding and to rule out other congenital anomalies. Cleft palate may be repaired in two steps by 12 to 16 months; or repair of the soft palate may proceed in 6 to 18 months and repair of the hard palate, as late as age 5. Timing of the procedures is related to normal growth changes, and repair usually takes place before speech development.

2. Proper feeding technique helps maintain the infant's nutritional status without complications.

3. Introducing new care techniques a few days before surgery helps the infant adapt to restrictions.
• Teaching the parents how to feed the infant by non-nipple devices prevents injury to the surgical site.

• Restrictive positioning prevents disturbance of the suture line.

• The back position is the position of choice to maintain respiratory function after surgery.

4. Providing information helps dispel the parents' anxiety and promotes compliance.
• Cleaning the incision helps the suture line heal.
• Dietary modifications help meet the infant's nutritional needs while maintaining integrity of the suture line.
• Sucking and blowing put stress on the suture line.

• Inserting objects into the mouth could traumatize the suture line.
• Rinsing the oral cavity removes residual food or fluids, which are possible sources of irritation and infection.

5. Refer the parents to community and home health care resources.

6. Use pamphlets to illustrate the procedure, suture lines, fading scar, and appliance used (Logan bow).

7. Additional individualized interventions: _____

5. Referrals help the parents and family with continued physical and emotional support outside the hospital.

6. Illustrations show what to expect and possible outcomes.

7. Rationales: _____

Documentation checklist

During the hospital stay, document:

❑ patient status and assessment findings, especially nutritional status, weight, intake and output, respiratory status, and status of oral cavity and mucous membranes
❑ changes in patient status
❑ pertinent laboratory and diagnostic findings
❑ patient's response to treatment
❑ patient's ability to bottle-feed or breast-feed
❑ family's reaction to cleft lip or cleft palate
❑ parent-infant interaction
❑ family teaching guidelines, especially for feeding techniques
❑ discharge planning guidelines.

Associated plans and appendices

❑ Postoperative care
❑ Preoperative care
❑ Fluid and nutritional needs in infancy (appendix G)
❑ Parent teaching guides (appendix J)

Additional nursing diagnoses

❑ Altered home maintenance related to care of infant with defect
❑ Dysfunctional grieving (parental) related to loss of the perfect child
❑ Ineffective infant feeding pattern related to physical defect
❑ Risk for altered parenting related to crisis of having infant with defect or interruption in parental bonding process
❑ Risk for infection related to trauma to oral mucosa as result of improper feeding technique

Congenital heart disease

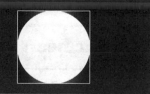

Definition

Congenital heart disease (cardiovascular malformation at birth) is found in 8 to 10 of every 1,000 neonates. About one-third of these infants also have noncardiac anomalies. In infants who weigh less than 5 lb, 8 oz (2,500 g) at birth, the incidence of congenital heart disease runs as high as 16%.

The cardiac defects most commonly identified during the first weeks of an infant's life are transposition of the great arteries, hypoplastic left heart syndrome, tetralogy of Fallot, pulmonary atresia, patent ductus arteriosus (PDA), coarctation of the aorta, ventricular septal defect (VSD), and combined defects. Noncardiac anomalies associated with cardiac defects include chromosomal syndromes, such as trisomy 13, 18, or 21; Turner's, Hunter's, DiGeorge's, Marfan's, Williams, or Laurence-Moon-Biedl syndrome; abnormalities of the skeleton, skin, muscles, GI tract, or renal system; and visceral malformations and malpositions.

Heart defects are classified as cyanotic (high-risk infant) and acyanotic (low-risk infant). Cyanotic defects interfere with or shunt pulmonary blood flow, resulting in desaturation of hemoglobin because insufficient blood moves through the lungs to oxygenate the hemoglobin. This, rather than a lack of circulation to peripheral tissue, causes the infant's blue appearance. (For descriptions, see *Cyanotic heart defects,* page 186.)

More common than cyanotic defects, acyanotic defects allow oxygenated blood to flow through the body with no cyanosis because shunting either does not occur or occurs from a high-pressured left side to a low-pressured right side. When using this classification, keep in mind that lesions that may potentially cause cyanosis do not always do so. Acyanotic defects may cause no signs and symptoms if the defect is small and the heart can compensate for the increased workload. More severe defects may cause cyanosis if pulmonary vascular changes take place or if the infant has secondary defects. (For descriptions, see *Acyanotic heart defects,* page 187.)

Cyanosis that occurs during the first hours or days of life usually results from transposition of the great arteries, tricuspid atresia, tetralogy of Fallot, truncus arteriosus, heart failure that results from hypoplastic left heart syndrome, severe coarctation of the aorta, interrupted aortic arch, severe aortic stenosis, or a combination of shunt lesions.

This plan focuses on care of the infant with congenital heart disease and clinical manifestations specific to the particular defect before surgical correction or palliative intervention.

Etiology and precipitating factors

• Thought to result from multifactorial inheritance, which is a combination of genetic, environmental, and intrauterine factors, accounting for the higher risk among infants who have a parent or sibling with a congenital heart defect
• Associated with maternal diseases, such as rubella during the first 8 weeks of pregnancy, diabetes mellitus, and alcoholism
• Associated with the use of such drugs as hydantoin, alcohol, and trimethadione during pregnancy

Physical findings
Maternal history
• High-altitude birth
• Congenital heart disease or previous child with congenital heart defect
• Drug use during pregnancy
Infant status at birth
• Preterm or full-term, low birth weight, or small for gestational age
• Visible anomaly or deformity
• Cyanosis
• Heart murmur
• Possibly asymptomatic at birth

Behavioral findings
• Irritability
• Agitation
  (For assessment findings, see *Cyanotic heart defects*, page 186, and *Acyanotic heart defects,* page 187.)

Diagnostic studies
• Chest X-ray to reveal small ventricle
• ECG to detect abnormal changes
• Cardiac catheterization to determine abnormal communication between chambers, obstructions in vessels, chamber pressures, and oxygen saturation
• Doppler flow in color to evaluate ductus
• M-mode echocardiography to determine anatomy and function of the circulation, including valve motion, great vessel size and location, location and size of chambers, and left ventricle function
• Contrast echocardiography to determine location of right-to-left shunting in the heart

(Text continues on page 188.)

Cyanotic heart defects

The chart below describes the major cyanotic heart defects and associated assessment findings.

Defect	Description	Assessment findings
Tetralogy of Fallot	• Defect is a combination of four defects: ventricular septal defect (VSD), overriding aorta, pulmonic stenosis, and right ventricular hypertrophy. The heart is boot-shaped. • Unoxygenated blood shunts through VSD, mixing with oxygenated blood in left ventricle. Cyanosis results. • Pulmonary blood flow is restricted by pulmonic stenosis, causing increased pressure in and hypertrophy of right ventricle as it attempts to shunt blood through restricted pulmonary valve.	*If severe:* • Cyanosis with hypoxic spells (increases after PDA closes) • Murmur associated with blood flow through pulmonary valve • Aortic ejection click with larger aorta • Dyspnea on exertion • Limpness or seizures *Later:* • Dyspnea • Clubbing of fingers and toes • Tachypnea • Fatigue • Squatting position (to relieve respiratory distress) • Growth retardation • Systolic murmur • Single second heart sound on auscultation • Thrill palpated in left lower region of sternal border
Truncus arteriosus	• Single vessel overriding ventricles (caused by failure of aorta and pulmonary artery to separate) carries blood for pulmonary and systemic circulation. Vessel can be above or below diaphragm; position has implications for prognosis. • Both ventricles pump oxygenated and unoxygenated blood into common artery, causing cyanosis. • VSD also may occur.	• Cyanosis with ashen appearance • Fatigue • Dyspnea *Later:* • Systolic murmur at left lower sternal border • Single second heart sound • Tachypnea • Crackles • Growth retardation • Heart failure
Tricuspid atresia	• Tricuspid valve is absent. • Blood flow is diverted from right atrium to left atrium, resulting in mixing of arterial and venous blood in left ventricle. Entry of mixed blood into circulation causes cyanosis. • Pulmonary blood flows through patent ductus arteriosus (PDA), if present.	• Cyanosis • Dyspnea • Anoxic spells • Fatigue • Single first and second heart sounds • Absence of murmur • Pansystolic murmur with VSD • Heart failure
Transposition of the great arteries	• Aorta leaves right ventricle; pulmonary artery leaves left ventricle. • Systemic circulation bypasses lungs for oxygenation; pulmonary blood flows through heart and back to lungs without entering systemic circulation. • Condition previously referred to as transposition of the great vessels.	• Cyanosis, especially during or after feeding or crying • Tachypnea • Systolic murmur or heart failure with VSD • Metabolic acidosis from hypoxia • Abnormal heart sounds, depending on type of defect
Hypoplastic left heart syndrome	• Left ventricle is nonfunctional. • Pulmonary blood returns to left atrium through atrial septum to right atrium. Systemic output, carried by right-to-left flow of blood through PDA, is restricted by normal PDA closure after birth.	• Marked cyanosis • Respiratory distress with grunting • Worsening of symptoms as PDA narrows • Heart failure • Death within 1 week unless wide-open PDA and atrial septal defect are present

Acyanotic heart defects

The chart below describes the major acyanotic heart defects and associated assessment findings.

Defect	Description	Assessment findings
Ventricular septal defect	• Ventricular septum has abnormal opening. • Oxygenated blood from left ventricle shunts through abnormal opening and then mixes with unoxygenated blood in right atrium.	*If small:* • Murmur *If large:* • Tachypnea • Irritability • Tachycardia • Difficulty feeding • Slight cyanosis from heart failure • Dyspnea with feeding • Growth retardation
Atrial septal defect	• Atrial septum has abnormal opening (caused by improper closure of foramen ovale or atrial septal wall). • Blood passes from left atrium to right atrium through abnormal opening. • Defect occurs in three types: ostium secundum, ostium primum, and sinus venosus.	• May be asymptomatic • Dyspnea on exertion • Fatigue • Orthopnea • Transient cyanosis *Later:* • Soft, pulmonic midsystolic murmur • Growth retardation
Patent ductus arteriosus	• Defect represents failure of vascular conduit between descending aorta and pulmonary artery to close after birth. • Blood shunts from aorta to pulmonary artery.	• Continuous murmur at second and third left intercostal spaces • Widening pulse pressure • Tachycardia • Difficulty feeding • Fatigue • Weak cry *Later:* • Dyspnea
Coarctation of the aorta	• Aorta is narrowed. • Defect may be preductal (in front of area of ductus arteriosus) or postductal (behind area of ductus arteriosus).	• Increased blood pressure and bounding pulse proximal to defect • Decreased blood pressure and weak pulse distal to defect • Dizziness • Headache • Fainting • Epistaxis • Discoloration of legs • Cold feet *If severe:* • Poor weight gain • Difficulty feeding • Heart failure • Possibly murmur at sternal border
Pulmonic stenosis	• Blood flow from right ventricle to lungs is obstructed. • Obstruction may be above or below pulmonic valve, or defect may occur as stenosis of valve. • Resistance to blood flow, (caused by stenosis) leads to right ventricular hypertrophy.	• Dyspnea • Fatigue • Cold arms and legs • Peripheral cyanosis • Systolic ejection murmur over second left intercostal space, accompanied by systolic thrill with murmur radiating over precordium and back • Less distinct second heart sound (may disappear)
Aortic stenosis	• Aortic valve is narrowed, causing obstruction of blood flow from left ventricle and persistent fetal circulation.	*If severe:* • Faint peripheral pulses • Tachycardia • Fatigue on exertion • Pale skin • Irritability • Syncope • Angina pectoris • Diaphoresis • Epistaxis

- Two-dimensional or real-time ultrasound echocardiography to reproduce intracavitary angiograms
- Hyperoxygenation test to rule out heart disease; partial pressure of oxygen must exceed 100
- Arterial blood gas (ABG) measurements to determine levels of pH, partial pressure of arterial carbon dioxide

($Paco_2$), partial pressure of arterial oxygen (Pao_2), and bicarbonate and changes resulting from cardiac or pulmonary disease
- Electrolyte analysis (of potassium, sodium, and chloride) to detect changes in heart failure

COLLABORATIVE PROBLEM

Risk for complications related to congenital heart disease (two expected outcomes)

Expected outcome 1

The infant at risk for a cardiac condition will demonstrate no signs or symptoms of complications related to the condition.

Interventions

1. Assess the risk for congenital heart disease by checking for the following factors:
- maternal history of congenital heart defects and such conditions as diabetes, rubella, and infections early in pregnancy; maternal history of drug use
- birth at high altitude
- presence of other congenital abnormalities.

2. Assess the infant at low risk for cardiac conditions, making sure to:
- review X-ray and echocardiography results
- identify murmur and note its location
- note difficulty feeding (lack of energy and pauses to rest)
- note pale or mottled skin
- observe for dyspnea
- note developing heart failure (if defect is severe).

3. Assess the infant at high risk for cardiac conditions, making sure to note:
- X-ray, ECG, echocardiography, cardiac catheterization, and hyperoxygenation test results
- generalized cyanosis
- respiratory distress and tachypnea
- skin mottling
- poor pulse rate and blood pressure changes
- hypotonia
- heart failure with weight gain and increased central venous pressure (CVP); cool, cyanotic arms and legs; periorbital edema; and hepatomegaly
- soft murmur with single second heart sound
- ABG measurements, with hypoxemia and, possibly, mild hypercapnia generally indicating primary heart disease.

4. Additional individualized interventions: _____

Rationales

1. Assessment provides information about possible defects, if the infant appears asymptomatic, or about the risk for developing congenital heart disease.

2. Of infants with congenital heart diseases, 30% to 40% have VSD. Less common, but important within the low-risk group, are atrial septal defect and PDA. Pulmonic and aortic stenoses and simple coarctation of the aorta usually are not symptomatic in the first months of life; signs and symptoms depend on the severity of the defect.

3. Presenting signs and symptoms of severe cardiac disease in the infant depend on the defects. Cyanosis results from intracardiac or intrapulmonary shunting of blood from right to left and indicates low arterial oxygen saturation. Respiratory distress results from pulmonary hypertension and congestion; tachypnea results from hypoxemia and acidosis. Heart failure may occur with either right- or left-sided heart failure in the infant with hepatosplenomegaly and in the infant with systemic venous congestion. Low cardiac output causes skin mottling, poor pulse rate, hypotonia even when the infant is asleep, and cyanosis because of increased oxygen extraction in peripheral tissues.

4. Rationales: _____

Expected outcome 2

The infant shows no signs of heart failure.

Interventions

1. Prepare and provide continued support for the infant undergoing cardiac tests and procedures.

2. Prepare and administer I.V. glycoside and diuretic as appropriate and prescribed, and accurately monitor fluid intake and output.

3. Continuously monitor the infant's heart rate and rhythm with an oscilloscope and ECG; discuss changes with the doctor.

4. Monitor CVP and maintain it at 3 to 8 cm H_2O, unless otherwise ordered.

5. Monitor arterial blood pressure; note changes and discuss them with the doctor.

6. Monitor ABG levels, and discuss changes in Pao_2 and $Paco_2$ levels with the doctor.

7. Administer oxygen by hood, nasal continuous positive airway pressure, or endotracheal tube.

8. Place the infant in semi-Fowler's position.

9. Maintain the infant's temperature at 98.6° F (37° C).

10. Prepare the infant for surgery if it needs an emergency procedure.

11. Additional individualized interventions: _____

Rationales

1. The caregiver's presence and continued physical support of cardiac status during diagnostic procedures decreases the potential for complications.

2. These drugs improve myocardial function and decrease fluid retention (see the "Heart failure" plan, page 221, for complete care of this complication).

3. Hemodynamic changes in CVP, pulse rate, and blood pressure and cardiac arrhythmias must be noted and reported as soon as they occur to prevent complications in severe cases and in infants who need surgery.

4. Evaluating CVP helps assess changes in fluid volume status. CVP monitoring is not a standard procedure because of the difficulty in obtaining reliable readings; it requires an umbilical venous catheter in addition to the umbilical artery catheter.

5. Blood pressure changes must be assessed for indications of heart failure.

6. Changes indicate the potential for hypoxemia and acidosis and determine whether the problem is cardiac or pulmonary.

7. Oxygen therapy may be necessary to relieve respiratory distress and improve ventilation and perfusion.

8. Semi-Fowler's position is more comfortable and promotes diaphragmatic movement and lung expansion.

9. Maintaining a neutral thermal environment prevents excessive oxygen consumption.

10. An infant with a life-threatening condition related to a heart defect may need immediate surgery (see the "Preoperative care" plan, page 284).

11. Rationales: _____

NURSING DIAGNOSIS

Altered nutrition: less than body requirements related to poor feeding as a result of lack of energy

Expected outcome

The infant exhibits signs of adequate nutrition.

Interventions

1. Use a soft nipple with larger holes.

2. Feed the infant for a short time in the upright position; pause, continue to feed, and then pause again for short periods.

3. Feed for 30 minutes; if the infant cannot finish, discontinue bottle feedings and initiate gavage feedings.

4. Additional individualized interventions: _____

Rationales

1. A soft nipple allows for increased flow and reduces the need for the infant to suck hard to feed (causing fatigue).

2. Shortened feeding periods allow the infant to rest between sucking and expending energy. Upright positioning promotes lung expansion.

3. Gavage feedings assure adequate nutrition for the infant whose long-term outcome may be growth retardation.

4. Rationales: _____

NURSING DIAGNOSIS

Risk for activity intolerance related to fatigue and dyspnea on exertion

Expected outcome

The infant is active and rests according to its limitations.

Interventions

1. Take measures to minimize the infant's energy expenditure:
• Do not handle the infant more than required.
• Do not wake the infant for feedings or care procedures.
• Anticipate the infant's needs to minimize crying.
• Allow rest periods during feeding and other essential care.
• Cluster care to disturb the infant as little as possible.

2. Additional individualized interventions: _____

Rationales

1. Energy expenditure affects cardiac output and increases the metabolic demand for oxygen.

2. Rationales: _____

NURSING DIAGNOSIS

Anticipatory grieving (parental) related to potential loss of infant

Expected outcome

The parents develop strategies to cope with their grief.

Interventions

1. Allow the parents to express their feelings, concerns, fears, anger, and guilt; allow for shock, denial, and feeling of loss of the "perfect child" envisioned during pregnancy.

Rationales

1. Expressing feelings helps the parents acknowledge shock, promotes the normal grieving process for the potential loss of the infant, and prepares the parents for long-term care and responsibilities.

2. Identify signs and symptoms of anticipatory grieving, including:
• feelings of sadness
• irritability
• crying or depression
• inability to eat or sleep
• constant thinking about the infant
• withdrawal.

3. Provide a quiet, accepting environment, using listening and touch techniques when appropriate.

4. Offer open visiting privileges, and allow the parents to participate in care, if feasible.

5. Provide information about the infant's condition, care, progress, and potential outcomes.

6. Provide support from clergy or others with similar problems, as acceptable to the parents.

7. Avoid judgmental attitudes when interacting with parents who are angry, critical, or sad.

8. Additional individualized interventions: _____
_____

2. These signs and symptoms indicate that the grief process is taking place.

3. A quiet, attentive atmosphere shows caring and fosters trust.

4. Open visitation promotes bonding and the infant-parent relationship and offers needed time with the infant.

5. This helps allay the parents' fear of the unknown and reinforces the hope for recovery.

6. Empathetic support helps the parents through the grieving process.

7. A nonjudgmental attitude assures the parents that their behaviors are normal.

8. Rationales: _____
_____

NURSING DIAGNOSIS

Knowledge deficit (parental) related to lack of information regarding the infant's condition, long-term care, and treatment

Expected outcome

The parents receive appropriate information to ensure safe short-term and long-term infant care and express an understanding of that information.

Interventions

1. Identify the parents' knowledge needs, interest in learning, and readiness and capability to learn.

2. Provide information regarding:
• infant's condition and progress
• possibility of immediate surgery
• possible surgery at a later date, depending on the defect and the infant's condition (noting that plans may change)
• infant's need for rest and sleep
• need to minimize the infant's fatigue and exertion, including directives to feed slowly and frequently with rest periods
• need to observe for cyanosis and dyspnea
• need to avoid exposing the infant to respiratory tract infections.

3. Impart accurate and complete information about the defect and what is and is not known about its cause.

Rationales

1. Learning assessment provides the basis for developing a teaching plan appropriate to the parents' abilities and needs.

2. Information makes the parents feel more secure in caring for the infant and reduces their anxiety about the infant's future. Long-term care may place the parents in a chronic crisis situation.

3. The parents may feel responsible for the infant's cardiac defect.

4. Teach the parents how to administer the glycoside and diuretic; make sure they know:
• name of the medication, how to measure it, and the amount to give
• how to add the drug to formula, which formula to purchase, and how to prepare the formula
• the importance of withholding the glycoside if the infant's heart rate drops below specified rate (usually 90 to 100 beats/minute)
• the importance of recording the infant's fluid input and output and weight daily
• the importance of reporting adverse effects, including nausea, vomiting, diarrhea, and dermatitis, and of stopping the drug if these effects occur.

5. Use visual aids and pamphlets to assist in teaching; write information in the parents' language.

6. Allow for questions and clarifications, including opportunities to prepare medications and to plan care.

7. Arrange for social services, community services, and home health care follow-up.

8. Additional individualized interventions: _____

4. Teaching promotes safe drug administration and prompt reporting of effects to the doctor.
• Knowing the drug name, dosage, and form is fundamental to safe administration.
• Infant medications should be given in liquid form.

• A decreased heart rate is a sign of drug toxicity.

• These actions help monitor the diuretic effect and fluid balance status.
• These are common responses to diuretic therapy, and the doctor should be made aware of them.

5. These teaching methods reinforce learning.

6. Repeating information may be necessary while parents are in crisis.

7. These referrals provide parents and family with continued support before and after discharge.

8. Rationales: _____

Documentation checklist
During the hospital stay, document:
❑ patient status and assessment findings, especially cardiorespiratory status, presence of murmurs (including quality, loudness, and location), presence and time of occurrence of cyanosis, and location and degree of edema
❑ changes in patient status
❑ pertinent laboratory and diagnostic findings, especially chest X-rays, echocardiography, ABG analysis, and electrolyte levels
❑ nutritional status
❑ activity tolerance
❑ patient's response to treatment or surgery or both
❑ family's reaction to diagnosis of congenital heart disease
❑ parent-infant interaction
❑ family teaching guidelines
❑ discharge planning guidelines.

Associated plans
❑ Heart failure
❑ Postoperative care
❑ Preoperative care
❑ Sexually transmitted diseases

Additional nursing diagnoses
❑ Altered peripheral tissue perfusion related to unoxygenated blood supply reaching arms and legs
❑ Decreased cardiac output related to malfunction of heart and impaired blood flow as result of defect
❑ Ineffective infant breathing pattern related to dyspnea or tachypnea as result of fluid accumulation in lungs
❑ Ineffective individual coping (parental) related to chronic situational crisis
❑ Ineffective infant feeding pattern related to lack of energy and fatigue
❑ Risk for altered parenting related to interruption in bonding process
❑ Risk for injury related to invasive diagnostic procedures

Developmental dysplasia of the hip

Definition

Developmental dysplasia of the hip (DDH, formerly called hip dysplasia) is a congenital malformation of the hip that can result in various degrees of deformity. DDH can result in the complete or partial displacement of the femoral head from the acetabulum (socket). These displacements are grouped into three types:

• *Preluxation,* the mildest form, does not involve actual dislocation but is a delay in acetabular development (oblique and shallow, with the femoral head remaining in the socket but susceptible to dislocation by manipulation).

• *Subluxation,* the most common form, is an incomplete dislocation. The femoral head remains in contact with the acetabulum, but a stretched capsule allows the femoral head to become partially displaced.

• In *dislocation,* the most severe form, the femoral head is not in contact with the acetabulum but becomes displaced backward and upward around the rim.

The incidence of congenital DDH is about 10 in 1,000 live births. About 60% of cases involve the left hip, 20% involve the right hip, and 20% involve both hips. The abnormality has a tendency to run in families and occurs more frequently in girls, firstborns, and those born by breech delivery. Early detection is vital for a successful outcome; the prognosis varies if the defect is not detected early on. This plan focuses on early identification and care of the neonate with DDH and on prevention of complications resulting from treatment.

Etiology and precipitating factors

• Actual cause unknown
• Possibly genetic association because of familial tendency
• Possibly result of fetal position in utero or breech birth
• Possibly result of pelvic laxity caused by maternal hormones secreted late in pregnancy to prepare for labor

Physical findings

Maternal and family history

• Other members of family with DDH

Infant status at birth

• Infant's presentation at delivery (DDH more common in breech births)
• Other congenital abnormalities, such as renal and other musculoskeletal anomalies
• Hip joint laxity in one or both hips

Musculoskeletal

• Failure to extend legs in breech presentation; possibly joint abscess if pain is present
• Ortolani's sign with reduction of femur—a palpable, audible click can be felt and heard when the affected limb is abducted; the femoral head can be felt to slip forward into the socket on pressure from behind, indicating dislocation
• Barlow's sign, indicating an unstable hip—the femoral head can be felt to slip over the lip of the acetabulum on pressure from the front and to slip back into the acetabulum on release of pressure (Barlow's maneuver)
• Allis' sign, indicating a shortened limb on the affected side
• Restricted abduction of the affected hip; asymmetry of thighs and gluteal folds may be apparent at birth

Diagnostic studies

• X-ray (when examination discloses problem) may reveal femur out of acetabulum, although femur may slip in or out with maneuvering.
• Ultrasonography of hips helps determine abnormalities.

NURSING DIAGNOSIS

Risk for injury related to delayed care or failure to provide appropriate care (two expected outcomes)

Expected outcome 1

The infant with hip dislocation will be recognized.

Interventions

1. Assess for partial or complete dislocation, as follows.

• Inspect the infant for laxity in one or both hips and for restricted hip abduction.
• Perform Barlow's maneuver by placing the infant on its back with hips flexed to a right angle and knees flexed; then place your middle finger over the greater trochanter and your thumb over the inner thigh. Make sure the infant's knees are midabducted, and press the hips forward and backward. Listen and feel for Ortolani's sign—a palpable and audible click when the femur moves in or out of the acetabulum.
• Inspect for Allis' sign by placing the infant's feet flat on the bed, with its knees flexed, and noting whether one knee is lower than the other. Also inspect for asymmetry of thighs and gluteal folds.
• Inspect for a broadened perineum if the infant is a girl.

2. Additional individualized interventions: _____

Rationales

1. Early diagnosis and treatment (before age 2 months) are important; otherwise, the hip will develop an abnormal configuration because the femoral head fails to remain in the hip socket as growth and ossification occur.
• Laxity indicates possible dislocation.

• This maneuver identifies subluxation of the hip if the femoral head can be heard and felt slipping into the acetabulum on pressure from behind (Ortolani's sign) or if the femoral head slips back into place on pressure from the front (Barlow's sign).

• Shortening of the limb and asymmetry on the affected side indicate hip displacement.

• This sign is found in bilateral dislocation.

2. Rationales: _____

Expected outcome 2

The infant exhibits correct hip positioning.

Interventions

1. Apply a device for reduction of hip, as follows:

• Apply two or more cloth diapers to achieve abduction, pinning them snugly from front to back.
• Apply a Frejka pillow splint over the diapers, and secure it at the shoulders in a snug—not tight—position; cover this with plastic, and remove and reapply it at each diaper change.
• Apply a Pavlik harness (most commonly used type).
• Prepare for and assist with hip spica cast application, if indicated.

2. Care for the device or cast as follows.
• Apply a plastic or waterproof substance around the edges of the cast that are near the perineal area.
• Remove and wash protective materials daily.
• Report damage to the cast, such as cracks or breaks.

3. Additional individualized interventions: _____

Rationales

1. Various methods of hip reduction are used, depending on the severity of dislocation.
• Diapers help maintain the femoral head in the acetabulum and are used for borderline subluxation.
• The splint maintains the thighs in flexion, abduction, and external rotation; the plastic covering reduces soiling of splint appliances.

• The harness splints the legs while maintaining the thighs in position.
• A hip spica cast may be used to treat DDH when other methods of maintaining reduction fail.

2. Plastic prevents soiling or damage to the cast or device that may alter its effectiveness; regular washing keeps the cast or device clean; reporting damage ensures cast effectiveness by maintaining proper joint immobility.

3. Rationales: _____

Nursing diagnosis

Risk for impaired skin integrity related to pressure and irritation from reduction device or cast

Expected outcome

The infant exhibits good skin integrity.

Interventions	Rationales
1. Assess the infant's skin for the following: • cleanliness, wetness, or soiling from elimination (urinary and fecal) • redness, excoriation, abrasions, coolness, pallor, paresthesias, and pulselessness • pressure against the skin around cast edges (tightness) • neurovascular changes in the legs (nail beds and toes) every 2 to 4 hours.	**1.** Regular assessment promotes measures to prevent skin irritation and relieve pressure. Pressure may decrease circulation to tissues, leading to skin breakdown and, possibly, infection.
2. If the infant is in a cast, petal sharp cast edges and protect the edges with plastic.	**2.** This technique prevents the cast from rubbing on skin; the plastic shields the cast from moisture and soiling.
3. Apply foam rubber around the edges of the cast.	**3.** Foam rubber provides cushioning and reduces pressure and irritation from the cast.
4. Turn the infant in a cast or an appliance every 2 hours (every 4 hours during the night). Support with pillows.	**4.** Turning and support prevent prolonged pressure on one area and promote proper positioning.
5. Change diapers frequently.	**5.** Frequent diaper changing minimizes the risk of skin irritation and breakdown.
6. Additional individualized interventions: _____	**6.** Rationales: _____

Nursing diagnosis

Altered peripheral tissue perfusion related to constriction of cast or reduction device

Expected outcome

The infant maintains good peripheral circulation.

Interventions	Rationales
1. Assess for signs and symptoms of circulatory impairment, including: • tightness of the cast or apparatus • coolness and duskiness of toes (if in a cast).	**1.** Assessment promotes interventions to prevent complications. Changes in color and temperature of the arms and legs indicate impaired circulation.
2. Check neurovascular signs every 2 hours.	**2.** Checking neurovascular signs helps evaluate circulation to the arms and legs. Changes in signs may indicate compromised status, requiring prompt interven-
3. Additional individualized interventions: _____	**3.** Rationales: _____

NURSING DIAGNOSIS

Knowledge deficit (parental) related to deformity and care of infant

Expected outcome

The parents receive appropriate information about the infant's condition and care and express an understanding of that information.

Interventions

1. Identify what the parents' need to learn, their interest in learning, and their readiness and ability to learn.

2. Inform the parents that treatment may take some time and that they will need patience in caring for their infant.

3. Encourage the parents to fondle, hold, and cuddle the infant, regardless of the cast or appliance.

4. Provide information about:
• the infant's condition
• effects of early treatment
• how to apply the appliance (if used) and how to remove it for bathing and diaper changes
• cast care (if used)
• skin protection
• how to apply diapers if they are used as a splint (snug but not tight)
• how to feed the infant, keeping it in the supine position with its hips and legs supported on a pillow at the mother's side or, if the mother is breast-feeding, holding it like a football with its legs behind the mother
• how to obtain a car seat compatible with the appliance or cast
• importance of follow-up care.

5. Allow for questions, clarifications, and demonstration of care techniques.

6. Refer the parents to community and home health care.

7. Additional individualized interventions: _____

Rationales

1. This provides the basis for a teaching plan appropriate to the parents' needs and abilities.

2. Restrictive movement may make the infant irritable; it will need help to adjust.

3. Contact with parents promotes the infant's development and provides stimulation.

4. Providing information assures safe infant care and maintains correct hip positioning.

5. These measures reinforce learning and decrease anxiety.

6. Referrals provide continued support and instruction, promoting compliance with therapy and follow-up.

7. Rationales: _____

Documentation checklist

During the hospital stay, document:
❏ patient status and assessment findings, especially Ortolani's sign and Allis' sign (if present), results of Barlow's maneuver, family history of DDH, and peripheral perfusion if the patient is in traction or a cast
❏ changes in patient status

❏ pertinent laboratory and diagnostic findings, especially X-rays or ultrasound of hip
❏ patient's response to treatment
❏ family's reaction to diagnosis
❏ parent-infant interaction
❏ family teaching guidelines, especially for supportive devices to be used for hip stability
❏ discharge planning guidelines.

Associated plans and appendices
❏ Spinal cord defects and hydrocephalus
❏ Talipes deformity
❏ Parent teaching guides (appendix J)

Additional nursing diagnoses
❏ Altered growth and development related to physical disability and stimulation deficiencies
❏ Impaired physical mobility related to cast
❏ Ineffective family coping: compromised related to congenital defect
❏ Risk for altered parenting related to lack of knowledge, lack of support from significant other, and unrealistic expectations for infant
❏ Sleep pattern disturbance related to cast or reduction device

Drug addiction and withdrawal

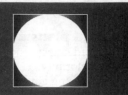

Definition

Mothers addicted to such drugs as heroin, morphine, methadone, and barbiturates deliver infants who are passively addicted to the same drug and who display withdrawal symptoms. Depending on the type and quality of the drug used, symptoms may appear as early as 12 to 24 hours after birth or as late as 2 to 4 weeks after birth. Symptoms may last for 6 to 8 weeks (hyperirritability, 3 to 4 months), with the most pronounced symptoms occurring between 48 and 72 hours after birth. Most symptoms appear in the first 24 hours of life.

Long-term effects on the infant suffering from drug withdrawal are not known. Concerns focus on the importance of safe care in the home after discharge by a mother who can function, who is dependable, and who is following a treatment program. Social services must provide supervision and home health care personnel must make home visits when an infant is discharged in the mother's care. If this is not possible, the infant must be placed in foster care until the parent or family achieves stability.

This plan focuses on care of the infant who displays signs and symptoms of drug withdrawal and on recognizing the potential for inappropriate care or neglect by the mother after discharge.

Etiology and precipitating factors

• Maternal addiction to drug (heroin, methadone, amphetamine, cocaine, or other substance)
• Maternal treatment for seizure condition with phenobarbital

Physical findings

Maternal history

• Drug addiction or dependence: name of drug used, time of last dose, length of time addicted, and route; names of drugs given intrapartally
• Inadequate or no prenatal care (note type and length)
• Prenatal conditions associated with pregnancy, such as placenta previa and hypertension
• Prenatal disorders, such as bacterial infection, toxoplasmosis, rubella, cytomegalovirus, herpes simplex, other sexually transmitted diseases, human immunodeficiency virus (HIV) seropositivity, and poor nutrition
• Participation in drug treatment or rehabilitation program
• Previous addiction to narcotics because effect on infant (growth deficiency) may extend beyond addiction

• Alcohol abuse
(*Note:* Because an addicted mother may be an unreliable information source, you may need to interview another family member to confirm history.)

Infant status at birth

• Low Apgar score, indicating possible asphyxia in utero
• Infant small for gestational age (SGA) if maternal nutrition is poor or if mother uses heroin, cocaine, or morphine
• Infant large for gestational age with maternal use of methadone
• Preterm birth
• Cardiovascular disorders
• Cleft lip or cleft palate

Gastrointestinal

• Low birth weight, with difficulty gaining weight or weight loss
• Poor feeding resulting from uncoordinated sucking and swallowing
• Vomiting or regurgitation after feeding caused by hyperactivity; overfeeding from constant need for sucking
• Abdominal cramps, diarrhea caused by GI hyperactivity

Integumentary

• Redness; abrasion marks on knees, elbows, or face caused by constant restlessness, kicking, and hyperactive movements associated with rubbing against sheets or clothing
• Jaundice with maternal use of methadone
• Slight to excessive sweating and flushed appearance
• Sudden circumoral pallor
• Excoriated buttocks
• Facial scratches

Neurologic

• Restlessness, hyperactivity from drug effect on central nervous system (CNS) functioning
• Hypertonicity, hyperactive reflexes, hyperreflexic arms and legs, kicking at times when mother would be due for drugs
• Seizures

Pulmonary

• Excessive mucus, stuffy nose, sneezing
• Tachypnea, chest retractions
• Periods of apnea

Cardiovascular

• Tachycardia

Behavioral findings
- Decreased sleep and lengthened awake periods
- Dislike for cuddling and close contact
- Frequent or prolonged sneezing or yawning
- High-pitched or weak cry, inconsolability
- Irritability

Diagnostic studies
- Toxicology screen identifies drug and drug levels in mother's and infant's blood and urine.
- Serum electrolyte levels detect losses from vomiting and diarrhea and determine other causes of neurologic symptoms or seizures, such as hypocalcemia.
- Serum glucose test determines decreases, if the cause of neurologic symptoms or seizures is hypoglycemia.
- Capillary blood gas (serial) studies identify changes in partial pressure of oxygen and pH, increased partial pressure of carbon dioxide from hypoxia, and metabolic acidosis as the need for oxygen increases during withdrawal because of irritability, crying, and tachypnea.
- Complete blood count (CBC) detects decreased white blood cell count, changes in ratio of immature to mature neutrophils, and decreased platelet count (with sepsis); decreased hematocrit, hemoglobin level, and red blood cell count indicate anemia (these abnormal measurements result from conditions acquired in utero or intrapartally).
- Blood culture identifies sepsis.
- HIV antigen test identifies HIV exposure (especially if the mother used I.V. drugs).

COLLABORATIVE PROBLEM

Neurologic and respiratory instability related to withdrawal from drug exposure (two expected outcomes)

Expected outcome 1

The infant withdraws from drug exposure with minimal distress.

Interventions

1. Assess for withdrawal symptoms, including:
- restlessness or wakefulness
- irritability; excessive yawning; high-pitched, shrill cry; hyperpyrexia
- hyperactivity, hypertonicity, poor coordination, tremors
- seizure activity or twitching
- vomiting or diarrhea.

2. Ask about maternal use of drugs during pregnancy (names, time, route, and amount of last intake) and review serum and urine toxicology screen for drug identity.

3. Provide calming techniques, including:

- holding, vertical rocking, and cuddling the infant; do not rock, talk to, and look at the infant at the same time

- touching, patting, smiling, and talking to the infant. Use an infant carrier for closeness.
- limiting or increasing contact, depending on response

- tightly swaddling the infant in the side-lying position and supporting its back with a small pillow

Rationales

1. About 90% of infants of addicted mothers display signs and symptoms of withdrawal as early as 12 hours after birth. Early recognition allows for early interventions and prevention of complications. Early signs of withdrawal include irritability and hyperactivity. Later manifestations of withdrawal include seizures and GI responses.

2. The severity of the drug's effect on the infant depends on the degree of abuse, time of last dose, and possible use of more than one drug. Because a history taken from the mother may be unreliable, more objective data are necessary to assess neonatal involvement.

3. Calming techniques help soothe the infant and reduce irritability and hyperactivity.
- Cuddling quiets and comforts the infant. Vertical rocking provides vestibular stimulation; providing too much stimulation together—such as the human face, which is very stimulating to an infant, combined with rocking—overwhelms the infant.
- These actions provide contact.

- Close contact may increase or decrease infant irritability.
- Positioning provides a restful environment to discourage hyperactivity and increase comfort while reducing stimuli.

• providing a dimly lighted, quiet environment for sleep
• clustering care between rest periods and limiting procedures whenever possible.

4. Prepare to give ordered medications for withdrawal symptoms and to evaluate their adverse effects.
• Paregoric may be given by mouth with formula or in water. The drug dosage is decreased over 2 to 4 weeks.

• Chlorpromazine (Thorazine) may be given by mouth with formula or I.M. in the vastus lateralis.

• In the unstable infant, phenobarbital may be given I.V. initially until oral drugs can be introduced.

• Phenytoin (Dilantin) may be given I.V. if phenobarbital fails to stop seizures; then give I.V. or by mouth for maintenance.
• Diazepam (Valium) may be given I.V., but it is not the drug of choice because it displaces bilirubin from its albumin binding sites.

5. Monitor serum glucose and calcium levels for decreases.

6. Additional individualized interventions: _____
_____

• A dimly lighted, quiet environment reduces external stimuli that may increase the infant's irritability.
• Clustering care allows for needed rest and reduces external stimuli.

4. Pharmacologic agents alleviate withdrawal symptoms.
• By increasing the smooth-muscle tone of the GI tract (which in turn decreases digestive secretions), paregoric decreases GI tract motility and peristalsis.
• Chlorpromazine controls vomiting, producing sedation by acting on the hypothalamus and reticular formation.
• Phenobarbital controls hyperactivity, irritability, and seizures. It acts to interfere with impulse transmission of the cerebral cortex by inhibiting the reticular activating system.
• Phenytoin acts to reduce the voltage, frequency, and speed of electrical discharges in the motor cortex.

• Diazepam is given if respiratory status is controlled and the infant is not preterm or jaundiced. It acts at limbic and subcortical levels of the CNS, with a shorter duration than chlorpromazine.

5. This can rule out hypoglycemia and hypocalcemia, which can cause symptoms similar to those of withdrawal, such as tremors, irritability, tachypnea, and seizures.

6. Rationales: _____
_____

Expected outcome 2

The infant does not experience injuries or complications.

Interventions

1. Assess the infant's respiratory status and airway clearance, noting the following:
• respiratory rate, depth, and effort; location and severity of chest contractions; and nasal flaring

• increased secretions, stuffy nose

• bluish tint to face, trunk, nail beds, arms, legs, and mucous membranes
• crackles heard on auscultation

• Apgar score or apneic periods; the infant may be placed on an apnea monitor or cardiopulmonary monitor.

Rationales

1. Assessment provides data related to respiratory function and airway patency.
• Respirations often are depressed with narcotic addiction. Tachypnea of 60 breaths/minute or more indicates distress. The normal respiratory rate for an infant ranges from 30 to 50 breaths/minute.
• Secretions cause respiratory difficulty because the infant can breathe only through its nose.
• Cyanosis is a sign of hypoxia and requires immediate attention.
• Auscultation allows for comparison of breath sounds to identify abnormalities.
• A low Apgar score at birth may indicate asphyxia and hypoxia. The cause of apnea must be established because sepsis, a birth-related respiratory condition, or preterm status may complicate withdrawal from drug addiction. Monitoring the infant at risk for severe respiratory distress allows for rapid detection of distress.

2. Carefully suction mucus from the infant's nose and mouth, as needed.

3. Position the infant with its head slightly elevated or use an infant seat.

4. Assess for signs of seizures, including:
• twitching movements (as opposed to tremors)
• uncoordinated movements of the mouth or tongue, such as thrusting tongue, sucking, or chewing
• muscle rigidity, with arching of back
• nystagmus, blinking, and staring.

5. Identify potential HIV seropositivity. Use standard precautions in caring for the infant. Carry out other protective procedures for the infant and personnel according to agency protocols or those recommended by the Centers for Disease Control and Prevention.

6. Additional individualized interventions: _____

2. Suctioning clears the nose and makes breathing easier, especially during feedings.

3. This position improves breathing by promoting lung expansion.

4. The infant undergoing withdrawal is at risk for seizures because of CNS involvement. Tonic seizures are more common in preterm infants; clonic seizures, in full-term infants. Carefully observing the infant for these signs allows for immediate treatment to prevent injury.

5. If the mother is an I.V. drug user, her infant is at risk for developing acquired immunodeficiency syndrome.

6. Rationales: _____

NURSING DIAGNOSIS

Altered nutrition: less than body requirements related to poor or low intake because of lack of coordination in sucking or swallowing and because of vomiting

Expected outcome

The infant develops improved nutritional status.

Interventions

1. Assess the infant's nutritional status and needs, including:
• gestational age and weight

• uncoordinated sucking and swallowing

• gag reflex in response to secretions

• vomiting, regurgitation, and diarrhea (compare output with intake if the infant is on oral feedings)

• daily intake (I.V., oral, or gastric gavage), including calorie count

• serum glucose review.

Rationales

1. The infant's nutrition in utero may reflect poor maternal nutrition.
• Infants of drug-addicted mothers often are SGA with low birth weight, or they may be preterm from poor nutrition during the prenatal period, causing the number of organ cells to be reduced.
• CNS stimulation causes hyperactivity, which leads to poor feeding.
• In preterm infants, the gag reflex may not be completely developed.
• CNS stimulation causes GI hypermotility and irritation, which may result in an inability to retain or absorb nutrients, a later manifestation of withdrawal.
• I.V. fluids should probably be given until the infant is stable because feeding an irritable infant at risk for seizures might foster aspiration. The infant may not tolerate full-strength feedings and may need to increase its strength gradually when fed orally or by gastric gavage.
• The serum glucose test identifies hypoglycemia caused by inadequate reserves or maternal malnutrition.

2. Provide appropriate nutrition as follows:

• If the infant is unstable, assure proper administration of the I.V. infusion and delay feedings.
• When the infant is stable, start feedings at half-strength, 10 ml every 3 hours.
• Check the residual after an oral feeding; if the residual is high, reduce the amount at the next feeding. Then, increase as tolerated to 5 to 10 ml hourly if hyperactivity is decreasing.
• Place the infant on its right side, supporting its back with a small pillow or towel, or place the infant on its abdomen after feedings, once they have been started.
• If the infant receives gastric gavage (intermittent or continuous):
– Insert the tube through the mouth and confirm placement.
– Administer the measured amount as ordered or by gravity or volumetric pump.

– Position the infant on its right side with the head slightly elevated for 1 hour or as tolerated.
– Evaluate the infant's tolerance of feedings and record any emesis.

– Evaluate residual feeding amount before next feeding. Hold feedings if the residual amount exceeds the infant's acceptable quantity.

3. Measure the infant's abdominal girth every 2 hours and compare with past measurements.

4. Weigh the infant daily and record its weight on a flow sheet for comparison; monitor fluid intake and output.

5. Provide a dimly lighted, quiet environment.

6. Provide a pacifier for sucking when the infant is not feeding.

7. Allow the mother to feed the infant, and help her offer food slowly and calmly while holding the infant.

8. Additional individualized interventions: _____

2. A full-term infant needs 100 to 200 calories/kg daily. An SGA infant needs more, based on age and projected daily weight gain.
• These actions avoid aggravating the GI problem if the infant cannot tolerate feedings.
• Smaller feedings improve nutritional intake if the GI tract can accept the feeding.
• This action prevents vomiting from overfeeding while still providing I.V. fluids according to the infant's tolerance.

• This action prevents vomiting or aspiration after feedings and may prevent accumulating residuals and distention.
• Gastric gavage is an alternate feeding route when the infant cannot tolerate oral feedings.
– The route is used because the infant breathes through its nose, which may be stuffy.
– Gravity administration permits slow instillation, minimizing gastric distention; use of a volumetric pump allows the feeding to be given at a controlled rate over a specified time, eliminating the risk of overfeeding.
– Positioning prevents vomiting or aspiration.

– Evaluating how the infant tolerates the feedings helps to determine if changes in feeding are required. Feedings are increased to provide calculated caloric needs; the in fant may vomit 1 to 2 ml.
– Residual feedings may indicate the infant's failure to digest or tolerate feedings and may lead to abdominal distention. With a 10-ml feeding, a residual of 2 ml or more after 3 hours is significant.

3. Widening girth indicates distention. This test may be done with oral feedings too.

4. Weighing reveals gains or losses and the need for feeding changes; monitoring fluid intake and output helps evaluate fluid balance.

5. A dimly lighted, quiet environment reduces external stimuli, which may increase hyperactivity and irritability, thus increasing caloric and metabolic needs.

6. A pacifier helps quiet the infant by satisfying its sucking need.

7. The mother's participation encourages the bonding process, giving support and confidence to the mother while preventing overfeeding.

8. Rationales: _____

NURSING DIAGNOSIS

Risk for fluid volume deficit related to diarrhea or vomiting

Expected outcome

The infant maintains fluid and electrolyte balance.

Interventions

1. Assess for signs of fluid or electrolyte imbalance; include the following:
• intake (oral and I.V.)
• urine output (weigh diapers: 1 g = 1 ml)

• fluid loss from phototherapy to treat jaundice or from a radiant warmer
• vomiting or diarrhea

• urine specific gravity

• dry skin and mucous membranes, sunken fontanels, weight loss
• abnormal serum electrolyte levels.
2. Monitor and evaluate administration of I.V. fluids.

3. Additional individualized interventions: _____

Rationales

1. Imbalances may occur from inadequate fluid or nutritional intake.
• Comparisons determine whether an imbalance exists.
• Normal urine output for a neonate is from 2 to 3 ml/kg hourly; the first voiding may occur as late as 24 hours after birth.
• Heat sources may promote fluid losses.

• Vomiting and diarrhea — later symptoms of withdrawal related to GI hypermotility — subject the infant to fluid loss as well as loss of such electrolytes as potassium and chloride.
• Normal specific gravity is 1.001 to 1.020, with increases being an indication of concentrated urine as a result of decreased output caused by fluid loss. Increases could indicate dehydration.
• Dryness indicates dehydration from fluid or electrolyte loss.
• GI fluid losses may cause hypokalemia.
2. Fluids and electrolytes are replaced by I.V. infusion with 10% to 20% increases based on severity of fluid loss
3. Rationales: _____

NURSING DIAGNOSIS

Risk for impaired skin integrity related to perianal irritation from diarrhea and rubbing against sheets because of hyperactivity

Expected outcome

The infant maintains good skin integrity

Interventions

1. Inspect the skin frequently for areas of redness or irritation.
2. Clean the perianal area gently, and apply soothing cream with each diaper change.
3. Pad the infant's knees and elbows, cover its hands with mittens, and place soft sheepskin under its face.

Rationales

1. Frequent inspection promotes early detection and prevention of skin breakdown.
2. Cleaning and applying cream prevent irritation and, possibly, skin breakdown from frequent diarrhea.
3. Padding prevents skin contact with linens and thus possible irritation; covering the hands with mittens prevents the infant from scratching the skin.

4. Provide the infant with a waterbed mattress.

5. Additional individualized interventions: _____

_____

4. A waterbed mattress reduces pressure on skin surfaces.

5. Rationales: _____

_____

Nursing diagnosis

Ineffective individual coping (maternal) related to drug abuse or inability to care for the infant

Expected outcome

The mother identifies coping skills, verbalizes the need to make changes in her lifestyle, and demonstrates appropriate parenting skills and an adequate support system.

Interventions

1. Assess the mother's mental state; include the following:

• individual and family stressors; use of coping mechanisms, both constructive and destructive; the mother's behavior and comments regarding the infant; and the mother's reaction and willingness to participate in the infant's treatment
• feelings of vulnerability

• mother's anxieties and fears regarding infant care and her need to participate in a drug rehabilitation program.

2. Help the mother identify coping skills she needs and available support systems: family, church groups, drug assistance groups such as Born Free, and parenting classes.

3. Assess the need for a protected environment, such as a halfway house, supportive follow-up at home with social service, home health care visits, foster home for the infant, or hospital-based boarder infant program. Make appropriate referrals.

4. Additional individualized interventions: _____

_____

Rationales

1. Assessment provides information about the mother's ability to care for the infant and to pursue drug rehabilitation.
• Assessment offers clues to potential problems leading to infant neglect.

• Assessment allows for expression of concerns and reveals the mother's ability to assume responsibility for the infant.
• Assessment allows the mother to understand her own needs to change her lifestyle.

2. This helps the mother determine her need for help with drug addiction and infant care.

3. Follow-up care offers support and help to the mother undergoing treatment and provides safe infant care.

4. Rationales: _____

_____

Nursing diagnosis

Knowledge deficit (parental) related to emotional inadequacy and lack of exposure to information about infant care

Expected outcome

The parents receive appropriate information about safe infant care and demonstrate their understanding of that information.

Interventions

1. Identify what the parents need to learn, their interest in learning, and their readiness and ability to learn.

2. Provide information about:
• the infant's condition, signs of infant withdrawal, and rationale for treatment

• the need for infant stimulation as well as rest periods, depending on responses

• how drugs can pass to the infant through breast-feeding if the mother is taking drugs; encourage bottle-feeding unless abstinence is assured
• physical care of the infant (feeding, bathing, clothing, and holding).

3. Have social services arrange for home care, if needed, and follow-up.

4. Advise the mother of the possibility of foster care for the infant while the mother receives drug treatment and rehabilitation.

5. Teach the parents how to give medication with feedings, including times, amounts, and adverse effects.

6. Additional individualized interventions: _____

Rationales

1. This provides the basis for developing a teaching plan appropriate to the parents' abilities and needs.

2. Parents need information to care for the infant safely.
• Understanding the infant's condition, signs of withdrawal, and reasons for treatment help the parents provide better care.
• Diversity provides the infant with needed rest and activity and promotes maternal-infant bonding without overtaxing the infant.
• Breast-feeding prolongs the infant's addiction.

• This helps the mother give infant care safely and increases her feeling of competence in parenting.

3. Social services' participation ensures follow-up and safety of the infant while it is in the mother's care.

4. Foster care may be an alternative until the mother's situation stabilizes.

5. This ensures safe administration of medications given for withdrawal (if needed after discharge).

6. Rationales: _____

Documentation checklist

During the hospital stay, document:
❏ patient status and assessment findings, especially signs of withdrawal, cardiopulmonary status, abrasions on skin, diarrhea or vomiting
❏ changes in patient status
❏ pertinent laboratory and diagnostic findings, especially toxicology screen; electrolyte, serum glucose, and blood gas levels; CBC with differential; HIV antigen test and blood culture results, and urine specific gravity
❏ nutritional status
❏ neurologic status
❏ patient's response to treatment
❏ family's reaction to the diagnosis
❏ parent-infant interaction
❏ stability and safety in the home environment
❏ family teaching guidelines
❏ discharge planning guidelines.

Associated plans and appendices
❏ Acquired immunodeficiency syndrome — infant
❏ Cleft lip and cleft palate
❏ Congenital heart disease
❏ Fetal alcohol syndrome
❏ Inappropriate size or weight: small for gestational age
❏ Intracranial hemorrhage

❏ Preterm infant
❏ Sexually transmitted diseases
❏ Substance use and fetal and neonatal abnormalities (appendix C)
❏ Aspects of psychological care — maternal (appendix D)
❏ Parent teaching guides (appendix J)

Additional nursing diagnoses
❏ Activity intolerance related to neurologic irritability
❏ Diarrhea related to GI hypermotility
❏ Impaired home maintenance management related to inadequate support system, insufficient financial resources, and continuation of drug abuse patterns
❏ Ineffective breathing pattern related to decreased lung expansion, depressed respirations, apnea associated with prematurity, respiratory disorders, and nasal stuffiness affecting airway clearance
❏ Ineffective family coping: disabling related to intolerance, rejection, and ambivalent family relationships
❏ Risk for altered parenting related to previous lifestyle associated with drug abuse and unrealistic expectations of self and infant
❏ Risk for aspiration related to diminished gag reflex and poor swallowing and sucking
❏ Sleep pattern disturbance related to neurologic irritability

Fetal alcohol syndrome

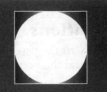

Definition

Fetal alcohol syndrome (FAS) in the neonate results from the mother's chronic or periodic ethanol intake during pregnancy. A related disorder, fetal alcohol effect typically causes less severe signs and symptoms; it may result in only cognitive and behavioral problems without the physical effects caused by FAS. The severity of the effects of FAS on the infant depends on the degree and timing of alcohol consumption. Because no one knows what constitutes a "safe" level of alcohol consumption during pregnancy or when alcohol consumption may cause the most harm to the fetus, pregnant women are advised to abstain from alcohol consumption throughout pregnancy.

Neonates damaged by their mother's alcohol abuse may be physically and mentally deficient and may display multiple congenital abnormalities. Diagnosis is based on a cluster of findings rather than a single, isolated finding. Perinatal mortality is about 20%.

This plan focuses on caring for the neonate who displays signs of withdrawal and on preparing the mother to care for her infant after discharge.

Etiology and precipitating factors

• Chronic maternal alcoholism
• Social drinking
• Binge drinking (taking large amounts periodically)

Physical findings

Maternal history

• Alcohol consumption and possibly use of street, scheduled, or prescription drugs
• Participation in Alcoholics Anonymous or another treatment program or support group
• Possibly at high risk for human immunodeficiency virus (HIV) seropositivity
• At risk for sexually transmitted infections

Infant status at birth

• Small for gestational age (SGA) with low birth weight and height
• Congenital cardiac defects, joint contractures, or malformations
• Facial abnormalities, such as microcephaly, short eye slits, midfacial hypoplasia, thin upper lip, and smooth philtrum

Neurologic

• Abnormal reflexes, including hyperactive rooting and increased sucking
• Irritability, poor coordination, hyperactivity from effect of drug on central nervous system (CNS) functioning, neonatal abstinence syndrome
• Tremors, seizures

Behavioral findings

• Sleeplessness
• Inconsolability
• Easily hyperstimulated by noise, light, and touch
• Exhibits activity with little ability to remain alert and attentive to environment

Diagnostic studies

• HIV seropositivity test (if indicated by history)
• Toxicology screen for alcohol or other drugs in maternal or infant blood
• Serum glucose levels to determine hypoglycemia in infant who is SGA

COLLABORATIVE PROBLEM

Risk for neurologic instability (short-term) and mental deficiency (long-term) related to alcohol addiction

Expected outcome

The infant withdraws from alcohol exposure with minimal distress.

Interventions

1. Assess the infant for withdrawal, including:

• maternal use of alcohol during pregnancy, time and amount of last intake, and other drugs taken

• irritability, hyperactivity, tremors, restlessness, or poor coordination
• results of the toxicology screen to identify alcohol or other drugs.

2. Provide calming techniques:
• Hold, rock, and cuddle the infant. If possible, have volunteers perform these activities.
• Touch, pat, smile at, and talk to the infant; use an infant carrier for closeness.
• Swaddle the infant in the side-lying position, supporting its back with a small pillow. Provide a quiet, dimly lighted environment for sleep.
• Cluster care between rest periods and limit procedures if possible.
• Do not disturb the infant if it is quiet.

3. Prepare to give medications ordered for withdrawal symptoms and evaluate their adverse effects.
• Give paregoric with formula or water by mouth with dose based on the infant's reactions.

• Give I.V. phenobarbital initially to the unstable infant until an oral drug can be introduced.

4. Recognize the long-term effects of alcohol addiction. Assess for congenital anomalies, including microcephaly, cardiac defects, and musculoskeletal abnormalities.

Rationales

1. Signs of alcohol withdrawal usually appear within 12 hours of birth; however, if exposed only to alcohol and not other drugs, most infants do not display withdrawal patterns.
• The severity of effects on the neonate depends on the degree of the mother's abuse; the infant's withdrawal may be delayed if intake occurred just before birth.
• Monitoring the degree of these signs helps determine whether treatment is reducing withdrawal responses.
• The mother may be an unreliable source of information about her alcohol and drug habit.

2. These techniques soothe the infant.
• Holding helps sooth the infant and reduces irritability and hyperactivity.
• Touching quiets and comforts the infant while providing personal contact.
• A restful, restricted environment reduces hyperactivity and provides comfort while reducing external stimuli.

• Careful scheduling reduces external stimuli, which increase irritability.
• This allows for needed rest and sleep.

3. Pharmacologic agents help reduce withdrawal symptoms.
• Paregoric treats withdrawal symptoms (see the "Drug addiction and withdrawal" plan, page 198, for actions and adverse effects).
• Phenobarbital controls hyperactivity, irritability, and seizures (see the "Drug addiction and withdrawal" plan, page 198, for actions and adverse effects).

4. Infants with FAS continue to have difficulties with growth and development throughout childhood. Neonates affected by FAS may have anomalies; 50% are estimated to have mental deficiencies.

NURSING DIAGNOSIS

Altered nutrition: less than body requirements related to lack of nutritional reserves and to poor or low intake

Expected outcome

The infant demonstrates improved nutritional status.

Interventions

1. Assess the infant's nutritional status and needs; include the following:
• gestational age and weight

• sucking or swallowing coordination; ability to swallow secretions without gagging

Rationales

1. Determining a baseline nutritional status helps identify how best to meet the infant's needs.
• Infants of alcoholic mothers are commonly SGA with low birth weight.
• Hyperactivity from CNS stimulation causes poor feeding.

• daily intake (by I.V. or oral route or gastric gavage), including calorie count

• serum glucose levels.

2. Provide appropriate nutrition:

• Assure proper administration of the I.V. infusion; delay feedings if the infant is unstable.

• Start oral feedings at half-strength: 10 ml every 3 hours.
• Check for residual feeding after oral or gavage feedings, and reduce the amount of next feeding if residuals are high; increase feedings gradually, as tolerated, to 5 to 10 ml hourly, while increasing the strength of feedings.
• Place the infant on its right side, supporting its back with a small pillow, or place it on its abdomen when feedings begin.
• Monitor gastric gavage (intermittent or continuous).

• Have suction equipment on hand and ready for use.

3. Weigh the infant daily, and record its weight on a flow sheet for comparison.

4. Provide a pacifier for nonnutritive sucking when the infant is not feeding.

5. Provide a dimly lighted, quiet environment.

6. Allow the mother to feed the infant; help her feed slowly and calmly, holding the infant while feeding.

7. Additional individualized interventions: _____
_____

• The infant will probably need I.V. fluids until it stabilizes; it may not be able to tolerate full-strength feedings initially, so increases may have to be gradual.
• The SGA infant with low nutritional reserves may be hypoglycemic. Ethanol intake causes hypoglycemia, which is passed on to the infant because ethanol is metabolized like sugars.

2. The full-term infant needs 100 to 200 calories/kg daily; the SGA infant needs more, based on age and projected daily weight gain.
• I.V. fluid administration ensures nutrition; delayed feedings prevent complications when the infant cannot tolerate feedings.
• Half-strength feedings provide nutritional intake if the infant cannot tolerate full-strength feeding.
• Monitoring for residuals prevents overfeeding or vomiting after feedings.

• This positioning prevents overfeeding and vomiting.

• Gavage feeding provides an alternate feeding route when the infant cannot tolerate oral feedings (see Interventions for gastric gavage in the "Drug addiction and withdrawal" plan, page 198.)
• Suction may be needed in case of aspiration.

3. Weighing reveals gains or losses and the need for changes in feedings.

4. A pacifier helps to quiet the infant by satisfying its need for nonnutritive sucking.

5. A dimly lighted, quiet environment reduces external stimuli, which may increase hyperactivity and irritability, thus increasing caloric and metabolic needs.

6. The mother's participation encourages the bonding process; it also gives support to the mother while preventing overfeeding.

7. Rationales: _____
_____

Nursing diagnosis

Risk for altered parenting related to previous lifestyle associated with alcohol abuse or to unrealistic expectations of self and infant (two expected outcomes)

Expected outcome 1

The mother makes appropriate lifestyle changes.

Interventions

1. Assess the mental status of the mother, including:
• individual and family stressors
• mother's behavior toward and comments about the infant
• mother's reaction to the infant's possibly long-term treatment
• developmental stage
• use of coping mechanisms.

2. Offer information about parenting classes and alcohol rehabilitation programs; encourage attendance.

3. Help the mother identify support systems, including family, spouse, and church as well as support groups such as Born Free, Alcoholics Anonymous, and Al-Anon.

4. Additional individualized interventions: _____
_____

Rationales

1. Assessment provides information about the mother's ability to pursue treatment for alcohol abuse and offers clues to potential problems that may lead to infant neglect.

2. To change her lifestyle successfully, the mother needs support groups and rehabilitation.

3. Support systems provide long-term assistance and decrease maternal fear and guilt.

4. Rationales: _____
_____

Expected outcome 2

The mother demonstrates appropriate parenting skills and an adequate support system.

Interventions

1. Encourage the mother to express her expectations, both realistic and unrealistic, and feelings about the infant and her own capabilities.

2. Help the mother identify realistic expectations and develop strategies to fulfill them.

3. Allow for discussion of alcohol abuse and rehabilitation needs.

4. Refer the mother to social services for community and home health care resources.

Rationales

1. This provides information about the mother's expectations, coping skills, fears, and anxieties.

2. Success is more likely if the mother is involved in decisions.

3. Self-assessment of alcohol abuse and the need for change may promote realistic decisions about infant care.

4. Such resources provide continued support before and after discharge and promote compliance with follow-up regimen.

Nursing diagnosis

Knowledge deficit (parental) related to lack of information about infant care

Expected outcome

The parents receive appropriate information about and express their understanding of safe infant care practices.

Interventions

1. Identify what the parents need to learn, their interest in learning, and their readiness and ability to learn.

Rationales

1. This provides the basis for developing a teaching plan appropriate to the parents' abilities and needs.

2. Provide information about the infant's condition, signs of infant withdrawal, and the rationale for treatment as well as:
• need for increased or decreased stimulation, depending on the infant's reactions
• how alcohol can pass to the infant during breast-feeding if the mother still drinks
• mental and, possibly, behavioral effects on the infant of alcohol exposure
• how to provide physical care, including how to feed, bathe, dress, and hold the infant.

3. Determine whether the parents have adequate clothing and safe baby equipment for their child.

4. Refer the parents to social services for community resources and home health care.

5. Additional individualized interventions: _____
_____

2. Such information will help the parents understand the infant's behavior and care for the infant who has prolonged signs of withdrawal.
• The infant's responses to stimuli may be increased or decreased during withdrawal
• Continued alcohol intake will prolong the breast-fed infant's addiction.
• Alcohol addiction causes mental and growth restriction in infants.
• This information helps the parents safely care for the infant and increases their feelings of competence in parenting.

3. Alcoholic parents may not have planned for their infant's care needs after homecoming.

4. Such resources provide emotional and physical support, promoting compliance with the follow-up regimen.

5. Rationales: _____
_____

Documentation checklist
During the hospital stay, document:
❐ patient status and assessment findings
❐ changes in patient status
❐ pertinent laboratory and diagnostic findings, especially toxicology screen, HIV antigen testing, and serum glucose level
❐ patient's response to treatment
❐ family's reaction to the diagnosis
❐ parent-infant interaction, especially appropriateness of the mother's interaction
❐ stability and safety of the home environment, determined through discussions with the parents
❐ family teaching guidelines
❐ discharge planning guidelines.

Associated plans and appendices
❐ Acquired immunodeficiency syndrome —infant
❐ Congenital heart disease
❐ Drug addiction and withdrawal
❐ Hypoglycemia
❐ Inappropriate size or weight: small for gestational age
❐ Intracranial hemorrhage
❐ Parent teaching guides (appendix J)

Additional nursing diagnoses
❐ Activity intolerance related to neurologic hyperirritability
❐ Altered growth and development related to maternal alcohol use and FAS
❐ Impaired home maintenance management related to continued alcohol abuse
❐ Ineffective family coping: disabling related to intolerance, rejection, and ambivalent family relationships

❐ Ineffective individual coping (maternal) related to anxiety, fear, guilt, inadequate support systems, excessive drinking (alcohol), and unrealistic expectations and perceptions
❐ Risk for aspiration related to uncoordinated sucking and swallowing
❐ Sleep pattern disturbance related to neurologic irritability

Full-term infant

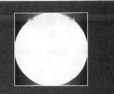

Definition

An infant born after the 38th and up to the 42nd week of gestation is considered full-term. At birth, it must leave the life-sustaining environment of the uterus and adapt to one that requires profound physiologic changes. Any interference with the infant's transition to extrauterine life affects its well-being. Some physiologic factors that can affect the transition include initiation of extrauterine cardiopulmonary function, thermoregulation, defenses against infection, neurologic impairment, fluid and nutritional deficits, congenital defects, and skin impairment.

The first 4 weeks, or 28 days, of life present the greatest risk to the infant. The incidence of death is highest during the 1st day, and two-thirds of all deaths during the 1st year of life occur within the 1st month.

In the first 24 hours, two periods of reactivity occur. The first period, lasting up to 30 minutes after birth, reveals an alert, open-eyed, vigorously crying, fist-sucking infant whose vital signs and bowel sounds increase while body temperature decreases. This is followed by a decrease in responses and vital signs and a sleep period lasting 2 to 8 hours.

The second period of reactivity starts when the infant awakens (4 to 8 hours after birth). It is alert, with an increase in vital signs, secretions, and gagging. This period lasts 2 to 5 hours, concluding when secretions decrease and hunger, sucking, and a sleep and activity pattern become established.

This plan focuses on nursing care of the full-term infant. It includes interventions for possible abnormalities (related to immature systems) and interventions for maintaining normal physiologic function and meeting the infant's needs.

Physical findings

Maternal history

- Prenatal care, age, and expected date of confinement
- Genetic profile and familial tendencies
- Abnormal conditions or disorders during pregnancy
- Use of medications, over-the-counter drugs, street drugs, alcohol, tobacco, or caffeine
- Test results: amniotic fluid; blood type; Rh factor; Coombs' test; screens for sexually transmitted diseases, sickle cell, and tuberculosis; and other screens
- Description of delivery, especially if difficult

Infant status at birth

- Gestational age 38 to 42 weeks
- Apgar score 7 to 10 at 1 minute and at 5 minutes after birth, indicating absence of abnormalities and normal adjustment to life
- Weight: 5 lb, 8 oz to 8 lb, 13 oz (2,500 to 4,000 g)
- Length: 19″ to 21″ (48 to 53 cm)
- Head circumference: 13″ to 14″ (33 to 35.6 cm), ¾″ to 1¼″ (2 to 3 cm) larger than chest

Cardiovascular

- Heart rate ranging from 110 to 160 beats/minute at apical site with regular rhythm; decreases during sleep and increases during crying
- Blood pressure ranging from 60 to 80 mm Hg systolic and 30 to 45 mm Hg diastolic
- Apical pulse at third to fourth intercostal space at sternal edge
- S_2 of higher pitch and sharper than S_1
- Possibly murmur because of functional vibrations within the heart or major arteries
- Pink nail beds with transient cyanosis

Gastrointestinal

- Intact mouth, lips, and palate; normal sucking, swallowing, gag, and rooting reflexes
- Stomach capacity about 90 ml
- Soft, cylindrically shaped abdomen
- Liver palpable; spleen not palpable
- With clamp in place, cord at umbilicus has two arteries and one vein
- Anus patent with meconium stool passing within 12 hours or history of meconium passage in utero

Integumentary

- Red (not beefy red) and smooth skin, changing to pink, dry, and flaky
- Edema and puffiness around eyes, face, arms, legs, and presenting parts
- Acrocyanosis
- Possibly petechiae, nevi, spots, ecchymoses, rash, milia, and mongolian spots
- Fingernails and toenails; lanugo and vernix caseosa
- Intact skin and mucous membranes

Musculoskeletal

- Normal range of motion in arms and legs with good muscle tone
- Flexion of head, arms, and legs
- Ear cartilage flexible
- Equal muscle tone with symmetry; resists flexion
- Creases on soles
- Possibly skeletal deformities resulting from fetal positioning

- Soft skull and rib bones with fontanels and separations at suture lines present in head (fontanels soft, flat, and firm)
- More cartilage than ossified bone

Neurologic
- Bilateral and equal Moro's, plantar, palmar grasp, and Babinski's reflexes; loud and lusty cry
- Eyes usually closed, with vision the least developed sensory function and touch the most developed; infant can taste, smell, and hear
- Startle, blinking, pupillary, crawling, yawn, and cough reflexes apparent
- Daily sleep and activity patterns: 1 to 4 hours of alertness, activity, and crying; 4 to 5 hours of regular sleep; 12 to 15 hours of irregular sleep
- Skin temperature of 97° to 98.6° F (36° to 37° C); rectal temperature 1° F (0.6° C) degree higher

Pulmonary
- Nasal patency and nasal breathing, thin white mucus, and sneezing
- Respiratory rate ranging from 40 to 60 breaths/minute; chiefly abdominal breathing with slight sternal retractions during inspiration
- Bronchial breath sounds bilaterally, with possible transient tachypnea and slight nasal flaring
- Possibly crackles for short period after birth
- Possibly irregular respirations or periodic breathing

Renal
- Pale yellow urine, with voiding occurring within 24 hours after delivery
- Volume of 200 to 300 ml voided every 24 hours, with bladder capacity of about 15 ml causing involuntary emptying
- Kidneys palpable

Reproductive
- Girl: larger labia minora than labia majora; edema of labia and clitoris
- Boy: palpable testes in scrotal sac; scrotum edematous, large, and hanging with rugae present; urethral meatus at tip of penis

Behavioral findings
- Alternates among behavioral sleeping and waking states
- Habituates to environmental stimuli
- Responds to visual and auditory stimuli
- Shows motor maturity within normal limits
- Self-quiets effectively

Diagnostic studies
- Tests determined by findings of physical examination or observable changes in infant status
- Possible blood tests include serum bilirubin levels, complete blood count, electrolyte analysis, blood type and Rh factor, and Coombs' test
- Chemstrip or Dextrostix testing to determine glucose levels (followed by serum glucose study if glucose levels are low)
- Guthrie blood test to identify possible phenylketonuria (PKU; part of multiple screenings for metabolic defects)
- Hepatitis B screen and culture for Group B streptococcus on mother

NURSING DIAGNOSES

Ineffective breathing pattern related to irregular periodic breathing episodes and increased mucus secretion

Expected outcome

The infant exhibits good respiratory efforts and a patent airway.

Interventions

1. Assess the infant's respiratory rate, regularity, depth, and ease every 15 minutes to 2 hours as appropriate. Auscultate for breath sounds.

2. Assess for increased mucus production and for fluids, such as blood and amniotic fluid, swallowed during birth. Gently hand-suction oronasal areas as needed.

Rationales

1. An infant with an Apgar score between 7 and 10 at 1 and 5 minutes usually breathes at a rate ranging from 40 to 60 breaths/minute, with some irregularity, brief periods of transient crackles, and breathing rate changes followed by a period of sleep. Changes in breath sounds may indicate changes in respiratory status.

2. Hand-suctioning removes accumulated mucus and fluids and prevents aspiration. Parasympathetic nervous system stimulation increases saliva production, which is followed by gagging and vomiting. Increases in mucus and saliva occur by 6 hours after delivery.

3. Position the infant on its back or side with the head slightly lower or on its back supported by a small padded roll.

4. Assess the infant for tachypnea, nasal flaring, grunting, retraction, crackles, rhonchi, cyanosis, and tachycardia.

5. Keep the infant's clothing, diaper, and blanket loose.

6. Have oxygen on hand to be administered if needed.

7. Additional individualized interventions: _____

3. This position promotes chest expansion and mucus drainage.

4. These are signs of respiratory distress; normal breathing is diaphragmatic and abdominal. The normal infant respiratory rate ranges from 40 to 60 breaths/minute.

5. This action prevents constricted chest movement.

6. Oxygen should be available in case of respiratory distress.

7. Rationales: _____

NURSING DIAGNOSIS

Risk for altered body temperature related to fluctuations caused by the environment and increased activity

Expected outcome

The infant maintains a stable temperature within a neutral thermal environment.

Interventions

1. Initially, assess the infant's core temperature and skin temperature by the appropriate method (per institutional policy) every 30 to 60 minutes and then every 2 to 4 hours for 8 to 12 hours.

2. Monitor the ambient nursery temperature and humidity.

3. Maintain temperature stability by:

• drying the infant immediately after birth with a warm towel
• wrapping the infant in a warmed blanket and placing the infant on a warm surface
• allowing the mother to cuddle the infant or maintain skin-to-skin contact (kangaroo care) to provide warmth

• placing the infant under a radiant warmer and avoiding drafts, cold surfaces, or other exposure to cold
• placing a cap on the infant's head

• postponing bathing and other procedures until the infant's body temperature stabilizes (about 4 hours after birth)
• dressing the infant appropriately and covering the infant if it is placed in a bassinet.

Rationales

1. Optimal skin temperature is 97.7° to 98.6° F (36.5° to 37° C) for minimal oxygen consumption, with core (rectal) temperatures about 1° F (0.6° C) higher. After birth, the infant's body temperature falls; then it rises during periods of increased muscle activity and alertness because of sympathetic stimulation.

2. Infants lose body heat to surrounding areas by convection. The ambient nursery temperature should be 75° to 78° F (24° to 25.6° C), and humidity should be 40% to 50%.

3. The objective is to minimize heat loss by conduction, evaporation, radiation, and convection after delivery by providing warmth when the temperature decreases.
• Drying the infant helps to prevent body heat loss from evaporation.
• Warm blankets and surfaces conserve the infant's body heat and minimize heat loss from conduction.
• When the mother cuddles her infant or provides skin-to-skin contact, her body acts as a heat source. Cuddling and skin-to-skin contact also promote bonding.
• These actions help to prevent heat loss from evaporation and radiation.
• The large surface area of the infant's head may promote heat loss if the head remains uncovered.
• These actions prevent heat loss.

• These actions provide warmth for the infant.

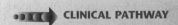

CLINICAL PATHWAY

Normal newborn

	Delivery to 1 hour	Transition to 12 hours
Consults	• Normal newborn nursery (at delivery) • Regional newborn intensive care nursery (at delivery)	
Tests	• Umbilical cord blood drawn for typing and other tests • Umbilical cord gases drawn to assess oxygenation • Check blood glucose level within 30 minutes if infant is small for gestational age or large for gestational age and symptomatic, weighs 9 lb (4,080 g) or more, is preterm or postterm, has low Apgar scores or an unstable temperature, or is in respiratory distress or if mother has insulin-dependent diabetes mellitus gestational diabetes mellitus on insulin or diet-controlled	• Blood group • Rh factor • Coombs' test (if Rh-negative mother) • Check blood glucose level per policy (normal: ≥40)
Activities and safety	• Put identification bracelets on infant • Take infant's footprints	• Check infant's identification bracelets on transfer • Make sure full-face photograph is taken
Nursing assessments	• Within 30 minutes, assess: temperature (normal: 97.5° to 99.5° F [36.4° to 37.5° C]), pulse (normal: 100 to 160 beats/minute), respirations (normal: 28 to 60 breaths/minute) • Assess Apgar scores at 1 and 5 minutes • Weigh infant (normal: >6 to <9 lb [>2,700 to <4,080 g]) • Assess maternal/infant interaction • Assess general appearance (gestational age [GA]) and perform risk assessment for respiratory distress, birth trauma, and other complications	• Assess temperature, pulse, and respirations (TPR) every hour for first 2 hours, then in 4 hours, then every 8 hours (normal: vital signs within normal limits [WNL]; temperature stable) • Within 3 hours of birth, assess blood pressure, perform physical examination, assess GA and perform risk assessment • Assess color, tone, and activity • Assess intake and output (I & O): feedings, urine, stool (normal: tolerates feedings)
Treatments	• Begin pulse oximetry if indicated	• Bathe as needed • Provide cord care • Circumcision may be performed 4 to 6 hours after delivery if infant is stable
Nutrition	• Initiate breast-feeding immediately after delivery or when stable (if breast-feeding)	• Feed on demand or every 2 to 4 hours • Note formula type (if bottle-feeding) • Offer sips of water before first formula feeding (if bottle-feeding)
Medications	• Instill erythromycin into infant's eyes	• Inject vitamin K
Education	• Teach mother about newborn reactivity and feeding cues	• Within 6 hours of delivery, teach mother about newborn reactivity, feeding cues, frequency of early feedings, positioning of infant, latching on (if breast-feeding)
Possible treatments	• Hepatitis B screen (on mother) • Group B streptococcus culture (on mother) • Prophylaxis for mother (if needed, based on specific indication) • Infant transferred to nursery • Other treatments as needed	• Hepatitis B immune globulin and hepatitis vaccine within 12 hours (if mother positive for hepatitis B) • Hepatitis vaccine within 12 hours (if results pending) • Circumcision evaluation form completed (if applicable)
Discharge planning		• Send social service referral • 50% diet consumed

12 to 24 hours	24 hours to discharge
• Lactation consultant referral (Inpatient/outpatient)	• Discharge outcome • Pediatrician completes physical examination
• Bilirubin level (if indicated)	• Metabolic diseases, phenylketonuria, and hyperthyroidism (MDPH) screen 24 hours after birth • If MDPH screen performed within 24 hours birth, outpatient redraw is scheduled
	• Verify and remove one identification bracelet • Complete infant identification form
• Assess TPR every 8 hours until 24 hours (normal: vital signs WNL) • Assess I & O (normal: voids and passes stool at least once within 24 hours of birth) • Weigh daily • Assess color, tone, and activity • Check circumcision site every 15 minutes for first 30 minutes, then at 1 and 2 hours, then with routine assessments (normal: no active bleeding or signs of infection)	• Assess TPR twice a day until discharge (normal at discharge: vital signs WNL) • Weigh infant (normal: weight loss <10% of body weight) • Assess I & O (normal: voids and passes stool at least once) • Assess circumcision site (normal: no bleeding or signs of infection)
• Bathe as needed • Remove cord clamp if dry • Provide cord care • Apply petroleum jelly to circumcision for 24 hours (if applicable)	• Cord clamp off • May be discharged 2 hours after circumcision if stable
• Feed on demand or every 2 to 4 hours (normal: feeds without difficulty and tolerates feedings)	• By discharge, infant feeds without difficulty, demonstrates latching on and active sucking (if breast-feeding), nurses at least 5 minutes each breast (if breast-feeding)
• Between 6 and 24 hours after birth, teach breast-feeding mother about milk supply, importance of avoiding artificial nipples, symptoms of letdown	• By discharge, mother demonstrates understanding of diaper changing, feeding frequency, milk supply and engorgement (if breast-feeding), community resources, when to call infant's doctor, when to call her doctor.
	• Infant discharge to mother • Critical indicators checked

Adapted with permission from Murray, Kathleen, 5th Medical Group/SGAL.

4. Provide a neutral thermal environment with a radiant warmer or an incubator. Use a Servo-Control device to monitor skin temperature if appropriate.

5. Assess for cold skin on the infant's trunk; a drop in temperature; pallor, cyanosis, or redness; edema or mottling of the arms and legs; bradycardia; feeble cry; lethargy; flaccid movements; slow, shallow, irregular breathing with expiratory grunting; poor feeding; vomiting; abdominal distention; and diminished activity or reflexes.

6. Additional individualized interventions: _____

_____

4. A neutral thermal environment maintains optimal core temperature with minimal oxygen consumption if the infant's temperature is not stable.

5. These are signs of cold stress and should be reported to the doctor at once.

6. Rationales: _____

_____

Nursing diagnosis

Altered nutrition: less than body requirements related to high caloric requirement because of increased metabolic rate

Expected outcome

The infant maintains adequate nutrition.

Interventions

1. Assess the infant's bowel sounds, clearing of mucus, and passage of meconium.

2. Weigh and measure the infant, and calculate nutritional requirements, even though the infant takes what is needed with each feeding.

3. Perform a Chemstrip or Dextrostix test to establish the infant's glucose level as ordered. Follow the test with a serum glucose test if the glucose level is less than 40 mg/dl.

4. Assess for signs of readiness to feed:
• active bowel sounds
• absence of abdominal distention
• lusty cry that diminishes with rooting or sucking behaviors when a stimulus is placed near the lips.

5. Start feedings with a small amount (about 15 ml) of 5% glucose in water if the infant's gag and swallowing reflexes are normal. Some infants start feedings with formula (based on doctor preference); if tolerated, these formula feedings may be repeated. If the infant will be breast-fed, its first attempt should take place during its first reactive period immediately after birth.

6. If the infant tolerates glucose and water, start feeding with formula. Breast-feeding may start soon after birth or when the infant can nurse.

Rationales

1. These processes usually occur between 2 and 6 hours after delivery and indicate possible readiness for feeding.

2. Daily caloric needs are based on the infant's weight and expected weight gain. Initially, infants lose weight because of the physiologic changes required to adapt to extrauterine life and because they are poor feeders for the first day or two.

3. The infant's glucose stores are quickly depleted and must be replaced by feedings or by dextrose 10% in water given I.V., if necessary; early feedings increase the glucose level after the initial drop.

4. Readiness to feed enhances feeding and helps prevent complications.

5. Initial feeding with sterile water allows absorption of water by lung tissue if aspiration occurs. Feedings may be given at birth or 4 to 6 hours later as tolerated. Because the infant's stomach capacity averages 90 ml (about 2¾ oz), with an emptying time of 2½ to 3 hours, frequent small feedings are better tolerated.

6. Early feedings are advised, with breast-feeding preferred. (See appendix G, Fluid and nutritional needs in infancy, and appendix J, Parent teaching guides, for more information.) Breast-feeding soon after birth stimulates milk production, promotes maternal-infant attachment, and enhances success of breast-feeding.

7. Offer feedings every 3 to 4 hours, according to the infant's demand and needs.

7. Breast milk (or formula closely resembling breast milk in content) is given. Special formulas may be prescribed for special deficiencies.

8. Assess for regurgitation, choking, fatigue during feeding or refused feedings, abnormal stools, respiratory changes, and irritability.

8. Regurgitation caused by reverse peristalsis results in caloric loss. Feeding may also be affected by other conditions. Stool color normally changes from greenish meconium, to greenish brown or yellowish brown, and then to light yellow in bottle-fed infants and yellow-mustard and pasty in breast-fed infants.

9. Position the infant on the right side after feeding.

9. This position promotes drainage and gastric emptying.

10. Additional individualized interventions: _____

10. Rationales: _____

NURSING DIAGNOSIS

Risk for fluid volume deficit related to sensible and insensible losses

Expected outcome

The infant maintains fluid and electrolyte balance.

Interventions

1. Calculate fluid requirements based on the infant's weight, even though full-term infants tend to restrict their own fluids initially and regulate their own needs.

2. Monitor fluid intake and output accurately, and include all sources of intake and losses.

3. Assess the infant's first voiding and subsequent voiding pattern.

4. Assess for the absence of voiding, poor skin turgor, edema, and depressed fontanels.

5. Additional individualized interventions: _____

Rationales

1. Fluid requirements depend on the infant's weight and condition (see appendix G, Fluid and nutritional needs in infancy, for information on fluid needs).

2. Kidney function in the infant is immature, affecting concentration and reabsorption of water and electrolytes.

3. The first voiding occurs within 24 hours and is limited until fluid intake has been initiated. Bladder capacity averages 15 ml; voidings range from 2 to 3 ml/kg/hour or more with an approximate total of 170 ml daily. By age 3 days, the infant may void 10 to 20 times in 24 hours.

4. These are signs of dehydration, which may be caused by warmers or phototherapy, vomiting, or poor feedings. These signs are seen between ages 3 and 7 days, not at birth or shortly thereafter.

5. Rationales: _____

NURSING DIAGNOSIS

Risk for impaired skin integrity related to rash, irritation, or use of skin-damaging substances

Expected outcome

The infant maintains intact skin, free from injury or irritation.

Interventions

1. Assess all bony prominences for redness and pressure and buttocks and perineal area for erythema (redness) and rash.

2. Avoid using tape on skin.

3. Clean the infant's skin with water-soaked gauze initially after delivery and at each diaper change thereafter.

4. Bathe the infant during the 1st week with warm water. After this, bathe the infant with soap and water (about once or twice weekly), using a low-alkaline, unscented soap, such as Neutrogena, Aveeno, or Oilatum.

5. Avoid using perfumed lotions, powders, and creams.

6. Use only warm water if the infant's skin is irritated or abraded.

7. Additional individualized interventions: _____

Rationales

1. These areas are prone to injury because of the infant's inability to change position and because of irritation from urine and stool.

2. Removing tape from the infant's fragile skin may damage or actually remove the skin.

3. This promotes cleanliness and comfort without using irritating substances.

4. Bathing is limited for the first few days to retain the acid mantle (pH) of the skin for its bactericidal action. Alkaline soaps destroy this mantle by changing the pH for 1 hour after use (see Appendix 12: Parent Teaching Guides, for more information on infant bathing).

5. Most lotions, powders, and creams may be absorbed into the skin and even cake on the skin, creating irritation and a medium for microorganism growth.

6. Using any substance on irritated skin increases the possibility of infection.

7. Rationales: _____

NURSING DIAGNOSIS

Risk for infection related to transmission of microorganisms to infant, umbilical cord stump, or circumcision

Expected outcome

The infant exhibits no signs of infection.

Interventions

1. Assess the infant daily for skin breaks, rashes, and lesions.

2. Assess the umbilical cord and circumcision areas for redness, drainage, and foul odor. Observe also for edema and decreased urine output.
• Keep the umbilical area clean and dry; as ordered, apply alcohol or other preparation, such as triple dye or iodine-based solution (for instance, Betadine).
• Fold diapers below the umbilical area.

3. Exclude infants with infections from the nursery; isolate those with suspected infections.

4. Wear gloves to care for infants with skin breaks or wounds. Discourage parents from kissing infant on the lips. Use proper hand-washing methods when handling infants. Discourage others who may have or carry infections, such as family members, from handling the infant directly.

5. Follow hand-washing protocols before and after handling the infant.

Rationales

1. Breaks in the body's first line of defense, the skin, expose the infant to infection.

2. These are indications of infection.

• These agents promote drying. Iodine-based solutions also provide a bactericidal effect.

• Wet or soiled diapers slow the drying process and increase the risk for infection.

3. Isolation prevents the exposure of infection-free infants to infectious agents.

4. An immature inflammatory response and phagocytic activity increase the infant's susceptibility to infection.

5. Hand washing removes transient flora and prevents cross-contamination.

6. Follow the protocol for care of equipment and supplies in the nursery. Maintain an individual unit and supplies for each infant.

7. Observe the infant for lethargy, poor feeding, apnea, tachypnea, hypothermia, weight loss, hypotension, jitteriness, hypertonia, hypotonia, jaundice, and vomiting.

8. Administer erythromycin ointment to the infant's eyes. This can be done after deliver or later in the nursery.

9. Additional individualized interventions: _____
_____

6. These measures prevent cross-contamination from infant to infant.

7. These are signs and symptoms of sepsis and other infectious processes.

8. Prophylaxis against gonorrheal infection is required by law. Medication may be given later to allow for eye contact and bonding after birth.

9. Rationales: _____
_____

Collaborative problem

Risk for complications (such as metabolic disorders, including hypoglycemia, hypocalcemia, and PKU, and other disorders, such as anemias, hypothyroidism, hyperbilirubinemia, and drug addiction) that may lead to brain damage

Expected outcome

The infant exhibits no signs of metabolic problems.

Interventions

1. Perform a heelstick test or test capillary blood for hemoglobin, bilirubin, glucose, and calcium levels; red blood cell count; and hematocrit, based on presenting symptoms.

2. Perform blood tests for neonatal screening, PKU, and hypothyroidism.

3. Perform a drug screen to determine blood alcohol or drug content if the mother's history warrants the test or the infant manifests withdrawal signs.

4. Carry out interventions specific to the abnormal condition as presented in individual plans. Base your interventions on test results and the infant's signs.

5. Administer vitamin K by injection, as ordered.

6. Additional individualized interventions: _____

Rationales

1. These tests identify abnormal levels of substances that may lead to shock, seizure activity, and subsequent brain cell damage (see plans for individual conditions for complete care of infant).

2. These are common neonatal screenings. Some states require them by law.

3. A drug screen identifies the drug responsible for the infant's condition. This information is needed to determine treatment.

4. Care is specific to the particular cause of the disorder.

5. Vitamin K protects against prolonged bleeding time and possible hemorrhage.

6. Rationales: _____

NURSING DIAGNOSIS

Knowledge deficit related to infant care

Expected outcome

The parents receive information and instruction and express understanding about how to care for their infant.

Interventions

1. Inform the parents about their infant's condition, progress, and behaviors and about various changes that take place.

2. Give information appropriate to the parents' level of understanding and readiness to learn.

3. Instruct the parents about bathing, feeding, holding, and clothing the infant and trimming the nails.

4. Inform the parents about caring for the umbilical cord and circumcision site.

5. Inform the parents why an infant cries. Explain that holding and rocking calm the infant.

6. Use several teaching methods, including discussion, printed materials, videotapes, and demonstrations.

7. Explain the importance of calling the doctor if necessary and of visiting the doctor at prescribed times.

8. Additional individualized interventions: _____

Rationales

1. Knowledge decreases the parents' anxiety about caring for their infant.

2. Information given at an appropriate level and in small amounts can be better accepted and understood.

3. Specific instruction about normal infant care relieves anxiety and promotes a feeling of adequacy and independence. See Appendix 12: Parent Teaching Guides for a complete set of guidelines to help parents care for an infant.

4. Parents may fear causing their infant pain if they touch these areas.

5. Giving information about crying and how to manage it will allay parental fears that the infant is ill.

6. Using a variety of teaching methods reinforces learning for those who learn best from different forms of teaching or from a combination of methods.

7. Follow-up care is essential to ensure a well baby and to prevent complications.

8. Rationales: _____

Documentation checklist

During the hospital stay, document:
❏ patient status and assessment findings
❏ appearance of the umbilical cord, especially signs of infection
❏ changes in patient status
❏ pertinent laboratory and diagnostic findings
❏ neonatal screening tests that were performed
❏ patient's response to treatment
❏ family's reaction to the birth
❏ parent-infant interaction
❏ family teaching guidelines
❏ discharge planning guidelines.

Associated plans

All plans have applications for caring for the full-term infant who may develop abnormal conditions or have congenital abnormalities. For specific information, refer to the appropriate plans.

Additional nursing diagnoses

❏ Altered family processes related to infant feeding schedule
❏ Altered parenting related to the addition of new family member
❏ Family coping: potential for growth related to adjustment to new family member
❏ Hypothermia related to cold stress

❏ Ineffective family coping: compromised related to temporary family disorganization and role changes and possibly to situational crisis of new baby
❏ Risk for altered parenting related to lack of support from significant others, lack of knowledge, and unrealistic expectations for self and infant

Heart failure

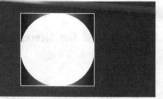

Definition

Heart failure is the heart's inability to pump and circulate the oxygen and nutrients needed to maintain the metabolic requirements that sustain life. In an infant, this condition usually results from a congenital defect that causes fluid overload or left-to-right shunt through the ductus or from surgical correction of the defect. The onset may occur soon after birth or in the 1st month or year, depending on the cause. A weak myocardium that cannot meet normal demands as a result of asphyxia is the usual cause of heart failure in the first few days after birth. Such defects as a narrowed passage or an obstruction, a fistula, and a shunt lesion hinder blood flow and increase the heart's workload, causing heart failure in the first few weeks after birth.

Cardiac dysfunction activates sympathetic nervous system compensatory mechanisms, producing peripheral vasoconstriction, which diverts blood from the skin and renal circulation to the heart and brain. The decrease in renal perfusion activates the angiotensin-aldosterone mechanism, causing hyperaldosteronism. The results are sodium and water retention and increased blood volume.

Ventricular dysfunction increases end-diastolic pressure and produces systemic venous or pulmonary venous engorgement, depending on which ventricle is affected. The ventricles dilate and hypertrophy. Because an infant's myocardium is less compliant (able to comply with changes in volume and pressure) and contains less contractile mass, a small increase in ventricular volume increases the pressure, but the ventricles may be unable to hypertrophy in response to the increased pressure. This produces signs and symptoms of heart failure (most often both left- and right-sided heart failure) with both systemic and venous engorgement resulting. Deterioration occurs more rapidly in a preterm infant than in a full-term infant because a preterm infant has even less compliance and less contractile mass than a full-term infant.

Prompt treatment of heart failure is necessary to maintain systemic perfusion. This plan focuses on early identification, prevention, and treatment.

Etiology and precipitating factors
• Congenital heart defects, such as transposition of the great vessels, severe coarctation of the aorta, hypoplastic left or right heart syndromes, severe aortic stenosis, interrupted aortic arch, and combined defects that cause increased pressure

• Conditions such as anemia, hypoglycemia, hypocalcemia, hypomagnesemia, and hypokalemia because they affect cardiac muscle fiber contractility; respiratory distress syndrome (RDS) with hypoxia because the lungs cannot keep up with tissue demands for oxygen

• Handling and repair of the heart (for correction of tetralogy of Fallot or truncus arteriosus) in an older infant; temporary surgeries, such as creative shunts and pulmonary artery banding, performed on a neonate

Physical findings
Infant status at birth
• Prematurity
• Low Apgar score (1 to 4) with hypoxia and bluish skin
• Congenital heart defect
Cardiovascular
• Tachycardia with rates as high as 200 beats/minute
• Peripheral vasoconstriction with cool arms and legs
• Increased central venous pressure
• Distended neck and, occasionally, superficial veins
Gastrointestinal
• Poor feeding with prolonged feeding time and poor sucking
• Propensity to fall asleep during feedings because of exhaustion
• Vomiting after feedings
• Gastric distention
• Hepatomegaly or splenomegaly with palpable liver in severe instances
Integumentary
• Pale or mottled skin and nail beds
• Cyanosis
• Periorbital edema and, possibly, peripheral edema on the backs of the hands and feet; dependent edema on the flank and scalp
Neurologic
• Restlessness and irritability
• Lethargy
Pulmonary
• Tachypnea and dyspnea with rates as high as 100 breaths/minute
• Intercostal muscle retractions
• Rhonchi and crackles on auscultation
• Possibly carbon dioxide retention in the preterm infant receiving ventilation therapy
Renal
• Oliguria or reduced urine output despite adequate fluid intake

Behavioral findings
- Irritability
- Agitation
- Lethargy
- Difficulty bonding and interacting with parent

Diagnostic studies
- Echocardiography, phonocardiography, and vectorcardiography to identify heart abnormalities
- ECG to identify arrhythmias (after controlling heart failure)
- Cardiac catheterization to determine heart abnormalities

- Chest X-ray to show heart enlargement in response to increased workload
- Hemoglobin (Hb) values and hematocrit (HCT) — decreases suggest anemia
- Serum glucose analysis and reagent strip testing for blood glucose levels — decreases suggest hypoglycemia
- Cardiac glycoside serum level — determines therapeutic levels of digitalis
- White blood cell count, platelet count, and neutrophil studies — may indicate infection
- Arterial blood gas (ABG) studies — may show acidosis
- Electrolyte analysis — identifies serum sodium and potassium levels

COLLABORATIVE PROBLEM

Decreased cardiac output related to decreased cardiac muscle contractility, causing heart failure (three expected outcomes)

Expected outcome 1

The patient at risk for or with heart failure will be identified as evidenced by oliguria, pallor, cyanosis, dependent edema, tachypnea, and tachycardia.

Interventions

1. Assess risk factors related to developing heart failure, including:
- prematurity
- RDS and hypoxia
- congenital heart defects (note type and severity)
- surgery for heart defect
- hypoglycemia, hypocalcemia, hypokalemia, anemia, and hypomagnesemia.

2. Assess for signs and symptoms of heart failure, including:
- tachycardia as high as 200 beats/minute with gallop rhythm

- oliguria (urine output range of less than 0.5 to 1 ml/kg)
- pale or mottled skin and nail beds; cool arms and legs

- tachypnea and dyspnea (as high as 60 or more breaths/minute)

- intercostal muscle retractions

- crackles and rhonchi on auscultation

Rationales

1. Risk factors and subtle signs of impending abnormal conditions, such as decreased HCT and serum glucose, calcium, and Hb values, are a warning of heart failure.

2. Identifying impending heart failure allows for immediate intervention.
- Tachycardia results from sympathetic nervous system stimulation and renal compensatory mechanisms (impaired cardiac output [CO] and renal perfusion); CO varies with the infant's weight but normally is about 200 ml/kg/minute.
- Renal perfusion is impaired because of decreased CO, causing reduced urine output.
- These signs result from peripheral vasoconstriction and the diversion of blood to vital organs.
- These changes result from pulmonary venous engorgement, causing decreased lung compliance. Tachypnea results from decreased oxygenation; dyspnea results from the decreased ability of the lungs to distend, creating the need for added respiratory effort (retractions).
- Retractions result from increased effort to take in oxygen.
- Abnormal breath sounds indicate fluid accumulation in the lungs, indicating pulmonary edema.

• cyanosis

• frothy sputum

• hepatomegaly (palpable liver below the right costal margin)

• periorbital edema and edema on the backs of hands and feet
• restlessness, irritability, and lethargy

• tiring during feeding, causing prolonged feeding time and low intake
• gastric distention or vomiting after feedings.

3. Additional individualized interventions: _____

• Cyanosis results from low oxygen saturation and decreased blood volume.
• Frothy sputum results from pulmonary effusion of fluid in the alveoli.
• Hepatomegaly results from systemic venous engorgement, which increases central venous pressure and causes liver congestion
• Edema results from fluid retained in tissues as renal perfusion is affected by decreased CO.
• Restlessness and irritability stem from oxygen and nutrient deprivation of the tissues and organs.
• Sucking and breathing efforts increase metabolic demands for oxygen and exhaust the infant.
• Distention or vomiting results from air swallowed during feeding and from rapid breathing.

3. Rationales: _____

Expected outcome 2
The patient will show no signs of excess intravascular fluid or cardiac compromise.

Interventions

1. Prepare and administer cardiac glycosides, such as digoxin or digitoxin, I.V

2. Assess serum digoxin levels for evidence of toxicity and ECG changes for bradycardia. Depending on institutional policy, withhold the dose and report a heart rate of less than 100 beats/minute.

3. Prepare and administer a diuretic, such as furosemide (Lasix), to promote diuresis in the infant with heart failure.

4. Assess for the effects of the diuretic and for electrolyte losses. Note:

• administration time and degree of response
• decreases in serum sodium, chloride, and potassium levels

• increased carbon dioxide levels, as indicated by ABG or venous blood gas analysis.

Rationales

1. Cardiac glycosides increase the force of contractions, decrease heart rate, slow impulse conduction by way of the atrioventricular node, and increase renal perfusion and urine output — all of which decrease heart size, venous pressure, and edema. However, their use in preterm infants is controversial; use may be reserved for infants ages 1 to 12 months rather than neonates.

2. The therapeutic serum digoxin level ranges from 1.1 to 2.2 ng/ml (SI: 1.1 to 2.2 nmol/L). Toxicity is more common in preterm infants than in full-term infants because digoxin has a longer half-life in preterm infants. The dosage is determined more by clinical signs than by serum levels.

3. Diuretic therapy helps reduce fluid retention. In a preterm or full-term infant, diuretics may be preferred to digoxin during the 1st week after birth because of the risk of digoxin toxicity

4. The assessment data reflect the patient's response to therapy, indicate whether the dosage needs to be adjusted, reveal deteriorating patient condition, and suggest whether the drug should be given I.V.
• This information reveals the effect of the drug.
• Decreases result from electrolytes lost because of diuresis and indicate the need for interventions to maintain electrolyte balance.
• Changes in electrolyte levels may predispose the infant to acid-base imbalances. Hypochloremia causes an increase in base bicarbonate (alkalosis), and hypokalemia causes increased renal excretion of hydrogen ion (acidosis); together, they may cause metabolic alkalosis or acidosis.

5. Have sodium chloride or potassium chloride on hand to prevent hypochloremia or hypokalemia.

5. These medications are used to prevent metabolic alkalosis and replace electrolytes. *Warning: Do not administer I.V. potassium chloride rapidly because rapid administration may cause death.*

6. Prepare and administer a sympathomimetic drug, such as dopamine (Intropin) or dobutamine (Dobutrex), to treat low CO.

6. An inotropic agent improves urine output (in lower doses) or increases heart rate and contractility (in higher doses).

7. Prepare and administer sodium nitroprusside (Nitropress) or nitroglycerin (Nitro-Bid) I.V. Either may be given with dopamine.

7. A vasodilator treats severe heart failure by decreasing the heart's workload, thereby improving myocardial performance.

8. Assess patient response, and prevent adverse reactions to sympathomimetic and vasodilation therapy.
• Continuously monitor the infant's heart rate and rhythm electronically.
• Monitor blood pressure by umbilical artery catheter and transducer with continuous readings on a screen. Keep the alarm on at all times.
• Administer nitroprusside through a volume-control set with the tubing covered, and change the solution every 4 to 6 hours. Do not mix with other drugs. Change the tubing without interrupting administration.
• Make dosage changes one drug at a time.

• Have volume expanders on hand to be given I.V. during vasodilation therapy.
• Monitor serum thiocyanate levels every 2 days for nitroprusside toxicity. Also review platelet and clotting factors.

8. Continual assessment prevents adverse effects of drugs and treatment.
• Inotropic agents and vasodilators may cause tachycardia or arrhythmias.
• Accurate monitoring helps prevent hypotension from excessive vasodilation.

• A volume-control set provides safe drug administration according to agency policy.

• This action allows assessment of the patient's response to each drug.
• Volume expanders treat hypovolemia.

• Nitroprusside breakdown produces thiocyanate and cyanide, decreasing platelet count and, thus, the blood's clotting ability. The toxic level for thiocyanate is 10 mg/dl.

9. Additional individualized interventions: _____
_____

9. Rationales: _____
_____

Expected outcome 3

The patient will have a decreased cardiac and respiratory demands.

Interventions

1. Limit the infant's physical activity by minimizing handling and performing as few procedures as safely possible.

2. Maintain a neutral thermal environment by:
• monitoring temperature radially or electronically
• providing a radiant warmer or an incubator.

3. Maintain optimal respiratory function by:
• elevating the infant's head to semi-Fowler's position or using an infant seat if appropriate
• providing supplemental warmed and humidified oxygen by mask, with nasal prongs, for an adequate fraction of oxygen in inspired air
• placing a padded roll under the infant's shoulders for support.

Rationales

1. Limited handling preserves the infant's energy (needed for feeding), minimizes metabolic oxygen demands, and prevents dyspnea, which occurs with exertion.

2. Because an infant has little subcutaneous fat to maintain its body temperature, a neutral thermal environment reduces the infant's need to consume more oxygen to maintain body temperature.

3. Semi-Fowler's position decreases the infant's breathing effort by allowing greater chest expansion. Oxygen relieves cyanosis and respiratory distress, and padding beneath the infant's shoulders extends the airway to ease breathing.

4. Additional individualized interventions: _____
_____

4. Rationales: _____
_____

NURSING DIAGNOSIS

Fluid volume excess related to compromised cardiac function

Expected outcome

The patient will maintain fluid balance as evidenced by good urine output, no edema, and no sudden weight gain.

Interventions

1. Assist in promoting and assessing fluid loss by:
• weighing the infant once or twice daily at the same time and on the same scale, noting a weight gain or loss of 50 g or more
• measuring and recording fluid intake and output (including weighing diapers)
• including all methods of fluid intake and output in comparisons
• assessing the infant's response to the diuretic, noting time and amount of diuresis.

2. Limit fluid intake, if appropriate, scheduling amounts to be given.

3. Additional individualized interventions: _____
_____

Rationales

1. Daily weight is a good indicator of fluid balance. Including insensible losses, I.V. fluids given, and urine output improves your assessment. Evaluating all aspects together produces an accurate picture of the infant's fluid status.

2. Heart failure may result in fluid retention. Limits on oral and I.V. fluid intake may be required to prevent additional fluid retention.

3. Rationales: _____
_____

NURSING DIAGNOSIS

Altered nutrition: less than body requirements related to inability to ingest feedings because of dyspnea or exhaustion

Expected outcome

The patient will maintain adequate nutritional intake as evidenced by ability to take oral feedings, steady weight gain, and no increase in respiratory effort.

Interventions

1. Offer small feedings when the infant appears hungry or after rest periods.

2. Limit feedings to 30 minutes. Use a soft nipple with large holes.

3. If the infant on fluid restriction is stable enough to eat, a low-sodium formula may be indicated.

4. According to the infant's condition, provide calorie additives in oral feedings if fluid intake is restricted.

Rationales

1. Sucking requires exertion, which causes dyspnea, making feeding more difficult. Small feedings require less energy.

2. Shorter feeding times and a soft nipple allow sucking with less effort; lengthy feeding sessions stress and exhaust the infant.

3. Low-sodium formulas reduce sodium and fluid retention, although urine output and sodium excretion should occur.

4. Providing adequate calorie intake when fluids are restricted is difficult; high-calorie formulas reduce feeding volume and provide additional calories for growth and repair.

5. If the infant cannot tolerate oral feeding, prepare and administer gavage feedings until the infant's condition stabilizes enough for oral feedings.

6. Provide a pacifier during gavage, if the infant tolerates the pacifier.

7. Additional individualized interventions: _____
_____

5. Because the infant's respiratory rate may be increased or the infant may be exhausted from trying to suck, a method such as gavage might be used to meet the infant's calorie demands (see the "Respiratory distress syndrome" plan, page 297, for more information on the gavage procedure).

6. A pacifier enhances digestion, thus promoting nutrition.

7. Rationales: _____
_____

Nursing diagnosis

Ineffective family coping: compromised related to guilt and emotional crisis associated with infant's illness

Expected outcome

The parents will demonstrate appropriate coping behaviors as evidenced by decreased anxiety, ability to openly express feelings, and participation in care.

Interventions

1. Assess the parents' verbal and nonverbal expression of their anxieties and fears as well as their use of coping mechanisms.

2. Help the parents express their feelings about the intensive care nursery, neonatal care, treatments, and the acuity of their infant's condition.

3. Encourage the parents to have contact with their infant, touching it and providing care as appropriate.

4. Keep the parents updated about their infant's condition and progress.

5. Additional individualized interventions: _____
_____

Rationales

1. This assessment helps all parties identify coping strategies and develop more constructive ones.

2. Helping the parents express their feelings and concerns promotes trust and demonstrates your acceptance of their concerns and fears.

3. Parental participation in care promotes bonding.

4. Knowledge about what is happening to their infant may help decrease the parents' anxiety.

5. Rationales: _____
_____

Nursing diagnosis

Knowledge deficit (parental) related to the infant's condition, treatment, and progress

Expected outcome

The parents will receive appropriate information about their infant's condition, progress, and long-term care and express an understanding of that information.

Interventions

1. Inform parents of the following:
• heart failure's possible cause, stressing how little is known about its actual cause
• infant's condition
• current treatment and its effect
• condition's seriousness
• infant's progress.

Rationales

1. This information may relieve possible parental guilt, anxiety, and concern that they caused the infant's illness.

2. Tell the parents about the infant's medication regimen, including:
- drug name and action
- dose and times to give the drug
- how to give the drug
- adverse reactions to watch for
- what to do if the infant vomits the drug
- where and how to store the drug safely.

Give them printed information on the drug regimen to reinforce their understanding.

3. Allow time for questions; clarify information given.

4. Refer the parents to community and home health care services.

5. Additional individualized interventions: _____

2. The infant may remain on a maintenance dosage of a cardiac glycoside and a diuretic. The parents need to know how to administer and monitor drug therapy when the infant goes home.

3. Explanations and clarification reinforce the learning process, enhancing understanding.

4. These services provide continued support for the parents and family before and after discharge.

5. Rationales: _____

Documentation checklist
During the hospital stay, document:
- ❏ patient status and assessment findings, especially cardiorespiratory status and fluid volume status
- ❏ changes in patient status
- ❏ pertinent laboratory and diagnostic findings, especially X-ray, echocardiography, HCT, complete blood count with differential, and Hb, serum glucose, electrolyte, blood gas, cardiac glycoside, and (if on a digitalis glycoside) digitalis values
- ❏ nutritional status, including feeding tolerance
- ❏ activity tolerance
- ❏ patient's response to treatment
- ❏ family's reaction to the diagnosis
- ❏ parent-infant interaction
- ❏ family teaching guidelines
- ❏ discharge planning guidelines.

Associated plans
- ❏ Congenital heart disease
- ❏ Hypothermia and hyperthermia
- ❏ Preterm infant

Additional nursing diagnoses
- ❏ Activity intolerance related to exertional dyspnea
- ❏ Anticipatory grieving (parental) related to potential loss of infant
- ❏ Fear (parental) related to possible death of infant
- ❏ Ineffective breathing pattern related to tachypnea, dyspnea
- ❏ Ineffective infant feeding pattern related to exertional dyspnea
- ❏ Risk for altered parenting related to interruption of bonding process

Hyperbilirubinemia

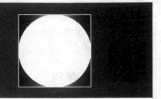

Definition

Hyperbilirubinemia is greater-than-normal amounts of bilirubin in the blood, which, when the level is high enough (5 mg/dl in a full-term infant), produces jaundice—a visible yellowing of the skin, mucosa, sclerae, and urine.

Hyperbilirubinemia results from an alteration in the normal pathways of bilirubin metabolism and excretion. Normally, after bilirubin is produced, it binds with albumin in plasma (8.5 to 17 mg of bilirubin to 1 g of albumin) and is transported to the liver in its unconjugated (indirect) form, where the enzyme glucuronyl transferase converts it to conjugated (direct) bilirubin. It is then excreted through the biliary tree into the duodenum; if serum levels become abnormally high, it is also excreted through the kidneys. In the intestine, the conjugated bilirubin is converted back to unconjugated bilirubin and absorbed by the intestinal wall into the enterohepatic circulation, which creates an additional load to be metabolized by the liver or excreted.

Because an infant's capacity to excrete bilirubin is only 1% to 2% of an adult's during the first few days of life, all infants have elevated bilirubin levels, with 25% to 50% of full-term infants and more than 50% of preterm infants experiencing jaundice.

Physiologic jaundice is the rise and fall in serum bilirubin (indirect) levels to 8 mg/dl (upper limit of 12 mg/dl) by the 4th day after birth, with a gradual decrease to less than 1.5 mg/dl by the 10th day in normal infants (about 80% of infants). Jaundice occurs from 24 to 48 hours after birth, usually because of a breakdown of erythrocytes, which have a shorter life span in an infant than in an adult (specifically, one-half to one-third that of an adult's), resulting in an increased load to the liver. In an infant, bilirubin production is 6.5 mg/kg daily, or 35 mg per breakdown of each gram of hemoglobin (Hb). Bilirubin that is not formed from erythrocyte breakdown results from the destruction of early red blood cell (RBC) forms within the bone marrow or shortly after release from the bone marrow. Deficiency of glucuronyl transferase and reabsorption of unconjugated bilirubin from the intestine may contribute to elevated bilirubin levels in physiologic jaundice.

Breast-feeding jaundice, another type of hyperbilirubinemia, occurs in 1% to 2% of breast-fed, full-term infants. It is thought to result from the inhibition of action of glucuronyl transferase by pregnanediol and a free fatty acid found in breast milk. This form of jaundice usually occurs by the 4th to 7th day after birth, with bilirubin levels rising to 15 mg/dl or more. Increased levels persist for 2 to 3 weeks before decreasing. The condition usually does not require the cessation of breast-feeding; if the infant is healthy, bilirubin levels tend to decrease without treatment and are not associated with toxic complications.

Pathologic jaundice results from conditions that increase the production of bilirubin or reduce its excretion. It usually occurs within 24 hours of birth or after the 4th day. Increased production results from hemolytic diseases, polycythemia, abnormal enterohepatic circulation, and extravascular bleeding. Decreased excretion results from decreased hepatic uptake of bilirubin, decreased bilirubin conjugation, impaired transport of conjugated bilirubin, and obstructed bile flow. Increased production and decreased excretion may result from prenatal infection or postnatal sepsis or from prematurity with associated serious illnesses. Infants of diabetic mothers may also have this condition because of the accelerated breakdown of excess RBCs produced during pregnancy. Bilirubin levels that exceed 12 mg/dl (or a much lower level in preterm infants) and that increase by 5 mg/dl or more daily (determined by gestational age and weight) indicate a pathologic process.

Bilirubin encephalopathy (*kernicterus*) results from deposits of unconjugated bilirubin in brain cells, which can result in mental retardation, behavioral disorders, delayed motor development, ataxia, and sensorineural hearing loss. Signs appear between the 2nd and 10th days after birth, with bilirubin levels exceeding 20 mg/dl in full-term infants and 10 mg/dl in preterm infants (15 mg/dl in larger preterm infants). Variations depend on prematurity and vulnerability, illness, and other factors. Exact levels at which brain damage results in any one infant cannot be determined.

This plan focuses on care of the infant who displays signs of hyperbilirubinemia with associated jaundice and on prevention of possible complications.

Etiology and precipitating factors
Physiologic jaundice

The following factors are believed to contribute to physiologic jaundice by presenting an increased load of bilirubin to the liver.
- Shortened RBC survival
- Destruction of early RBC forms
- Deficiency or decreased activity of glucuronyl transferase

• Enterohepatic reabsorption of indirect bilirubin from withholding of food and water or from late feedings, which causes intestinal stasis
• Hyperalimentation or intralipid administration

Pathologic jaundice
The following factors are believed to contribute to pathologic jaundice.
• Hemolytic diseases, such as ABO and Rh incompatibility and severe erythroblastosis, or use of certain drugs (such as vitamin K_3)
• Genetic disorders, such as galactosemia, enzyme defects, hemoglobinopathies, and spherocytosis
• Extravascular blood, such as blood swallowed during delivery, hematoma, petechiae, and cerebral hemorrhage
• Polycythemia from fetal transfusions or fetal hypoxia
• severe enterohepatic circulation from bowel obstruction or reduced peristalsis
• Decreased uptake of bilirubin by the liver, such as with decreased protein levels or from drugs competing for sites to bind to albumin (from maternal drug and alcohol abuse)
• Decreased conjugation of bilirubin from such drugs as sulfonamides, salicylates, corticosteroids, and chloramphenicol, or congenital decrease in enzyme activity
• Biliary obstruction from tumor, liver disease, or biliary atresia
• Infection in infant, perinatal or prenatal infection, toxoplasmosis, rubella, cytomegalovirus, herpes simplex, syphilis, hepatitis
• Preterm infant with or without serious illness
• Infant of diabetic mother

Physical findings
Family and maternal history
• Parent or sibling with neonatal jaundice or liver disease
• Possibly poor prenatal care
• Maternal diabetes mellitus
• Infections, such as toxoplasmosis, syphilis, hepatitis, rubella, cytomegalovirus, and herpes, which may be transmitted across the placenta during pregnancy
• Maternal or paternal use of I.V. street drugs
• Mother with Rh-negative blood and father with Rh-positive blood
• Past transfusions of Rh-positive blood if mother is Rh-negative, causing production of anti-Rh antibodies by mother's immune system
• Past abortions or deliveries of Rh-positive infant or fetus not followed by treatment with $Rh_o(D)$ immune globulin (RhoGAM) within 72 hours of delivery to destroy fetal RBCs passing into maternal circulation before they cause an immunogenic effect
• Treatment during pregnancy with $Rh_o(D)$ immune globulin if mother is Rh negative and father is Rh positive

• Medications, such as sulfonamides, nitrofurantoin, and antimalarials, taken during pregnancy
• Oxytocin-induced labor
• Vacuum extraction delivery
• Possibility that mother had phenobarbital 1 to 2 weeks before delivery to stimulate protein synthesis, provide increased binding sites, and increase activity of glucuronyl transferase (no longer considered appropriate therapy because disadvantages outweigh advantages)

Infant status at birth
• Prematurity or small for gestational age (SGA) or large for gestational age (LGA)
• Apgar score indicating asphyxia
• Delayed cord clamping
• Traumatic delivery with hematoma or injury
• Neonatal sepsis, presence of foul-smelling fluid
• Hepatosplenomegaly

Cardiovascular
• Generalized edema or decreased blood volume, leading to heart failure in hydrops fetalis

Gastrointestinal
• Poor oral feedings (refusal to take feeding or vomiting as bilirubin level rises)
• Weight loss of up to 5% in 24 hours caused by low caloric intake from delayed bilirubin conjugation
• Delay in passage of meconium or infrequent stools, causing increase in enterohepatic circulation of bilirubin
• Hepatosplenomegaly in severely affected infant with anemia or infection

Integumentary
• Jaundice (light to bright yellow hue) appearing within first 24 hours after birth (pathologic type), after first 24 hours (physiologic type), or after 1 week with breast-feeding; usually progresses from head to toe, with sclerae turning yellow before skin; in preterm infants, usually appears first on the trunk
• Pallor caused by anemia (occurs only with severe hemolysis of RBCs)

Neurologic
• Hypotonia
• Tremors, absent Moro's and sucking reflexes, diminished deep tendon reflexes with encephalopathy
• Downward gaze, irritability, elbows flexed with tight fists, rigid musculature, opisthotonic posture as central nervous system involvement progresses
• Seizures

Pulmonary
• Apnea, cyanosis, dyspnea later in kernicterus
• Asphyxia, pulmonary effusion in hydrops fetalis

Renal
• Dark-colored urine, which becomes more concentrated as bilirubin level rises

Behavioral findings
- Lethargy (kernicterus)
- Irritability (kernicterus)
- High-pitched cry (kernicterus)

Diagnostic studies
- Blood typing and Rh factor in mother and infant — to determine potential for incompatibility; the mother is screened at about 28 weeks' gestation and given $Rh_o(D)$ immune globulin if she is Rh negative
- Amniocentesis with amniotic fluid analysis — performed if indirect Coombs' test on the mother indicates increased anti-D antibody titer (1:32 or more in 4th to 5th month of pregnancy); bilirubin level in amniotic fluid increased to more than 0.28 mg/dl is considered abnormal (may indicate need for fetal transfusions)
- Coombs' test (direct) on cord blood after delivery — positive if antibodies (Rh positive anti-A or anti-B) are attached to the infant's RBCs
- Coombs' test (indirect) on cord blood — positive if antibodies (Rh positive anti-A or anti-B) are present in the mother's blood; may be done on the mother at intervals during pregnancy to measure increases in anti-D antibody titer, which suggest incompatibilities
- Serial total bilirubin levels — increase of more than 0.5 mg/hour to 20 mg/dl indicates risk for kernicterus and, possibly, the need for exchange transfusion, depending on the infant's weight and gestational age; cord bilirubin level is important, with increases of more than 4 mg/dl indicating the need for exchange transfusion, depending on whether the increase occurs 1 hour or 24 hours after delivery
- Direct bilirubin level — increased (above 1 mg/dl) with infection or severe Rh hemolytic disease
- Erythrocytes from peripheral smear — to determine numbers, immaturity, or abnormality revealing immaturity occurring with erythroblasts in Rh and spherocytes in ABO disorders
- Reticulocyte count — increased with hemolysis; level of 12% with hematocrit (HCT) of less than 40% indicates need for exchange transfusion
- Hb level and HCT — to determine concentration of Hb and percentage of RBCs in blood as Hb is released when RBCs are destroyed; HCT of less than 42% and Hb level of less than 14 g/dl with hemolysis result in anemia; Hb level in cord blood of less than 12 g/dl indicates need for exchange transfusion
- Total proteins — to determine decrease in binding sites
- White blood cell count — decreases of less than 5,000/mm³ or band forms increased to 2,000/mm³ indicate infection
- Urinalysis for specific gravity — to determine concentrating or reducing substance
- Urinalysis — to detect glucose, acetone, pH, urobilinogen, and creatinine levels

COLLABORATIVE PROBLEM
Increase in bilirubin level related to physiologic or pathologic conditions in newborn infant, placing infant at risk for long-term complications (two expected outcomes)

Expected outcome 1
The patient at risk for hyperbilirubinemia is recognized early to prevent long-term complications.

Interventions
1. Assess for infant at risk for hyperbilirubinemia, including:
- mother and infant blood types and Rh factors, Coombs' test results, prematurity, infant size (SGA or LGA), maternal illnesses or treatments that might affect the infant, traumatic delivery, severe infant illness (such as sepsis or asphyxia), family and maternal history, and infant's status at birth
- race or ethnicity

- color of amniotic fluid when membranes rupture

Rationales
1. The initial assessment performed for the infant at risk identifies abnormalities.
- Early identification of risk for hyperbilirubinemia allows preventive interventions and monitoring to ensure the infant's safety.

- Infants of Native American and Asian descent have higher mean bilirubin levels.
- Yellow amniotic fluid indicates significant hemolytic disease.

• cord bilirubin levels, reticulocyte count, HCT, and Hb levels

• Increases in the bilirubin level before 24 hours indicate pathologic hyperbilirubinemia; after 48 hours, physiologic hyperbilirubinemia. A serum bilirubin level increase of 5 mg/dl/day or more than 0.5 mg/hour or an increase in cord bilirubin level to 4 mg/dl indicates severe hemolysis or pathologic process. Increased reticulocytes and decreased Hb values and HCT are also significant and place the infant at risk.

2. Assess for physical signs of hyperbilirubinemia, including:
• jaundice (yellowish skin, sclerae, and mucosa); observe in daylight or under white fluorescent light, blanching the skin first over a bony prominence to remove capillary coloration; observe oral mucosa and conjunctival sac in dark-skinned infants
• delayed stools

2. Recognizing physical signs of hyperbilirubinemia permits timely intervention, preventing complications.
• Almost all infants develop some degree of jaundice from increased hemolysis of RBCs.

• Bilirubin that is not excreted in stool is reabsorbed and sent back to the liver in unconjugated form, creating an additional load to the liver.

• dark, concentrated urine

• Dark, concentrated urine may be observable in full-term infants with more mature kidneys as bilirubin levels rise.

• poor feeding, lethargy, tremors, high-pitched cry, and absent Moro's reflex
• vomiting, irritability, rigid musculature, opisthotonos, elbows flexed with tight fists, seizures.

• These are the first signs of bilirubin encephalopathy (kernicterus).
• These are later signs of encephalopathy, indicating the potential for permanent damage.

3. Evaluate physical signs, laboratory test results for bilirubin levels, and other changes; note whether the infant is full-term or preterm.

3. Laboratory results and signs in conjunction with infant maturity determine treatment; a full-term infant with a cord bilirubin level of 7 mg/dl at birth would be managed differently from a full-term infant with a cord bilirubin level of 7 mg/dl at 24 hours, for example.

4. Additional individualized interventions: _____

4. Rationales: _____

Expected outcome 2
The patient will exhibit no signs of complications from hyperbilirubinemia or its treatment.

Interventions

1. Provide phototherapy based on bilirubin levels, infant age (under or over 24 hours), and hospital protocol. A possible guideline is to use phototherapy for an infant less than 24 hours old if the bilirubin level is 5 to 9 mg/dl and for an infant more than 24 hours old if the bilirubin level is 10 to 14 mg/dl; check and update levels frequently.
• Note the length of time of the phototherapy as determined by the doctor, as well as the infant's age.

• Place the infant nude, except for a diaper, under special blue fluorescent lamps with a Plexiglas shield to protect the infant from ultraviolet rays.

Rationales

1. Phototherapy reduces bilirubin in the skin to a form that may be excreted in urine and feces by photo-oxidation of bilirubin to biliverdin, then to yellow pigments, and then to colorless, nontoxic compounds. Each hospital has its own protocol and guidelines for phototherapy indications.

• After an initial rise, bilirubin levels usually start to decrease after 2 to 3 days of treatment and show a steady decline.
• This setup emits the most effective wavelengths (420 to 460 nm) while reducing exposure to other light that does not treat jaundice.

• Cover the infant's eyes when under the light; remove the cover when not under the light. Use eye patches or a Bilimask; do not apply the mask too tightly.

• Monitor the energy delivered; record as watts/cm^2 over 420 to 475 nm. For a single light, measure photointensity once per shift; for two lights, check each light separately and then both lights together once per shift.

• If a fluorescent light is used, use 200 to 400 foot-candles. Turn the infant every 2 hours or as appropriate. Document the type and number of lamps, distance of lights from the infant, time of exposure, length of time each area is exposed, and the length of time the bulb is used.

• Continue with the feeding schedule.

• Remove the infant from the light when the mother visits or feeds the infant.

• Check the bilirubin level every 4 to 8 hours as ordered. (Some institutions require bilirubin checks every 2 hours.) Turn the light off when obtaining blood for testing; otherwise, a false low level may result.

2. Assess for adverse effects of phototherapy.

• Monitor temperature every 2 to 3 hours. If a thermistor probe is used, shield it from light. Use an Isolette for the infant.

• Weigh the infant every 8 hours; evaluate for a loss of 2% or more of body weight.

• Monitor urine output, specific gravity, and color every 1 to 4 hours.

• Clean the diaper area after the infant passes stool.

• Calculate fluid needs, and replace fluids according to weight loss and fluid input and output. Offer dextrose 5% in water by mouth between formula or breast feedings.

• Monitor stools for looseness and green color.

• Observe skin for color or rash every 4 hours, turning off the light to make an assessment.

• Remove eye patches every 4 hours for observation.

• Shield gonads (testes or ovaries) from light; make sure the infant has a clean, dry diaper.

• Monitor bilirubin levels as ordered after phototherapy.

• Monitor direct bilirubin levels before each phototherapy treatment, noting any increases. Report adverse effects of therapy to the doctor.

• High-density light may cause retinal injury and corneal burns. Irritation from patches may cause corneal abrasions and conjunctivitis.

• A relation exists between energy and mean rate in fall of bilirubin level.

• Types of light used vary according to effectiveness. Lamps that have been used longer than 200 hours may be ineffective.

• Feedings fulfill fluid and nutritional needs, and early feedings are thought to prevent delay in stool pattern.

• This encourages interaction and bonding between the mother and infant.

• Assessing skin jaundice alone is not accurate enough to evaluate bilirubin level decreases during phototherapy.

2. Phototherapy can cause fluid losses, hyperthermia, eye damage, and rashes.

• Elevated temperature may result from heat and dehydration.

• Weight loss may result from fluid loss from evaporation or loose stools.

• A desirable urine output ranges from 2 to 3 ml/kg/hour; green urine indicates photodegradation products that filter through the glomeruli; specific gravity indicates the degree of urine concentration.

• Phototherapy promotes the passage of stools, which can irritate the skin.

• Phototherapy lights may increase insensible fluid loss. Fluids keep the infant hydrated.

• Products of photodegradation are excreted in bile.

• Macropapular rash may occur from light.

• Phototherapy may cause conjunctivitis.

• Shielding protects the gonads from injury and skin irritation.

• The infant may have a rebound rise in bilirubin after phototherapy.

• Increased direct bilirubin level may indicate possible liver disease, which can result in bronze baby syndrome if the infant is exposed to lights. This syndrome results in bronze-tinted skin and urine; an infant with normal liver function recovers within several weeks.

3. Prepare for and assist with exchange transfusion based on bilirubin levels, infant age (less than or more than 24 hours), and hospital protocol. Check to make sure the doctor has obtained written informed consent. Possible guidelines for exchange transfusion are bilirubin levels of 10 to 14 mg/dl for an infant less than 24 hours old and bilirubin levels of 15 to 20 mg/dl for an infant more than 24 hours old.

• Assemble a disposable exchange setup with an appropriate-sized French catheter and cutdown set. Have an extra, unopened set and catheter available.
• Make sure all equipment and supplies are sterile, and maintain sterile technique during the procedure.
• According to policy, carefully check the type and Rh of donor blood for compatibility with the infant's blood. For Rh incompatibility, you may give the infant's type or type O, Rh-negative blood; for ABO incompatibility, you may give type O with the infant's Rh factor.
• Ensure that blood is less than 48 hours old and has a pH of 7.1.

• Remove cytomegalovirus-negative blood from the refrigerator 30 minutes before the transfusion and allow it to warm to room temperature. Use blood warmers to maintain blood at 98° F (3° C).
• Check the type of anticoagulant used: heparin or acid citrate dextrose (ACD)-preserved or citrate phosphate dextrose (CPD)-preserved blood.
• Have protamine sulfate ready to give at the end of the transfusion.

• Have calcium gluconate 10% ready to give (0.5 to 1.0 ml after each 100 ml of blood given) if ACD-preserved or CPD-preserved blood is used; give if irritability, tachycardia, or prolonged Q-T segment occurs.
• Have sodium bicarbonate available if needed.

• Restrain the infant with Circumstraint.

• Prepare a loading dose of albumin 25%.

• Observe as the catheter is placed in the umbilical vein or artery or the supraumbilical cutdown; X-ray verifies placement.
• Infuse a small amount of saline solution after the catheter is inserted.

• Assess bilirubin level, HCT, Hb level, and other test results on the first 10 ml of blood drawn.
• Begin with exchanges of 10 ml for the first 100 ml with increases to 15 to 20 ml if appropriate (computed by weight of the infant).
• At completion, withdraw blood for bilirubin, HCT, Hb, electrolyte, and calcium measurement and for crossmatching.

3. This process removes the infant's blood in small amounts and replaces it with compatible blood. Whole blood is given to remove circulating antibodies, replace sensitized erythrocytes, or remove bilirubin. Each hospital provides guidelines for exchange transfusion indications.

• This ensures that all necessary supplies are available.

• Sterility prevents contamination and potential sepsis or infection at the umbilical site.
• This prevents transfusion of mismatched blood and avoids hemolytic reaction.

• Older blood has high levels of potassium from hemolysis of old RBCs and may produce acidemia and cardiac arrest. Citrate content decreases pH of blood.
• Heating the blood instead of slowly bringing it to room temperature may traumatize and hemolyze RBCs close to the bag's surface. Maintaining blood at 98.6° F (37° C) prevents hypothermia or hyperthermia.
• Heparinized blood is preferred for acidosis or hypocalcemia; otherwise, ACD-preserved or CPD-preserved blood is preferred.
• Protamine sulfate is given if heparin anticoagulant is used to prevent hemorrhage from overheparinized blood.
• This prevents hypocalcemia during transfusion if symptoms appear.

• Sodium bicarbonate is given to correct acidosis if it should occur.
• Circumstraint immobilizes the infant during the procedure.
• A loading dose given 1 hour before transfusion increases the amount of bound bilirubin.
• Cutdown may be done if the catheter cannot be inserted or if infection exists in the umbilical area.

• Infusion clears the catheter and measures venous pressure, which should be 4 to 19 cm H_2O during transfusion.
• These levels must be measured before transfusion to establish a baseline.
• The total volume of blood used is twice the volume of the infant's blood; the procedure lasts for 1 hour. Blood volume at birth averages 90 ml.
• These levels must be assessed after transfusion; the bilirubin level should be half of what it was before the procedure.

4. Take measures to prevent complications of exchange transfusion.
• Use a radiant warmer and warm blankets (if needed) during the procedure, and monitor skin temperature.
• Remove stomach contents by nasogastric tube. Start an I.V. infusion of fluids.
• Attach blood pressure and heart rate monitors to the infant as indicated. Assess these signs every 10 minutes during the procedure and then every 15 to 30 minutes afterward.
• Maintain a closed system for transfusion. Monitor the stopcock for proper position during the procedure and before completion of the infusion.
• Have resuscitation equipment on hand (oxygen, suction, breathing bag, endotracheal tubes, and laryngoscope).
• Assess the infant for abdominal distention, bloody stools, pallor, hypotension, cyanosis, and vomiting, and report these signs as indicating a critical condition.
• Monitor the rate of infusion and amount infused. Adjust according to vital sign changes, and slow the rate of withdrawal and infusion if needed. If calcium is given, infuse slowly and assess for line patency.
• Assess the transfusion site for bleeding, redness, swelling, and drainage every 2 to 4 hours as needed. To prevent catheter dislodgment, restrain the infant if the catheter is left in place.
• Monitor bilirubin, glucose, and platelet values.

• Measure bilirubin levels every 4 hours after the procedure and HCT every 4 hours for 24 hours after the procedure and then every 8 hours.

• Resume feedings as soon as possible, or feed by nasogastric tube as prescribed.
• Assess for medications to be taken after transfusion.

5. Additional individualized interventions: _____
_____

4. Possibly life-threatening complications may result from the exchange transfusion.
• Extra warmth prevents hypothermia.

• Removing stomach contents prevents aspiration; I.V. fluids hydrate the infant when it is not taking feedings.
• Monitoring reveals abnormalities such as cardiac arrhythmias, signs of hypocalcemia, or hypervolemia resulting from the rate of infusion.

• A closed system prevents air from entering the catheter, possibly causing an air embolus.

• Equipment may be needed to treat cardiac arrest or another emergency.

• These are signs of intestinal perforation and, possibly, peritonitis as a result of catheter insertion.

• Too-rapid infusion or excessive replacement may result in heart failure from hypervolemia or arrhythmias from forceful infusion. Extravasation of calcium infusion causes tissue necrosis.
• These may be signs of infection, especially if the catheter is left in place for repeat exchanges; bleeding may occur with thrombocytopenia.

• The bilirubin level after the transfusion should be half of what it was before the transfusion. The platelet count is likely to decrease after the procedure. The glucose level decreases right after the procedure if heparinized blood is used and within 1 to 2 hours if ACD-preserved or CPD-preserved blood is used.
• Rebound effect caused by binding of bilirubin to fresh albumin may necessitate a repeat transfusion. Anemia may develop because remaining antibodies may continue to destroy cells.
• Feedings maintain the infant's caloric needs.

• Some medications (phenobarbital, ampicillin, and gentamicin) should not be given immediately after exchange.

5. Rationales: _____
_____

Nursing diagnosis

Altered parenting related to interruption in bonding between the infant and parents because of separation or critical condition of the infant

Expected outcome

The parents will exhibit appropriate bonding behavior as evidenced by their positive interactions with the infant, participation in care, and sensitivity to the infant's cues.

Interventions

1. Assess the parents' perception of the infant's condition and their expectations.

2. Help the parents identify and express feelings, needs, and fears.

3. Encourage the parents to visit and care for the infant as much as possible during treatment. Help them participate in:
• feeding
• holding and touching
• diapering and bathing.

4. Explain all procedures and treatments.

5. Additional individualized interventions: _____

Rationales

1. This allows you to determine their level of understanding and encourage them to set realistic expectations for the infant and themselves.

2. Discussing feelings provides an opportunity to offer emotional support to the parents and help them change parenting behaviors or interactions with the infant as needed.

3. Parental involvement reinforces bonding.

4. Information helps alleviate the parents' fear and assists with parental involvement.

5. Rationales: _____

NURSING DIAGNOSIS

Knowledge deficit (parental) related to lack of information about condition, treatments, and projected progress

Expected outcome

The parents will receive information about their infant's condition and needs and will express understanding of that information.

Interventions

1. Assess the parents' information needs and acceptance of the infant's condition.

2. Using language appropriate to the parents' level of understanding, provide information about the infant's condition, including causes, aspects of care, and expected progress.
• Explain phototherapy treatment, precautions taken, and results expected.

• Give the parents pamphlets and other written materials to improve understanding.
• Explain the need for exchange transfusion if indicated and subsequent care using monitoring devices.

• Explain that the blood to be transfused will be tested for human immunodeficiency virus.

• Keep the parents informed of daily improvements in the infant's condition.

Rationales

1. Parents may not know what information to ask for. Determining what they need to know helps you develop a realistic teaching plan.

2. This increases the parents' knowledge and understanding as well as their cooperation in the infant's care.

• Phototherapy decreases jaundice, and safety measures taken to protect their infant and prevent complications ease parental anxiety.
• Written information enhances learning and reinforces verbal instruction.
• The parents can more readily accept the need for more invasive procedures if they understand why they must be performed.
• Parental concern about acquired immunodeficiency syndrome is common when blood transfusion is mentioned.
• This promotes parents' trust in caregivers and allays their anxiety.

3. Allow time for questions and clarifications, and reinforce information if needed. Provide printed information at an appropriate level for the parents.

4. Teach the parents the signs of hyperbilirubinemia.

5. Teach the parents to use home phototherapy equipment, such as bilirubin lights and fiber-optic light blanket.

6. Refer the parents to a home health care agency for follow-up care of the infant.

7. Advise the parents to notify the doctor if jaundice appears within 4 to 7 days if the mother is breast-feeding. The condition resolves itself without complications.

8. Additional individualized interventions: _____

3. Large amounts of information may be difficult to absorb at one sitting. An opportunity to review information improves understanding, and printed material reinforces learning.

4. Learning to recognize signs improves the parents' ability to identify problems and notify the doctor.

5. Home phototherapy minimizes the need for hospitalization. Understanding the procedure and knowing how to use equipment maximize compliance.

6. Referral to a home health care agency allows additional support, follow-up, and instruction for parents.

7. Jaundice resulting from breast-feeding occurs later.

8. Rationales: _____

Documentation checklist

During the hospital stay, document:
- ❑ patient status and assessment findings, especially the appearance of jaundice, including degree and location
- ❑ changes in patient status
- ❑ pertinent laboratory and diagnostic findings, especially Rh factor; Coombs' test; serum bilirubin, glucose, total protein, and Hb levels; complete blood count; HCT; urine specific gravity and reducing substances; urinalysis for glucose, acetone, pH, urobilinogen, and creatinine levels
- ❑ patient's response to treatment
- ❑ family's reaction to the diagnosis and exchange procedure (if performed)
- ❑ parent-infant interaction
- ❑ family teaching guidelines
- ❑ discharge planning guidelines.

Associated plans and appendices
- ❑ Anemia
- ❑ Hypocalcemia
- ❑ Hypoglycemia
- ❑ Pregnancy complicated by diabetes mellitus
- ❑ Preterm infant
- ❑ Rh isoimmunization
- ❑ Sepsis neonatorum and infectious disorders
- ❑ Sexually transmitted diseases
- ❑ Normal laboratory values for the newborn (appendix I)
- ❑ Parent teaching guides (appendix J)

Additional nursing diagnoses
- ❑ Anxiety (parental) related to jaundice of infant, possible interruption of breast-feeding, potential for complications
- ❑ Diarrhea related to phototherapy
- ❑ Fear (parental) related to critical condition of infant at birth, possible death of infant from severe hemolysis and complications, acquired immunodeficiency syndrome exposure
- ❑ Ineffective family coping: disabled related to fear, guilt over condition of infant
- ❑ Risk for fluid volume deficit related to loss as result of phototherapy, reduced oral intake, vomiting, loose stools
- ❑ Risk for injury related to complications of encephalopathy leading to brain damage, adverse effects of phototherapy, complications of exchange transfusion

Hypocalcemia

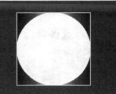

Definition

Hypocalcemia is an abnormally low level of serum calcium (7 mg/dl or less or 3.5 mEq/L or less), with symptoms occurring when levels drop below 7 mg/dl. Normally, calcium homeostasis begins soon after birth; hypocalcemia may result from the infant's reaction to stress and is usually related to normal physiology.

Hypocalcemia most commonly occurs during the first 48 hours after birth from low early-neonatal calcium levels. Preterm delivery, trauma during delivery, being small for gestational age (SGA), neonatal illness, neonatal asphyxia, and being born to a diabetic mother all increase an infant's risk for developing hypocalcemia. These conditions can result in a failure of homeostatic control of calcium partition between bone and serum.

Late-onset hypocalcemia may develop from 5 to 7 days after birth, typically from parathyroid disease. Less commonly, late-onset hypocalcemia results from hyperphosphatemia. Infants at risk for hyperphosphatemia include those taking a formula with a high phosphorus content and low calcium-phosphorus ratio (for example, unmodified cow's milk) and those with immature renal function resulting in phosphorus retention, which produces a disturbance in calcium homeostasis known as tetany of the newborn. This condition is rare because of breast-feeding and the availability of commercial formulas.

The calcium level of infants at risk for hypocalcemia should be tested daily; low levels may indicate the need supportive treatment. This plan focuses on care of the infant displaying signs of hypocalcemia, supportive treatment for symptomatic and asymptomatic hypocalcemia, and prevention of complications after discharge.

Etiology and precipitating factors

Early-onset hypocalcemia

• Preterm delivery, SGA, or low birth weight (infant has not accumulated calcium)
• Abnormal presentation, breech delivery, maternal hemorrhage, treatment with magnesium sulfate, birth by emergency cesarean section because of fetal distress, or trauma during delivery (such as use of forceps, vacuum extraction, pregnancy-induced hypertension).
• Asphyxia and associated I.V. sodium bicarbonate treatment for metabolic or respiratory acidosis (sodium bicarbonate decreases the ionized portion of serum calcium)
• Illnesses such as sepsis, hypoglycemia, cerebral injury, and respiratory distress syndrome (withholding food and water because of illness prevents oral intake of calcium)

• Diabetic mother (diabetes exaggerates the neonatal immaturity of the parathyroid because the mother has increased calcium levels that cross the placenta and increase the possibility of transient hypoparathyroid function in the infant)
• Hyperparathyroidism in the mother (causes hypocalcemia in the infant)
• Exchange transfusion with citrated blood (citrate combines with serum calcium, causing calcium to become nonionizable)

Late-onset hypocalcemia

• Use of formula with high phosphorus content and low calcium-phosphorus ratio
• Use of formula with butterfat (may cause calcium malabsorption)
• Phototherapy
• Maternal vitamin deficiency

Physical findings

Maternal history

• Prenatal conditions, such as diabetes mellitus and hyperparathyroidism
• Traumatic delivery
• Severe calcium and vitamin D deficiencies

Infant status at birth

• Preterm, SGA
• Apgar score indicating hypoxia and respiratory distress
• Transfusion of citrated blood, administration of sodium bicarbonate for acidosis, and other treatments
• Severe illness, delaying feedings
• Type of feeding (breast milk or formula)

Cardiovascular

• Arrhythmias with prolonged QT interval seen on electrocardiogram at early onset

Gastrointestinal

• Feeding intolerance or vomiting

Neurologic

• Jittery movements, hypertonicity, localized twitching, seizures
• Chvostek's sign (spasm of facial muscle elicited by light taps on facial nerve) over either cheek

Pulmonary

• Cyanosis, respiratory distress

Behavioral findings

• Irritability, high-pitched cry

Diagnostic studies
• Serum calcium level—7 mg/dl or less indicates hypocalcemia
• Ionized calcium level—decreased to less than 4 mg/dl

• Serum phosphorus level—increased in late-onset hypocalcemia to 8 mg/dl or more
• Total protein (refractometer) with serum calcium levels—increase may indicate hypocalcemia; should be measured daily in infant at risk

COLLABORATIVE PROBLEM

Risk for decreasing calcium levels and associated complications in infants at risk for hypocalcemia (two expected outcomes)

Expected outcome 1

The patient at risk for hypocalcemia will be identified early and not experience associated complications.

Interventions

1. Assess the infant for asymptomatic hypocalcemia, noting:
• maternal history and infant's status at birth

• prematurity, neonatal illnesses, traumatic delivery, maternal diabetes or hyperparathyroidism, asphyxia, and transfusion
• daily serum calcium, ionized calcium, and total protein levels.

2. Assess for signs of symptomatic hypocalcemia: irritability, vomiting, cyanosis or respiratory distress, seizure activity or twitching, incoordination of mouth and tongue movements, abnormal eye movements with blinking and staring, tonic posturing of a limb, and drooling. Review serum calcium and ionized calcium levels.

3. Additional individualized interventions: _____

Rationales

1. Infants at risk for hypocalcemia may need supportive treatment.
• Serum calcium levels fall after birth for 24 to 48 hours; then levels stabilize without symptoms.
• High-risk infants must be monitored for hypocalcemia so that they can receive supportive treatment as necessary.
• A calcium level of 7 mg/dl or less or an ionized calcium level less than 4 mg/dl with increases in total protein levels is an indication for treatment. The normal calcium level for a full-term infant ranges from 7 to 12 mg/dl (SI: 1.75 to 3 mmol/L); for a preterm infant, from 6 to 10 mg/dl (SI: 1.5 to 2.5 mmol/L). The normal ionized calcium level ranges from 4.4 to 4.8 mg/dl. The normal total protein level for a full-term infant ranges from 4.6 to 7.4 g/dl; for a preterm infant, from 4.3 to 7.6 g/dl.

2. Symptomatic hypocalcemia is life-threatening and requires immediate treatment. It is often accompanied by other problems. Serum calcium levels less than 7 mg/dl and ionized calcium levels less than 2.8 mg/dl cause signs of hypocalcemia.

3. Rationales: _____

Expected outcome

The patient exhibits normal calcium levels.

Interventions

1. Provide rest and minimize activity. Avoid suddenly moving the crib and handling or holding the infant.

Rationales

1. Unnecessary activity or stimuli may provoke tremors and seizures.

2. Prepare the asymptomatic infant for oral calcium replacements; administer calcium gluconate 10% (drug of choice) orally at a rate of 75 mg of elemental calcium/kg/day divided into six equal doses.

3. Prepare the infant with symptomatic hypocalcemia for infusion; use an infusion pump; do not mix with bicarbonate infusion. Immediate treatment consists of calcium gluconate 10% at less than 1 mEq I.V., repeated every 1 to 3 days.
• Calculate an accurate maintenance dosage if needed.

• Monitor heart and pulse rates during I.V. infusion. Discontinue infusion and notify the doctor if the infant vomits or its heart rate falls below 100 beats/minute.
• Monitor serum calcium levels daily.

4. Administer dietary calcium for prolonged or late-onset hypocalcemia, tapering off the supplement in 2 to 4 weeks. Calcium supplements of 35 to 70 mg/dl are provided in enteral feedings in the form of calcium lactate (13% calcium), calcium gluconate (9% calcium), or calcium glubionate (23% calcium) to raise the calcium-phosphorus ratio to 4:6.

5. Additional individualized interventions: _____

2. This is the treatment to replace calcium if serum calcium levels decrease to 7 mg/dl or ionized calcium levels fall below 4 mg/dl.

3. This treatment replaces calcium if levels decrease to 7 mg/dl or ionized serum calcium level falls below 2.8 mg/dl with associated symptoms.

• Treatment may continue with an I.V. infusion of up to 50 mg/kg daily for 3 days.
• Bradycardia is an adverse effect of calcium administration and indicates hypercalcemia.

• This allows detection of hypercalcemia from calcium administration.

4. Administration of calcium supplements ensures appropriate serum calcium levels.

5. Rationales: _____

NURSING DIAGNOSIS

Impaired tissue integrity related to tissue necrosis as a result of extravasation of chemical irritants from infusion

Expected outcome

The patient will exhibit no tissue damage from calcium administration.

Interventions

1. Monitor the infusion, noting:

• patency of infusion lines
• prolonged use of the same site

• precipitant in line
• movement of needle (secure with tape, if necessary).

2. Secure the line with a transparent occlusive dressing, and remove and replace the dressing carefully when changing the I.V. line (use as little tape as possible).

3. To discontinue the infusion, carefully remove the needle and apply pressure to the site for 1 minute.

4. Additional individualized interventions: _____

Rationales

1. Careful monitoring allows discontinuation as necessary to prevent tissue sloughing.
• A patent line ensures proper infusion.
• The site should be changed every 12 hours to prevent necrosis.
• Precipitant indicates incompatibility.
• Movement may cause leakage during infusion.

2. The dressing is a synthetic, transparent film that acts as a second skin, allowing view of site while protecting the skin.

3. This technique avoids extravasation of fluid into tissues during needle removal.

4. Rationales: _____

NURSING DIAGNOSIS

Knowledge deficit (parental) related to infant's condition and administration of calcium after discharge

Expected outcome

The parents will receive appropriate information about safe infant care and safe medication administration and will express their understanding of that information.

Interventions

1. Identify what the parents need to learn and their interest in and readiness for learning.

2. Provide information about:
• infant's condition and progress
• infant's need for rest (limit handling until calcium level is stable, then hold and feed)
• any supplies the parents may need to maintain the infant.

3. Teach the parents how to administer oral calcium. Make sure they:
• know the name of the medication, how to measure it, how to add it to formula or breast milk, and what formula to purchase
• understand the dosage schedule, including how to taper off the drug when discontinuing the medication
• know what adverse reactions to report, including vomiting and decreased heart rate, that may require stopping the drug
• understand that the drug may cause more frequent stools.

4. Allow for questions, clarifications, and opportunities to add the drug to formula and feed the infant.

5. Make sure the parents know how to recognize late-onset hypocalcemia. Tell them that this type of hypocalcemia seldom occurs when infants are breast-fed or receive formula that contains proper proportions of calcium. Explain that late-onset hypocalcemia:
• typically occurs 5 to 7 days after discharge
• causes twitching, hypertonicity, irritability, and abnormal eye and mouth movements.

6. Refer the parents to home health care for follow-up.

7. Additional individualized interventions: _____

Rationales

1. This provides a basis for developing a teaching plan appropriate to the parents' abilities and needs.

2. Information gives the parents confidence in their ability to care for their infant. Handling may provoke tremors and seizures.

3. Teaching promotes safe administration.

• This promotes safe administration; the drug should be given in formula.

• Abrupt discontinuation may cause rebound hypocalcemia.
• Knowing what adverse effects to report may prevent complications of hypercalcemia.

• Calcium administration commonly increases stool frequency.

4. Discussion and practice help reinforce instruction.

5. Recognizing signs helps prevent complications after discharge.

6. Referral to home health care provides parents with additional physical and emotional support and added instruction to promote compliance.

7. Rationales: _____

Documentation checklist

During the hospital stay, document:
- ❏ patient status and assessment findings
- ❏ changes in patient's status
- ❏ pertinent laboratory and diagnostic findings, especially serum calcium, phosphorus, glucose, and total protein levels
- ❏ patient's response to treatment
- ❏ family's reaction to the diagnosis
- ❏ parent-infant interaction
- ❏ family teaching guidelines
- ❏ discharge planning guidelines.

Associated plans and appendices

- ❏ Hypoglycemia
- ❏ Inappropriate size or weight: large for gestational age
- ❏ Inappropriate size or weight: small for gestational age
- ❏ Intracranial hemorrhage
- ❏ Pregnancy complicated by diabetes mellitus
- ❏ Preterm infant
- ❏ Fluid and nutritional needs in infancy (appendix G)
- ❏ Normal laboratory values for newborn infant (appendix I)
- ❏ Parent teaching guides (appendix J)

Additional nursing diagnoses

- ❏ Altered growth and development related to environmental and stimulation deficiencies or separation from significant others
- ❏ Ineffective family coping: compromised related to infant's condition
- ❏ Risk for altered parenting related to lack of information regarding infant care
- ❏ Risk for injury related to electrolyte imbalance

Infant

Hypoglycemia

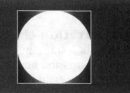

Definition

Hypoglycemia is a condition of abnormally low levels of serum glucose (25 mg/dl or less in preterm infants and 35 mg/dl or less in full-term infants). Signs can occur at or near these levels, usually between 24 and 72 hours after birth or within 6 hours of birth in a severely stressed infant. Practice dictates the need for immediate attention, either I.V. glucose administration or immediate feeding, in an infant with a serum glucose level less than 40 mg/dl. Serum glucose levels may be measured within 1 to 2 hours after birth or more frequently if the infant is determined to be at risk for hypoglycemia.

In the full-term infant, serum glucose levels usually fall to between 35 and 40 mg/dl 1 to 2 hours after birth and then rise to between 45 and 60 mg/dl within 6 hours of birth; hepatic glucose production ranges from 5 to 8 mg/kg/minute (25 to 45 calories/kg/hour). A glucose level of 40 mg/dl or more by 72 hours after birth is considered desirable, despite infant weight, gestational age, and other factors.

Hypoglycemia may be symptomatic or asymptomatic. Little correlation exists between indications and blood glucose level. Because each infant has his own "normal" level, assessment and treatment must be highly individualized to meet the infant's greater demand for glucose to maintain brain cells and decrease the risk of brain damage.

Transient hypoglycemia is common in intrauterine growth–restricted (IUGR) infants, those small for gestational age (SGA), those with erythroblastosis fetalis, preterm infants suffering from low energy reserves or an immature liver, and those with increased demands because of diseases or ineffective gluconeogenesis. IUGR infants and infants with erythroblastosis fetalis have hyperinsulinemia. These infants are screened and monitored for hypoglycemia and receive supportive treatment immediately after birth (if indicated) to reduce the potential for developing signs and complications. Hypoglycemia is also common in infants of diabetic mothers; such infants experience low glucose levels initially (1 to 2 hours after birth), followed by increases to acceptable levels by 4 to 6 hours after birth because of hyperinsulinism and increased number and activity of pancreatic beta cells. Fewer than 20% of these infants have symptoms.

The prognosis for hypoglycemia, if treated, is good; if hypoglycemia remains untreated or if the infant experiences seizures, significant sequelae can result, including cerebral damage and mental retardation. The prognosis for infants with asymptomatic hypoglycemia remains uncertain. Hypoglycemic infants with diabetic mothers do well and usually recover without complications.

Hyperglycemia may result from treatment of hypoglycemia and is defined as a glucose level of more than 150 mg/dl. It typically occurs in preterm infants receiving infusions of dextrose 10% or greater concentrations at 100 ml/kg/day. The result may be glucose levels as high as 450 mg/dl, causing osmotic diuresis or dehydration with intraventricular hemorrhage from brain volume changes (fluid shifts) and sepsis. Treatment and prevention consist of adjusting and carefully monitoring glucose infusion rates (not to exceed 8 mg/kg/ minute, as tolerated). Sick preterm infants may be given dextrose 2.5% instead of dextrose 10%; such infants have a poor insulin response to increased blood glucose levels.

This plan focuses on caring for the infant at risk for hypoglycemia after birth, providing supportive treatment, and preventing complications.

Etiology and precipitating factors

- Low economic status, little or no prenatal care
- Preterm delivery, SGA, large for gestational age (LGA), IUGR, low birth weight (infant has not had the benefit of storing glycogen)
- Illness, such as sepsis, respiratory distress, asphyxia, hemolytic disease, hypothermia, and galactosemia
- Diabetic mother
- Delayed feedings (glucose is not replaced)
- Pancreatic disorders, such as adenoma and nesidioblastosis, causing overproduction of insulin
- Administration of blood preserved with acid citrate dextrose (ACD)
- Adrenal insufficiency, causing inadequate carbohydrate-regulating hormone
- Cesarean delivery

Physical findings

Maternal history

- Little or no prenatal care
- Prenatal or gestational diabetes mellitus or pregnancy-induced hypertension (PIH)
- Poor nutrition during pregnancy
- Use or abuse of drugs, such as tolbutamide, chlorpropamide, alcohol, and street drugs, during pregnancy

Infant status at birth

- Preterm, SGA, LGA, IUGR
- Apgar score indicating asphyxia
- Such conditions as cold stress, congenital heart defects, sepsis, and central nervous system (CNS) injury
- Hypocalcemia

Gastrointestinal
- Poor or delayed feeding, refusal to suck

Neurologic
- Hypotonia, limpness
- Jittery movements, muscle twitching, tremors
- Hypothermia, diaphoresis
- Seizures

Pulmonary
- Cyanosis, respiratory distress, apnea, irregular respirations

Behavioral findings
- Lethargy
- High-pitched cry
- Irritability

Diagnostic studies
- Glucose reagent strip (as ordered) — color change indicates glucose level less than 40 mg/dl; reagent strip testing provides a more accurate glucose reading, followed by serum glucose test
- Serum glucose test — confirms concentrations by laboratory analysis of two specimens

COLLABORATIVE PROBLEM

Risk for decreasing glucose levels and associated complications in infants at risk for hypoglycemia (two expected outcomes)

Expected outcome 1

The patient at risk for hypoglycemia will be identified early and will experience no complications.

Interventions

1. Assess the infant for potential or actual hypoglycemia.

- Identify the infant's risk by assessing:
– maternal history, noting diabetes, PIH, level of prenatal care, and drug or alcohol use
– infant's status at birth
– parents' economic status.
- Assess physiologic factors that may cause hypoglycemia, including prematurity, SGA, LGA, IUGR, perinatal sepsis, neonatal illnesses, respiratory distress syndrome, asphyxia, cold stress, exchange transfusion with ACD-preserved blood, and multiple congenital anomalies.

- Warm the infant's heel to dilate vessels, and secure a capillary blood sample. Immediately test the sample with a glucose reagent strip or a reagent strip and an appropriate glucose-monitoring device.
- Test 1 hour after birth (when serum glucose levels fall) and secure blood for laboratory testing; test twice if levels are below a safe margin. If the infant is at risk, test right after birth.
- Repeat glucose level testing as indicated three times at 30-minute intervals, then two times at 2-hour intervals, and then before meals for the first 24 hours.

Rationales

1. An infant at risk for hypoglycemia may be given supportive treatment before signs appear or as indicated by assessment.
- These may identify factors that increase the infant's risk for developing hypoglycemia.

- These factors can all cause hypoglycemia. The preterm, SGA, malnourished, or sick infant has inadequate energy stores at birth. Abnormal conditions compromise or rapidly deplete an infant's existing energy stores. The LGA infant may have a mother with undiagnosed gestational diabetes or is not as easily recognized as being at risk for hypoglycemia. The preterm infant is usually the first to receive treatment for hypoglycemia.
- A sample from a cold heel may produce a falsely low glucose measurement because of stasis; levels may fall to 18 mg/dl/hour at room temperature.

- Repeat laboratory testing on an infant with a level less than 40 mg/dl provides a more accurate measurement. Relying on a glucose reagent strip alone can lead to difficulties.
- Repeat tests confirm a rise in glucose levels in a normal infant or a failure of levels to rise in a preterm infant, especially if food and water are withheld. Normal glucose levels range from 30 to 125 mg/dl in full-term infants and from 20 to 100 mg/dl in preterm infants; 40 mg/dl is the lowest level considered safe.

2. Assess for signs of hypoglycemia, including:
• irritability, tremors
• jittery movements, twitching
• lethargy or hypotonia
• irregular respirations, apnea, cyanosis
• refusal to suck, high-pitched or weak cry
• hypothermia, diaphoresis
• seizure activity with uncoordinated movements of mouth and tongue (chewing, sucking), abnormal eye movements with blinking, staring, tonic posturing of limbs, and drooling.

3. Additional individualized interventions: _____

2. The brain's requirement for glucose is continuous, decreases cause CNS symptoms and, if untreated, lead to cerebral damage and retardation.

3. Rationales: _____

Expected outcome 2

The patient will exhibit normal glucose levels and show no signs of complications.

Interventions

1. Provide early feedings. Allow the infant to breast-feed as soon as possible, and supplement breast milk with formula or an I.V. solution of dextrose 10% in water ($D_{10}W$). Offer the bottle-fed infant glucose 5% in water at birth or within 2 hours if the infant is preterm or suspected of being hypoglycemic.

2. Prepare the infant at risk for hypoglycemia for glucose infusion when indicated, using an infusion pump to regulate the rate.

3. Prepare the infant with acute hypoglycemia (a serum glucose level less than 30 mg/dl in a full-term infant) for a glucose infusion, using an infusion pump to deliver glucose at a steady rate. Administer an I.V. push dose of $D_{10}W$ at rate of 1 to 2 ml/kg (less if the infant has a diabetic mother), followed by an I.V. infusion of 100 to 200 ml/kg/day (glucose, 7 to 8 mg/kg/minute), with the rate increased according to glucose levels and the infant's response.

4. Using a reagent strip, glucose reagent strip, or serum glucose level, monitor glucose levels hourly or more frequently during therapy until the infant's condition stabilizes; verify levels every 4 to 8 hours with serum glucose measurement.

5. Maintain rest, reduce activity, and provide an optimal thermal environment with an Isolette or over-bed warmer.

6. Prepare for administration of steroids as an additional or alternative treatment; give glucagon as an emergency treatment, especially in the infant with a diabetic mother; and supply insulin I.V. as another alternative treatment.

Rationales

1. Early feedings and supplementation provide nutrition, serving as a preventive measure against hypoglycemia. If the infant is hypoglycemic, colostrum alone is inadequate for feeding.

2. Asymptomatic treatment is given to prevent hypoglycemia. Using an infusion pump to deliver glucose at a steady rate improves the response.

3. Symptomatic treatment is given for acute hypoglycemia.

4. Monitoring glucose levels prevents hyperglycemia while correcting hypoglycemia.

5. Rest and relaxation reduce the infant's energy requirements and need for increased glucose.

6. Steroids may be administered to stimulate gluconeogenesis in the liver; glucagon stimulates insulin release (usually a last-ditch effort); this is dangerous because glucose levels rise and then fall precipitously to lower levels than those measured initially. Administration of insulin would be the preferred treatment if more insulin were needed.

7. Additional individualized interventions: _____

7. Rationales: _____

NURSING DIAGNOSIS

Risk for injury related to hyperglycemic response

Expected outcome

The patient will exhibit no signs of hyperglycemia or its complications.

Interventions

1. Assess for risk factors, including:
• immaturity (less than 30 weeks' gestation with weight of 1.1 kg or less)
• age of 3 days or less
• infusion therapy with rate greater than 7 mg/kg/minute
• increased serum glucose level
• glycosuria (more than a trace).

2. Monitor infusion carefully by:
• using an infusion pump to regulate rate
• adjusting the rate to the infant's needs, usually 5 to 8 mg/kg/minute, as tolerated
• ensuring line patency and keeping the infusion site free of extravasation.

3. Monitor blood and urine glucose levels for changes.

4. Additional individualized interventions: _____

Rationales

1. Hyperglycemia is common in infants with illnesses and in immature infants who are receiving I.V. therapy because of slower insulin response and failure of decrease in liver glucose release. A serum glucose level of 130 mg/dl or more is considered hyperglycemic; a level of 450 mg/dl results in osmotic changes that lead to brain damage, intraventricular hemorrhage, and glycosuria.

2. These actions prevent hyperglycemia and tissue necrosis.

3. This is essential to determine safe glucose levels and the infant's response to glucose therapy.

4. Rationales: _____

NURSING DIAGNOSIS

Risk for altered parenting related to interruption in bonding between infant and parents caused by separation and concern over infant's condition and treatment

Expected outcome

The parents will exhibit appropriate bonding behavior.

Interventions

1. Assess the parents' perception of their infant's condition and what to expect.

2. Help the parents identify feelings, needs, and fears, and provide an opportunity for them to express their feelings.

3. Offer information about the infant's condition, progress, and behavior.

Rationales

1. Assessment clarifies what the parents need to know about their infant.

2. The parents may feel guilty, especially if the infant has other problems or abnormalities.

3. Providing timely information helps allay the parents' anxiety because the infant may not respond as they expect.

4. Allow maximal contact between the infant and parents.

5. Refer the parents to social service and community resources.

6. Additional individualized interventions: _____

_____

4. Touching and physical contact reinforce bonding.

5. The resources offer emotional and physical support.

6. Rationales: _____

_____

Documentation checklist
During the hospital stay, document:
- ☐ patient status and assessment findings
- ☐ changes in patient status
- ☐ pertinent laboratory and diagnostic findings, especially serum calcium, phosphorus, glucose, and total protein levels as well as glucose reagent strip or reagent strip results
- ☐ patient's response to treatment
- ☐ family's reaction to diagnosis
- ☐ parent-infant interaction
- ☐ family teaching guidelines
- ☐ discharge planning guidelines.

Associated plans and appendices
- ☐ Congenital heart disease
- ☐ Hypocalcemia
- ☐ Hypothermia and hyperthermia
- ☐ Inappropriate size or weight: large for gestational age
- ☐ Inappropriate size or weight: small for gestational age
- ☐ Intracranial hemorrhage
- ☐ Pregnancy complicated by diabetes mellitus
- ☐ Preterm infant
- ☐ Sepsis neonatorum and infectious disorders
- ☐ Fluid and nutritional needs in infancy (appendix G)
- ☐ Normal laboratory values for the newborn infant (appendix I)
- ☐ Parent teaching guides (appendix J)

Additional nursing diagnoses
- ☐ Altered nutrition: less than body requirements related to difficulty feeding
- ☐ Anxiety (parental) related to potential for complications
- ☐ Fear (parental) related to condition of infant at birth, potential loss of infant
- ☐ Ineffective family coping: disabling related to fear, guilt over condition of infant
- ☐ Knowledge deficit (parental) related to disease process

Hypothermia and hyperthermia

Definition

Hypothermia is an abnormally low body temperature (lower than 97° F [36.1° C]); hyperthermia is an abnormally high body temperature (higher than 99° F [37.2° C]). The risk for either condition depends on the neonate's age, weight, and general condition. Maintaining a normal body temperature is essential to extrauterine adaptation. Limited subcutaneous fat and a large body surface relative to mass predispose the neonate to an abnormal body temperature. Other factors also can alter body temperature, including an excessively warm or cold environment, insufficient brown fat, inability to shiver, reduced metabolism per unit area, and peripheral vessels that are dilated and close to the body surface.

Most of an infant's body heat is produced through nonshivering thermogenesis as a result of lipolysis of brown fat (2% to 6% of total body weight), which is located in the axillae, at the nape of the neck, around the adrenal glands, and around the great vessels. This fat has a greater concentration of energy-producing mitochondria in its cells, which enhances heat production. Full-term infants also generate heat by motor activity. Sick or preterm infants have little muscle activity; they cannot sustain contractions, have less muscle mass, and lack subcutaneous fat for heat production.

The infant's environment is affected by airflow, proximity to heat or cold, surrounding air temperature, and humidity. Heat may be lost from within the body to the body surface (internal gradient) and from the body surface to the environment (external gradient). The internal gradient may be altered by such physiologic control mechanisms as vasomotor changes, which deliver heat to the epidermis by way of blood flow from the core to subcutaneous tissues. The external gradient consists of heat loss through convection, radiation, evaporation, and conduction.

Excessive environmental temperature causes the infant's peripheral vessels to dilate, delivering heat to the skin to be lost through the body surface. The infant also attempts to remove excess heat by evaporation, through insensible water loss and visible perspiration. When the infant reaches the physiologic limits of heat loss, its temperature increases and hyperthermia results.

When the environmental temperature is too low, a normal neonate has three mechanisms to maintain its temperature: flexed fetal position (which decreases exposed surface area), peripheral vasoconstriction, and nonshivering thermogenesis. When these mechanisms fail, hypothermia results. A complication of hypothermia is cold stress. Occurring most commonly in the preterm infant, cold stress leads to hypoxia, hypoglycemia, and metabolic acidosis. These conditions are caused by the release of norepinephrine in response to chilling. Norepinephrine release stimulates the metabolism and uses oxygen and glucose to raise body temperature. Once these resources have been used up, glycogen is converted without oxygen, causing metabolic acidosis and pulmonary vasoconstriction, which lead to impaired pulmonary function from decreased blood flow and gas exchange. These conditions may be irreversible, even with rewarming. Untreated hyperthermia may lead to brain damage and death.

After birth, the infant's core temperature may drop as much as 0.2° F (0.1° C) a minute. Based on individual needs, the infant should have a neutral thermal environment, including a higher-than-normal room temperature, adjusted so that the infant has to use the least amount of oxygen and the fewest calories to maintain normal core temperature. This plan focuses on caring for the full-term and preterm infant at risk for altered thermoregulation and maintaining a neutral thermal environment.

Etiology and precipitating factors

Hypothermia
- Prematurity
- Asphyxia, with resuscitation procedures performed
- Sepsis
- Neurologic conditions, such as meningitis and cerebral hemorrhage
- Inadequate drying and warming of infant after birth (wet infant in cold environment)
- Exposure to cold environmental conditions

Hyperthermia
- Excessive environmental temperature
- Dehydration
- Infections
- Phototherapy
- Central nervous system (CNS) damage from trauma or drugs

Physical findings

Maternal history
- Difficult delivery with trauma to infant
- Drug use
- Type of anesthesia or analgesia used by mother

Infant status at birth
- Prematurity
- Low Apgar score
- Asphyxia with resuscitation
- CNS anomalies or damage
- Skin temperature lower than 97° F (36.5° C) or core temperature lower than 96° F (35.5° C) (hypothermia)
- Skin temperature higher than 99° F (37.2° C) or core temperature higher than 99.5° F (37.5° C) (hyperthermia)
- Maternal fever precipitating neonatal sepsis

Cardiovascular
- Bradycardia
- Tachycardia (hyperthermia)

Gastrointestinal
- Poor feeding
- Vomiting or abdominal distention
- Weight loss

Integumentary
- Central cyanosis or pallor (hypothermia)
- Bright (beefy) red color (hyperthermia)
- Edema of face, arms, and legs
- Cold to touch on trunk and extreme cold on arms and legs (hypothermia)
- Perspiration (hyperthermia)

Neurologic
- Feeble cry
- Decreased reflexes and activity

- Temperature fluctuations above or below normal range for age and weight

Pulmonary
- Nasal flaring or decreased, irregular, and shallow respirations
- Retractions
- Expiratory grunt
- Apneic episodes or tachypnea (hyperthermia)

Renal
- Oliguria

Behavioral findings
- Irritability
- Lethargy
- Restlessness

Diagnostic studies
- Serum glucose levels to identify decrease (glucose reserves are used in response to chilling)
- Arterial blood gas (ABG) studies to determine increased carbon dioxide and decreased oxygen levels, indicating potential for acidosis
- Blood urea nitrogen levels to identify increase, indicating impaired renal function and potential oliguria
- Electrolyte studies to identify potassium increases associated with impaired renal function
- Cultures of body fluids to identify infection

COLLABORATIVE PROBLEM

Abnormal temperature related to gestational age and weight, abnormal disorders at birth, and exposure to cool or warm environments (four expected outcomes)

Expected outcome 1

The patient at risk for potential or actual temperature instability will be identified early and demonstrate no wide temperature fluctuations.

Interventions

1. Assess risk factors for temperature fluctuations, including:
- prematurity
- sepsis and infections
- asphyxia and hypoxia
- CNS trauma
- fluid and electrolyte imbalance
- high or low environmental temperature
- trauma during delivery
- maternal drug use.

Rationales

1. Assessment offers an opportunity to detect temperature fluctuations and to intervene early to prevent complications.

2. Assess for potential or actual hypothermia or hyperthermia:
• Monitor the infant's core temperature according to institutional protocol. Take axillary temperature and apply a thermostatic skin probe. Monitor both axillary and skin temperatures every 30 to 60 minutes or as needed during rewarming or during cooling for hyperthermia, and then every 2 to 3 hours for 8 to 12 hours. Correlate axillary and skin temperatures to ensure accurate temperature readings.
• Monitor the environmental temperature hourly and record according to hospital policy, correlating the infant's temperature and the environmental temperature.

• Be alert for environmental factors that can cause infant heat loss, including cold sheets, scale, or table; wet linens or wet infant; placement near cold incubator sides or a window; exposure to drafts, cold environment, oxygen, or improper humidification.
• Check respiratory rate (tachypnea), depth, and ease.

• Observe skin for pallor, mottling, coolness, or warmth.
• Monitor for irritability, tremors, and seizure activity.

• Monitor for flushing, respiratory distress, apneic episode, skin moisture, seizure activity, fluid loss, elevated temperature, and hypotension.

3. Additional individualized interventions: _____

2. These assessment data indicate whether hypothermia or hyperthermia may develop.
• Optimal skin temperature ranges from 97.7° to 98.6° F (36.5° to 37° C) for minimal oxygen consumption, with core temperature about 0.9° F (0.4° C) higher. Axillary temperatures may be falsely high because of friction between skin and thermometer. A skin probe placed on the abdomen over the liver is the best indicator of cold stress because the probe responds to peripheral vasoconstriction.
• The nursery temperature should be regulated at about 77° F (25° C). The infant may lose heat by conduction, radiation, convection, or evaporation in response to the environmental temperature.
• These environmental factors cause heat loss from, respectively, conduction, evaporation, radiation, and convection.

• An increased respiratory rate occurs with an increased need for oxygen.
• Peripheral vasoconstriction causing these signs results from hypothermia.
• These signs of hypoglycemia result from increased use of glucose reserves.
• These signs of hyperthermia may indicate infection or overheating. An infant with an axillary temperature higher than 99.5° F (37.5° C) has hyperthermia.

3. Rationales: _____

Expected outcome 2

The patient will not exhibit wide temperature fluctuations.

Interventions

1. Carry out the following procedures at birth:
• Dry the infant immediately.
• Wrap the infant in a warmed blanket.
• Allow the mother to cuddle her infant to provide warmth.
• Place the infant under a radiant warmer; make sure it does not touch any metal or other surface until its temperature stabilizes. Do not place the infant in a draft.
• Transport the infant to the nursery in a warmed blanket or use an incubator if needed.
• Place the infant under a radiant warmer in the nursery.
• Place the preterm or full-term infant with an unstable temperature in an isolette. The infant should be naked with a warm cap on its head and a plastic wrap blanket around its body to reduce heat loss. A plastic wrap blanket prevents insensible water loss. If the infant is very immature, make sure the plastic wrap isn't sticking directly to the infant's skin.

Rationales

1. These procedures prevent heat loss, provide warmth, and prevent temperature fluctuations, especially if the nursery is a long distance from the delivery room. Core and skin temperatures decrease as much as 0.2° F (0.1° C) and 0.5° F (0.3° C) a minute, respectively, from evaporation as the infant's moist body is exposed to the cold air in the delivery room after birth.

2. To prevent heat loss while caring for the infant:
• Remove the infant from the radiant warmer and then dress it, place it in a bassinet, and cover it with blankets for 1 to 2 hours.
• Warm linens before use.
• Maintain hood temperature to deliver oxygen equal to the temperature in the Isolette.
• Dress the infant in a cap, diaper, booties, and shirt if observation is needed.
• Do not bathe the infant if it needs a heat source, or wait at least 3 hours before bathing if it does not need a heat source.
• Use portholes in the Isolette for access to the infant.
• Use an over-bed warmer with a probe when caring for the infant outside the Isolette.
• If the infant is in an open bassinet in the nursery, dress and cover it with two or more blankets.

3. Additional individualized interventions: _____

2. These measures maintain the infant's temperature and prevent cold or heat stress.

3. Rationales: _____

Expected outcome 3

The patient will maintain a normal body temperature in a neutral thermal environment.

Interventions

1. Place the infant under a radiant warmer and set the temperature dial to the desired temperature. Cover the infant with a plastic blanket when intubated, attaching a Servo-Control device to the infant's abdomen.

2. Place the naked infant in an incubator with an attached Servo-Control device.
• Warm the incubator before placing the infant in it, adjusting the temperature according to the infant's weight and age.
• Check the alarm function on the Servo-Control device, and attach the device to the infant's abdomen.
• Keep the portholes closed as much as possible.

3. If using a Servo-Control device, attach as follows:
• Place the device on the infant's abdomen (right upper quadrant) over the liver but not over bone.
• Use heat-reflective adhesive.
• Set the desired temperature.
• Keep the skin probe uncovered.
• If the infant lies prone (preterm), place the probe on the infant's back.
• Raise the incubator's side panels.

4. Alleviate hyperthermia by:
• reducing the environmental temperature
• reducing clothing and bundling
• sponging the infant gently with tepid water
• decreasing the temperature on the warming device.

Rationales

1. A neutral thermal environment permits optimal core temperature with minimal oxygen use. The amount of external heat needed depends on the infant's weight, age, maturity, and physical condition. A radiant warmer may be used for temporary warming and for procedures.

2. The incubator provides heat by convection and allows manual or automatic control of temperature. The Servo-Control device continuously monitors the infant's temperature.

3. This device is used in radiant warmers and incubators to control temperature and maintain a neutral thermal environment. It increases the environmental temperature if it detects a drop in skin temperature.

4. These measures provide cooling for the hyperthermic infant.

5. Provide an appropriate environment to prevent or alleviate hypothermia as follows:
• Move the infant from a radiant warmer to an incubator.
• Move the infant from an incubator to a bassinet or to a radiant warmer when performing procedures.
• Assess for optimal temperature hourly or as needed.
• Use a low-reading thermometer to measure the axillary temperature in a low-birth-weight infant.

6. Additional individualized interventions: _____

_____

5. Environmental support ensures a neutral thermal status.

6. Rationales: _____

_____

Expected outcome 4

The patient will not exhibit signs of cold stress.

Interventions

1. Assess the infant for signs of cold stress, including:
• drop in core temperature, as low as 90° F (32.2° C)
• early restlessness and irritability
• poor feeding and lethargy
• pallor, central cyanosis, or mottling
• skin cold to touch
• beefy red color
• bradycardia
• slow, shallow, irregular breathing with expiratory grunt
• diminished activity and reflexes
• flaccid movements and feeble cry
• vomiting and abdominal distention
• edema of face, arms, and legs.

2. Perform treatments for actual or potential cold injury as follows:
• Warm the infant slowly and record skin temperature every 15 minutes.
• Set the ambient temperature about 3° F (1.1° C) warmer than skin temperature.
• Prepare and administer plasma protein fraction (Plasmanate) over 30 minutes.
• Administer warmed and humidified oxygen.

• Monitor serum glucose levels to identify decreases.

• Prepare and administer sodium bicarbonate for metabolic acidosis.

• Withhold food and water; administer I.V. dextrose 10% in water, or supply gavage feedings until the infant's temperature reaches 95° F (35° C).

3. Additional individualized interventions: _____

_____

Rationales

1. These are signs of cold stress from extreme hypothermia. Although most signs of cold stress emphasize the infant's decreasing activity, early cold stress manifests itself in increased activity as the infant attempts to compensate with movement to increase heat production.

2. Cold stress increases oxygen and caloric metabolism.

• If the infant warms rapidly, apnea may result from increased oxygen consumption.
• This optimal ambient temperature prevents cold stress.
• Plasmanate is used when a volume expander is needed.

• This supplies oxygen if cold stress increases oxygen use.
• Detecting decreased glucose levels helps to identify hypoglycemia, which results in anaerobic metabolism; this condition in turn causes metabolic acidosis.
• Sodium helps correct metabolic acidosis and improve circulation if the infant is not responding to treatments to provide warmth.
• If the infant's temperature drops below 95° F (35° C), nothing-by-mouth status minimizes oxygen expenditure. Then alternative feeding methods provide nutrition and fluids.

3. Rationales: _____

_____

NURSING DIAGNOSIS

Knowledge deficit (parental) related to infant's condition and maintenance of appropriate body temperature

Expected outcome

The parents will receive information about the infant's condition and care needed and will express understanding of that information.

Interventions

1. Inform the parents about:
- causes of temperature fluctuation
- infant's condition
- temperature stabilization treatments
- length of time the infant is allowed out of the temperature-regulated environment
- appropriate covering and protection for infant when holding and visiting; emphasize the need to keep the infant away from drafts and to ensure that the infant wears a cap to prevent heat loss through the head's large surface area.

2. Teach the parents how to take axillary temperature and have them demonstrate the procedure.

3. If applicable, inform the parents that when the infant's weight and condition allow, it will be weaned from the incubator before going home.

4. Encourage questions, requests for clarifications, and demonstrations.

5. Additional individualized interventions: _____

_____

Rationales

1. Informing the parents helps relieve their anxiety and concern about their infant's condition. Teaching them heat conservation procedures ensures that the infant will be appropriately protected when they care for it.

2. This allows the parents to obtain an accurate temperature reading and thus monitor increases or decreases in temperature.

3. Weaning the infant from the incubator allows the infant's temperature to be reduced safely to that of the nursery.

4. Honest and open discussion promotes better understanding.

5. Rationales: _____

_____

Documentation checklist

During the hospital stay, document:
- ❏ patient status and assessment findings, especially temperature
- ❏ changes in patient status
- ❏ pertinent laboratory and diagnostic findings, especially serum glucose and electrolyte, ABG, and blood urea nitrogen levels and the results of any cultures that were done
- ❏ patient's response to treatment, including either cooling or rewarming
- ❏ family's reaction to the diagnosis
- ❏ parent-infant interaction
- ❏ family teaching guidelines
- ❏ discharge planning guidelines.

Associated plans

- ❏ Anemia
- ❏ Hypoglycemia

- ❏ Inappropriate size or weight: small for gestational age
- ❏ Intracranial hemorrhage
- ❏ Preterm infant
- ❏ Sepsis neonatorum and infectious disorders

Additional nursing diagnoses

- ❏ Altered peripheral tissue perfusion related to cold stress
- ❏ Hyperthermia related to exposure to hot environment
- ❏ Hypothermia related to exposure to cool environment, illness or trauma, inability to shiver
- ❏ Ineffective thermoregulation related to immaturity, fluctuating environmental temperature
- ❏ Risk for fluid volume deficit related to loss from radiant warmer

Inappropriate size or weight: Large for gestational age

Definition
Infants who are large for gestational age (LGA) include those with birth weights above the 90th percentile on the intrauterine growth chart at any gestational week, regardless of whether they are preterm, full term, or postterm. A full-term or preterm infant who weighs 8 lb, 13 oz (4,000 g) or more is considered LGA. The mortality rate is higher for LGA infants if delivery is difficult and cesarean birth is necessary, which may lead to trauma and other complications during birth. Postterm infants are those born after 42 weeks' gestation, regardless of birth weight. They appear long, thin, and wasted and resemble infants that are 1 to 3 weeks old. Cesarean birth or labor induction usually is performed to avoid the risks associated with overdue birth, including hypoxia and meconium aspiration associated with placental insufficiency.

This plan focuses on identifying and caring for the LGA infant and preventing complications associated with this condition.

Etiology and precipitating factors
• Mother with diabetes mellitus
• Large maternal size, overeating, excessive weight gain during pregnancy
• Genetic predisposition to large size
• Erythroblastosis fetalis, transposition of great vessels, Beckwith's syndrome (genetic condition associated with neonatal hypoglycemia and hyperinsulinism)

Physical findings
Maternal history
• Diabetes mellitus, pregnancy-induced hypertension, or vascular or renal disease
• Poor nutritional status (being overweight or having excessive weight gain during pregnancy)
• Multiparity or past delivery of LGA infants
• Possibly miscalculation of expected date of confinement (EDC)
Infant status at birth
• High birth weight or length or both
• Cesarean birth or oxytocin-induced labor
• Low Apgar score

• Asphyxia or use of resuscitation
• Birth trauma from use of midforceps and difficulty in delivery, causing shoulder dystocia, fractured clavicle, depressed skull fracture, facial paralysis, or brachial plexus palsy
• Congenital heart defect, including transposition of great vessels
• Congenital anomalies
Gastrointestinal
• Poor feeding and bloated, prominent abdomen
• Weight greater than 8 lb, 13 oz (4,000 g)
Integumentary
• Reddish complexion or possibly jaundiced appearance
• Obese, plump-looking, with generous fat deposits; plethoric fat deposits in infant of diabetic mother
• Loose, baggy look in postterm infant (from use of fat for energy)
• Dry, peeling, skin that is parchmentlike and long nails in the postterm infant
• Hematoma resulting from traumatic birth
Pulmonary
• Sighing respirations

Behavioral findings
• Listlessness

Diagnostic studies
• Glucose reagent strip or reagent strip by heelstick to identify glucose levels less than 40 mg/dl within 1 to 2 hours after birth; test repeated frequently for 2 days after birth
• Serum glucose measurement to identify and confirm decreases if glucose reagent strip or reagent strip results are below normal
• Serum bilirubin levels to check for increase resulting from additional load to liver caused by breakdown of blood from hematoma, hemorrhage caused by birth trauma, or polycythemia associated with hypoxia
• Serum calcium levels to check for decrease 1 to 3 days after birth

COLLABORATIVE PROBLEM

Risk for complications from physiologic changes associated with LGA status, with or without diabetic mother (two expected outcomes)

Expected outcome 1

The patient will exhibit no complications from being LGA.

Interventions

1. Assess the infant for risk factors, including:

• maternal diabetes mellitus, possibly miscalculated EDC, large maternal size, excessive maternal weight gain during pregnancy

• low Apgar score, asphyxia, respiratory distress syndrome, bone fractures, soft-tissue paralysis, and congenital anomalies

• increased bilirubin level and red blood cell count

• decreased glucose levels in capillary blood sample taken from lateral aspect of heel; to measure, warm heel for 15 minutes and test immediately with glucose reagent strip or reagent strip and meter, using fresh reagent strip and accurate glucometer; continue strip testing for 2 to 3 days after birth with serum glucose analysis if levels fall below 40 mg/dl

• signs of hypoglycemia, such as twitching, lethargy, irritability, apnea, hypothermia, and seizures

• decreases in serum calcium levels.

2. Additional individualized interventions: _____

Rationales

1. Because of their size, LGA infants often are not considered at risk for complications. However, they need careful assessment and close attention because their mortality rate is higher than that for average-size infants.
• LGA infants have a higher mortality rate and higher risk for complications; those with diabetic mothers also have a higher risk for abnormalities unless they are delivered before EDC.
• LGA infants are prone to these problems because of intrauterine stress caused by decreased placental efficiency and delivery difficulty because of their large size or premature status if delivered early (an elective procedure; may be used for the infant of a diabetic mother).
• Increases because of polycythemia in infants of diabetic mothers are thought to be associated with hypoxia, which causes blood hyperviscosity. This increases the risk for cardiopulmonary and circulatory congestion and emboli.
• A sample from an unwarmed heel may lead to an underestimation of the glucose level. Because of stasis, the level may fall as much as 18 mg/dl/hour at room temperature. When glucose reagent strip or reagent strip testing reveals glucose levels less than 40 mg/dl, glucose measurement should be repeated by laboratory analysis to confirm an accurate reading. This double testing should not delay treatment.
• In infants of diabetic mothers, a state of hypoglycemia exists 2 to 4 hours after delivery. When the glucose supply from the mother is removed at birth, insulin production continues and depletes the existing glucose level; these sudden drops may cause neurologic symptoms and central nervous system damage.
• Decreased calcium levels occur after delivery and may be accentuated in infants of diabetic mothers with asphyxia. A measurement of less than 7 mg/dl indicates hypocalcemia.

2. Rationales: _____

Expected outcome 2
The patient will maintain physiologic stability.

Interventions

1. Maintain respiratory function by:

• noting and reporting abnormalities in respiratory rate, depth, or ease; respiratory distress; and cyanosis

• suctioning nasopharyngeal area as appropriate

• providing vibration, percussion, and postural drainage if indicated
• providing warm, humidified oxygen

• monitoring arterial blood gas (ABG) results.

2. Maintain nutritional status by:
• initiating feedings, as tolerated, as soon as possible after birth
• weighing the infant daily and evaluating its weight in light of calorie intake and fluid intake and output

• providing treatment for hypoglycemia or hypocalcemia, as indicated, based on blood glucose and serum calcium levels.

3. Maintain a neutral thermal environment for the infant.

4. Take steps to prevent complications from birth trauma by:
• noting birth injuries, such as hematoma, paralysis, and fractures

• monitoring serum bilirubin levels for increases.

5. Additional individualized interventions: _____

Rationales

1. Maintaining adequate respiratory function prevents hypoxia.
• Infants who have asphyxia at birth or decreased surfactant levels or whose mothers have diabetes are more likely to have respiratory distress. The infant delivered by cesarean birth is at risk for wet lung.
• Suctioning ensures airway patency by removing potential obstructions.
• These interventions mobilize secretions for removal.

• This action promotes adequate oxygenation; humidified oxygen helps prevent drying of the mucous membranes; warm oxygen minimizes heat loss.
• Monitoring ABG levels identifies the potential for hypoxemia and hypercapnia, which lead to acidosis.

2. Physiologic stability requires adequate nutrition.
• Feedings prevent hypoglycemia and provide for nutritional needs.
• Monitoring the infant's weight and fluid intake and output ensures that calorie and fluid needs are met and helps prevent fluid imbalance.
• This prevents continuing decreases in glucose and calcium levels, which may lead to brain damage (see the "Hypoglycemia" plan, page 242, and the "Hypocalcemia" plan, page 237, for administration of medications and treatment).

3. A neutral thermal environment assures metabolic stability and prevents hypothermia and hyperthermia, both of which increase the infant's energy needs.

4. Birth trauma can cause physiologic complications.

• Most injuries caused by traumatic birth resolve within 2 to 3 days. Severe injuries that involve nerves or the spinal cord require more complex medical and nursing care.
• Hyperbilirubinemia is possible in infants with hematoma because the breakdown of blood from bleeding adds to the liver's bilirubin load.

5. Rationales: _____

Nursing diagnosis

Knowledge deficit (parental) related to infant's condition and care

Expected outcome

The parents will receive appropriate information about the infant's condition and growth pattern and will express understanding of that information.

Interventions

1. Inform the parents about:

• infant's condition and progress toward stability

• infant's feeding and nutritional needs

• effects of trauma during delivery; explain that effects usually are temporary.

2. Answer questions and clarify information as needed.

3. Encourage the parents to have physical contact with their infant, allowing them to participate in the infant's care.

4. Additional individualized interventions: _____

Rationales

1. Information allays parental anxiety and enhances infant care.
• Information about the infant's condition and progress reduces parental anxiety and concerns.
• This ensures that the parents will understand how to provide their infant with the proper nutrients to replace deficiencies.
• Obvious bruising, paralysis, or fractures increase parental fear about the loss of the "perfect child."

2. This promotes better understanding.

3. Contact with their infant reinforces bonding and increases their ability to care for the infant.

4. Rationales: _____

Documentation checklist

During the hospital stay, document:
❏ patient status and assessment findings, including pertinent maternal history and Apgar scores
❏ changes in patient status
❏ pertinent laboratory and diagnostic findings, especially serum glucose, calcium, and bilirubin levels and glucose reagent strip or reagent strip results
❏ patient's response to treatment
❏ family's reaction to the diagnosis
❏ parent-infant interaction
❏ family teaching guidelines
❏ discharge planning guidelines.

Associated plans

❏ Cesarean section birth
❏ Congenital heart disease
❏ Drug addiction and withdrawal
❏ Hyperbilirubinemia
❏ Hypocalcemia
❏ Hypoglycemia
❏ Hypothermia and hyperthermia
❏ Meconium aspiration syndrome
❏ Pregnancy complicated by diabetes mellitus

Additional nursing diagnoses

❏ Ineffective family coping: compromised related to fear, guilt
❏ Risk for impaired skin integrity related to trauma during difficult delivery
❏ Risk for injury related to difficult delivery of LGA infant

Inappropriate size or weight: Small for gestational age

Definition

A neonate is considered small for gestational age (SGA) if its birth weight is below the 10th percentile on the intrauterine growth chart at any week of gestation, whether preterm, full term, or postterm. A more definitive description of an SGA or intrauterine growth–restricted (IUGR) infant is based on deviation from mean weight, length, and head circumference for a particular gestational age, as follows:

• mild IUGR—weight more than two standard deviations below mean with a reduced weight-to-length ratio
• moderate IUGR—weight-to-length ratio greater than two standard deviations below mean
• severe IUGR—weight-to-length ratio and head circumference all greater than two standard deviations below mean. A full-term infant weighing 5 lb, 8 oz (2,500 g) or less fits into the IUGR category.

Early in fetal development, all growth is the result of increases in cell number (hyperplasia). Cells are fewer in number in IUGR but normal in size, causing below-normal growth. Later in fetal development, cells increase in size (hypertrophy) and are normal in number in IUGR and SGA infants. Outcome and appearance of the infant at birth depend on the period (early or late development) of intrauterine insult to the fetus.

Maternal, placental, and fetal factors may all contribute to SGA, low birth weight (LBW), and IUGR problems in newborn infants. Whether the infant is labeled as SGA, LBW, or IUGR is determined during the assessment for gestational age done on all neonates, using the Dubowitz or a similar system and plotting the information on the Denver intrauterine growth curve.

The prognosis depends on the cause, severity, and duration of the intrauterine insult to the fetus and on the care the infant receives after birth. The mortality rate decreases as gestational age increases and increases as birth weight decreases, except for postterm infants, whose mortality and morbidity increase greatly past 42 weeks.

This plan focuses on identifying and caring for the SGA infant and preventing complications associated with this condition. It also applies to infants who are LBW (less than 2,500 g) regardless of gestational age.

Etiology and precipitating factors

• Genetic factors (small or short parents, chromosomal abnormalities, multiple anomalies, anencephaly)
• Multiple fetuses
• Maternal malnutrition
• Maternal use of alcohol, cigarettes, or narcotics or mother living in high altitude
• Maternal infection, such as sexually transmitted infections
• Placental insufficiency caused by diabetes, renal disease, pregnancy-induced hypertension (PIH), hypertension unrelated to pregnancy
• Congenital anomalies
• Maternal use of medications, such as antimetabolites and anticonvulsants
• Congenital fetal infections and inborn errors of metabolism

Physical findings
Maternal history

• Small stature or history of SGA infants in family
• Mother's age (adolescent or advanced)
• Poor prenatal care or nutrition, low socioeconomic status
• Conditions such as diabetes, heart disease, renal hypertension, PIH, or sexually transmitted infections
• Such disorders as placenta previa and abruptio placentae
• Use of alcohol, cigarettes, narcotics, or other drugs in the past or during pregnancy

Infant status at birth

• One of multiple births
• Low Apgar score, asphyxia, use of resuscitation, acidosis
• Possibly wasted appearance, with smaller body parts and asymmetry
• Weight, length, and head circumference disproportionate
• Congenital or chromosomal anomalies

Gastrointestinal

• Sunken abdomen
• Possibly hungry appearance, with sucking of hands or clothing

Integumentary

• Pale, dry skin
• Sparse hair
• Loose, baggy skin and widened skull sutures

Musculoskeletal

• Lack of adipose tissue and poor muscle growth on trunk, arms, and legs, with long, thin appearance

Neurologic

• Possible flaccidity or activity
• Hypothermia

Pulmonary

• Tachypnea, gasping respirations, crackles, or cyanosis if meconium aspiration occurred

Behavioral findings
• Lethargy
• Vigorous cry
• Alertness

Diagnostic studies
• Chest X-ray to determine pulmonary complications associated with asphyxia, such as pneumonia, pneumothorax, or aspiration
• Nonstress test to monitor placental function (performed weekly)
• Maternal serial estriol levels — decrease if placenta is dying, resulting in poor intrauterine environment
• Heelstick glucose measurement — may drop to 40 mg/dl within 1 to 2 hours after birth and frequently for 2 to 3 days after birth; reagent strip testing with glucometer provides more accurate glucose measurements
• Serum glucose measurement — verifies heelstick measurement (should be performed on two specimens)

• Hemoglobin (Hb) level and hematocrit (HCT) — Hb level increases to 20 g/dl and HCT increases to 70% in polycythemia (increased viscosity)
• Bacterial and viral cultures and screen for sexually transmitted infections — may indicate infection
• Bilirubin levels — increase in polycythemia associated with hypoxemia
• Immunoglobulin (Ig; especially IgM and IgG) levels — may increase if infection is present; associated findings include a change in white blood cell count, decreased platelet count and, possibly, abnormal prothrombin time or partial thromboplastin time
• Arterial blood gas (ABG) levels — oxygen levels decrease and carbon dioxide levels increase in asphyxia
• Serum electrolyte levels — sodium and calcium levels may decrease

COLLABORATIVE PROBLEM

Risk for complications caused by physiologic changes associated with SGA infant (two expected outcomes)

Expected outcome 1

The infant at risk for being SGA will exhibit no complications.

Interventions

1. Assess the infant at risk:

• Review maternal history and delivery events.

• Note low Apgar score, asphyxia, meconium-stained skin, nails, or fluid (amniotic fluid or meconium in upper airway at birth); monitor respirations every 4 hours for tachypnea, gasping, and cyanosis, which indicate respiratory distress.
• Look for signs of hypoglycemia, such as twitching, lethargy, irritability, apnea, hypothermia, and seizure activity. Secure a blood sample for immediate glucose testing; to do so, warm the infant's heel for 15 minutes to dilate vessels and take the sample from the lateral aspect of the heel. Repeat the test every 3 to 4 hours.

• Assess for hypothermia by measuring axillary temperature every 2 to 3 hours; note cold skin, lethargy, and poor feeding.

Rationales

1. Anticipating and recognizing complications in an infant who is LBW, SGA, and IUGR allow for preventive measures to ensure the infant's stability.
• Maternal conditions predispose the infant to complications.
• Asphyxia may be due to hypoxia in utero or during labor, causing the fetus to pass meconium and producing meconium aspiration or other respiratory disorders. Preterm infants are not meconium-stained but still may have significant asphyxia.
• Lack of glycogen stores at birth may cause hypoglycemia within 48 to 72 hours. Glucose levels should be maintained between 40 and 120 mg/dl; if levels are low, two serum glucose tests should be done in laboratory for accurate assessment. Drops in glucose levels may cause neurologic symptoms and central nervous system (CNS) damage.
• Hypothermia may result from reduced glycogen and fat stores, decreasing the infant's ability to maintain normal heat and reducing its energy level.

• Measure red blood cell (RBC) count and HCT at birth and as needed, and check skin for pallor, petechiae, bruising, and bleeding at I.V. sites; these are indications of polycythemia.

• Check vital signs, peripheral pulses, and capillary refill.

2. Additional individualized interventions: _____

_____

• This potential complication is caused by a prolonged lack of oxygen in utero, sometimes creating a need for partial exchange or plasmapheresis transfusion using plasma in exchange for the infant's blood to reduce viscosity and maintain HCT below 65% on a central venous — not arterial — blood sample.
• Changes in vital signs and vascular status may signal complications.

2. Rationales: _____

_____

Expected outcome 2

The patient maintains physiologic stability.

Interventions

1. Maintain respiratory function by:

• preparing for immediate resuscitation at birth

• suctioning the nasopharynx, as needed

• providing warm, humidified oxygen with a hood, a mask, or mechanical ventilation, as appropriate
• monitoring ABG and pH levels

• providing chest physiotherapy and postural drainage.

2. Maintain nutritional status by:
• initiating feedings as soon as possible, within 4 hours after birth, if asphyxia is not present or if food and water have been withheld for 24 hours and the infant is receiving I.V. feeding
• weighing the infant at the same time on the same scale daily and comparing weight with caloric intake
• monitoring fluid intake and output at least every 4 hours
• preparing to give dextrose 10% to 12.5% I.V. to the infant with asphyxia who cannot be fed orally.

3. Maintain a neutral thermal environment by:
• placing the infant in an Isolette and checking and adjusting the temperature every 2 to 3 hours
• avoiding drafts and placing the infant on cold surfaces
• using additional blankets, if needed
• warming the infant gradually and monitoring for hyperthermia.

4. Maintain circulatory status by:
• preparing and assisting with exchange transfusion
• monitoring bilirubin level every 8 hours
• initiating phototherapy, if indicated (see the "Hyperbilirubinemia" plan, page 228).

5. Additional individualized interventions: _____

Rationales

1. Adequate respiratory function supports physiologic stability.
• Neonatal asphyxia is common in SGA infants, so anticipate respiratory distress in infants at risk.
• Suctioning ensures airway patency by removing potential obstruction.
• This action prevents gas exchange imbalances that could lead to respiratory acid-base problems.
• Monitoring identifies the potential for hypoxia, hypercapnia, and acidosis.
• Respiratory physiotherapy enhances mobilization and removal of secretions.

2. Adequate nutrition is essential to physiologic stability.
• Early feedings prevent continued weight decreases, with potential for hypoglycemia and hypocalcemia. The infant with asphyxia needs to rest the gut before feeding because it may have suffered an anoxic episode to the gut.
• Daily weighing measures whether caloric and fluid needs are being met.
• An accurate comparison is important to maintaining fluid balance with increased fluids.
• I.V. dextrose prevents hypoglycemia by maintaining the infant's glucose level.

3. These precautions prevent hypothermia by maintaining a temperature of 97° to 99° F (36.1° to 37.2° C). Because SGA infants do not have adequate fat stores and adipose tissue for insulation, they are prone to hypothermia, which produces feeding intolerance. Proper monitoring of temperature and equipment prevents hyperthermia. Thermoregulation is difficult because SGA infants cannot conserve body heat.

4. Polycythemia may result from stimulation of RBC production by a hypoxic condition. The increased production of RBCs increases the bilirubin load to the liver and causes jaundice with possible CNS involvement.

5. Rationales: _____

_____

Nursing diagnosis

Knowledge deficit (parental) related to infant's condition and care

Expected outcome

The parents will receive appropriate information about the infant's condition and growth patterns and will express understanding of that information.

Interventions

1. Keep the parents informed:
• Review the infant's condition and progress toward stability, and reinforce the doctor's teaching about the cause and effect of the underlying problem.
• Review the infant's feeding, nutritional needs, and potential for normal weight pattern.

• Give rationales for the treatments needed and for follow-up care.

2. Listen to parental questions and clarify information.

3. Encourage the parents to have physical contact with the infant, and allow them to participate in the infant's care.

4. Refer parents to community services for follow-up.

5. Additional individualized interventions: _____

_____

Rationales

1. Information about the infant reduces parental anxiety.
• Information about the SGA infant's condition, progress, and diagnosis helps reduce parental concern about the infant's welfare.
• Some SGA infants have a large initial weight deficit to make up in the first 6 months, unless a complicating condition exists.
• The infant may need follow-up care to maintain its status.

2. Information enhances parental understanding.

3. Participating in the infant's care reinforces bonding and increases the parents' confidence in their ability to care for their infant.

4. These services provide additional support before and after the infant's discharge.

5. Rationales: _____

_____

Documentation checklist

During the hospital stay, document:
❏ patient status and assessment findings — Apgar scores, weight, length, head circumference, skin and adipose tissue appearance, neurologic status, maternal history (height, family history of SGA infants, medications taken and infections contracted)
❏ changes in patient status
❏ pertinent laboratory and diagnostic findings — chest X-rays; heelstick glucose results; HCT; Hb, serum bilirubin, IgM, ABG, serum electrolyte, glucose, and calcium levels; complete blood count with differential; and viral and bacterial cultures for sexually transmitted infections
❏ patient's response to treatment
❏ family's reaction to diagnosis
❏ parent-infant interaction
❏ family teaching guidelines
❏ discharge planning guidelines.

Associated plans

❏ Heart disease
❏ Hyperbilirubinemia
❏ Hypoglycemia

❏ Hypothermia and hyperthermia
❏ Inappropriate size or weight: large for gestational age
❏ Meconium aspiration syndrome
❏ Multiple gestation
❏ Preterm infant
❏ Sexually transmitted diseases

Additional nursing diagnoses

❏ Altered nutrition: less than body requirements related to LBW, malnutrition, nothing-by-mouth status, I.V. fluid support, low glycogen and fat stores at birth
❏ Hypothermia related to malnutrition
❏ Impaired gas exchange related to altered oxygen supply (hypoxia)
❏ Ineffective family coping: compromised related to fear, guilt
❏ Risk for altered parenting related to infant's need for specialized care
❏ Risk for injury related to future growth patterns, immune factors leading to infection, abnormal blood profile leading to circulatory deficiencies, hyperbilirubinemia, altered clotting factors

Intracranial hemorrhage

Definition

Intracranial hemorrhage is bleeding within the cranium that affects the brain. Arising during the perinatal period, it typically occurs in preterm infants.

Periventricular/intraventricular hemorrhage (P/IVH) is bleeding from capillaries in tissue adjacent to the ventricular wall (germinal matrix) that remains in place or bursts into the cerebrospinal fluid (CSF) and circulates into the ventricular system. These fragile capillaries can rupture from hypoxia or ischemia in the brain. If CSF flow becomes obstructed, the ventricles dilate from the accumulation of fluid and pressure. If the obstruction is not relieved, hydrocephalus may result. The most common type of intracranial hemorrhage that arises during the neonatal period, P/IVH is a major cause of morbidity and mortality in infants. It is the most serious and most common neurologic disorder in preterm infants, seen almost exclusively in those who are born at less than 32 weeks' gestation or who weigh less than 3 lb, 5 oz (1,500 g).

Primary subarachnoid hemorrhage—bleeding into the subarachnoid space without involving other areas— occurs predominantly in preterm infants. The condition may be mild, with complete recovery expected within 1 week of life, or severe and associated with neural damage. The prognosis depends on the extent of the injury.

Subdural hemorrhage, occurring most frequently in the full-term infant 1 week or later after birth, is bleeding in the subdural space related to tearing of the dural sinuses or small superficial cerebral veins. Signs and symptoms may be mild or severe and are caused by the localized, space-occupying accumulation of subdural fluid. The prognosis depends on the severity and extent of tearing.

This plan focuses on caring for the infant with mild or severe intracranial hemorrhage and preventing neurologic damage.

Etiology and precipitating factors

- P/IVH
  - prematurity
  - hypoxia and ischemia to the brain from pregnancy-induced hypertension (PIH), maternal drug addiction or therapy, placental insufficiency, or birth trauma
  - respiratory distress syndromes, pneumothorax, sepsis, or positive-pressure ventilation, causing increased venous pressure
  - increased cerebral blood flow from excess fluid or volume expanders, vasopressors, surfactant, and hy-

perosmolar drugs, such as sodium bicarbonate, that cause fluid shift and pressure on cerebral capillaries when given in improper dilution
  - coagulopathies
- Subarachnoid hemorrhage
  - birth trauma
  - asphyxia
  - prolonged or difficult labor
  - fetal distress
- Subdural hemorrhage
  - mechanical trauma from difficult delivery of the head, causing tearing of the dural sinuses, superficial cerebral veins, or tentorium
  - bleeding from coagulation problems or thrombocytopenia
  - shaken baby syndrome

Physical findings

Maternal history
- Such conditions as diabetes and PIH
- Drug use, history of addiction

Infant status at birth
- Prematurity or postmaturity
- Low Apgar score showing asphyxia
- Head trauma from birth

Cardiovascular
- Decreased blood pressure in P/IVH
- Sudden decrease in hematocrit (HCT)

Integumentary
- Abrasions or hematoma on the head in subdural or subarachnoid hemorrhage

Neurologic
- Mild P/IVH
  - possibly asymptomatic
  - hypotonia or intermittent opisthotonos
  - focal seizures that pass rapidly
  - head enlargement with increase in circumference, tightness of anterior fontanel, or separation of sutures in 1 to 2 weeks
- Severe P/IVH
  - temperature difficult to maintain
  - cyanosis and severe hypotonia
  - increased intracranial pressure (ICP)
  - seizures after hemorrhage onset or within a few hours; the time of seizure onset tells if bleeding occurred before, during, or after birth
- Mild subarachnoid hemorrhage
  - possibly asymptomatic
  - hypotonia

- Severe subarachnoid hemorrhage
  - hypotonia, hyporeactivity
  - seizures for several days
- Subdural hemorrhage
  - usually asymptomatic in neonatal period

Pulmonary
- Apnea or cyanosis in severe P/IVH and, if infant is preterm, in subarachnoid hemorrhage
- Irregular breathing

Behavioral findings
- Lethargy
- Irritability
- High-pitched cry

Diagnostic studies
- Computed tomography (CT) scan — to reveal type of intracranial hemorrhage
  - In P/IVH, CT scan shows high-density cast. Lesions are graded from I to IV (least to most severe). The procedure necessitates moving the infant to the radiology department; if the infant is on a ventilator, this is inadvisable.
  - In subarachnoid hemorrhage, lumbar puncture reveals blood in the CSF. A CT scan reveals increased ventricular size.
  - In subdural hemorrhage, a CT scan reveals fluid accumulation.
- Transillumination — to reveal abnormalities
- Cranial ultrasonography (when P/IVH is suspected) — to detect bleeding; the test must be performed within 2 weeks of bleeding to detect it; otherwise, bleeding resolves, leaving no abnormality or increased ventricular size
- CSF studies identify bleeding; CSF may be red-brown, indicating old blood from past P/IVH
- HCT identifies falls from 20% to 60%, indicating P/IVH
- Arterial blood gas (ABG) studies detect hypercapnia and hypoxemia even with ventilatory support in P/IVH

COLLABORATIVE PROBLEM

Risk for neurologic impairment related to intracranial hemorrhage caused by trauma, asphyxia, hypoxia, or ischemia (three expected outcomes)

Expected outcome 1

The patient will exhibit no signs of intracranial hemorrhage or alterations in neurologic status.

Interventions

1. Assess the infant for changes in neurologic function, including:
- apnea or irregular respirations
- decreased activity or hypotonia
- decreased spontaneous and elicited movements
- opisthotonos and other abnormal positions
- lethargy
- tremors, shrill cry, or jittery movements
- cyanosis
- fixed and dilated pupils or pupil inequality or sluggishness
- unstable temperature
- variable heart rates or bradycardia
- increased ICP with tight, bulging anterior fontanel, separation of sutures, or head enlargement
- seizure activity with tonic manifestations, including horizontal deviation of eyes, blinking, limb posturing, staring, drooling, chin movements, chewing, and sucking.

2. Review CT scan, skull X-ray, CSF analysis, and other study results.

Rationales

1. Intracranial hemorrhages can occur without signs or symptoms, or they may appear and disappear intermittently (with P/IVH) until stopping or occur with more frequency than had been suspected. Recovery and survival are common.

2. Results may confirm hemorrhage and fluid retention.

3. Assess for other conditions that cause neurologic changes, such as seizures, including:
- hypoglycemia, hypocalcemia, and hypomagnesemia
- sepsis, meningitis, and encephalitis
- hyponatremia or hypernatremia
- hypoxia
- drug withdrawal
- brain tumor or malformation
- hyperbilirubinemia.

4. Review serum glucose, calcium, bilirubin, and magnesium levels; drug panel; culture results; CSF analysis; ABG measurements; and electrolytes, including Ca and Mg.

5. Additional individualized interventions: _____

_____

3. Assessment rules out other common conditions that can cause seizures.

4. Test results may indicate the abnormal conditions that are causing signs.

5. Rationales: _____

_____

Expected outcome 2

The patient will exhibit no neurologic impairment.

Interventions

1. Prepare and assist with serial lumbar punctures and intraventricular taps.

2. Prepare and administer I.V. anticonvulsants, as ordered:
- for mild and infrequent seizures: phenobarbital I.V. initially, with a repeat dose after 8 to 12 hours, followed by maintenance dose I.V. in two to three divided doses
- in refractory cases: phenytoin with phenobarbital I.V. initially, followed by a maintenance dose I.V., or orally in two separate doses.

3. Prepare and administer diazepam I.V., a muscle relaxant, as ordered.

4. Prepare and administer I.V. steroids, such as dexamethasone, as ordered, to reduce cerebral edema.

5. Review blood studies (phenobarbital and phenytoin levels) for possible drug toxicity, and observe for adverse reactions to anticonvulsants, including decreased activity, diarrhea, and increased motor seizures.

6. Additional individualized interventions: _____

Rationales

1. These procedures reduce pressure in the ventricles.

2. Phenobarbital is given for its sedative effect. Maintaining a therapeutic range of 20 to 30 mg/L for phenobarbital and 20 mg/L for phenytoin is essential for desired effect.

3. Diazepam is given when additional relaxation is needed, although it is not administered in jaundiced infants.

4. Although dexamethasone use is controversial, it may be ordered to reduce CSF levels.

5. Adverse reactions and inappropriate blood levels of drug necessitate discontinuing the medication and reporting the reaction to the doctor for possible medication or dosage changes. Decreased activity, diarrhea, and increased motor activity are adverse reactions to phenobarbital.

6. Rationales: _____

Expected outcome 3

The patient's ICP will remain within normal limits.

Interventions

1. Elevate the head of the bed slightly; place the infant in a prone or side-lying position, with the head midline or to the side. Do not flex the infant's neck.

2. If a phototherapy mask is ordered, make sure it is not tight.

3. Administer I.V. volume expanders, as ordered, at the prescribed rate; use an infusion-control device to prevent overly rapid infusion.

4. Continuously monitor the infant's vital signs, especially blood pressure.

5. Suction only as needed.

6. Avoid measures that may make the infant cry; minimize handling and manipulation.

7. Monitor ABG values.

8. Additional individualized interventions: _____

Rationales

1. Such positioning helps minimize ICP; placing the infant's head midline or to the side prevents cerebral blood flow obstruction.

2. Pressure on the occiput can increase ICP by impeding venous drainage.

3. Rapid increases in intravascular volume may rupture cerebral capillaries and increase ICP.

4. Changes in vital signs may indicate changes in ICP; early detection of such changes allows for prompt treatment.

5. Suctioning increases cerebral blood flow volume and raises ICP.

6. Crying can impede venous return and increase cerebral blood volume and ICP.

7. Acid-base imbalances can further impair the infant's compromised ability to regulate cerebral blood flow and ICP.

8. Rationales: _____

NURSING DIAGNOSIS

Anxiety (parental) related to infant's condition, prognosis, and risk for permanent brain dysfunction

Expected outcome

The parents will express minimal anxiety.

Interventions

1. Help the parents appraise the crisis in terms of their needs and the infant's needs.

2. Maintain a calm and accepting manner.

3. Encourage questions, give honest and accurate answers, and provide information about:
• cause and severity of the condition
• infant's status
• procedures and rationales
• possible prognosis and ongoing report of problem resolution
• rarity of permanent brain damage if condition is monitored and treated effectively while the infant is hospitalized (unless the infant's condition is severe).

Rationales

1. This helps them make necessary changes and develop strategies to cope with the crisis.

2. This allows the parents to feel comfortable expressing their feelings and asking questions.

3. Informative interaction promotes trust and lessens parental anxiety and fear, especially of the unknown. Parents often blame themselves for a sick infant or one with abnormal conditions or defects.

4. Allow the parents to visit and participate in the infant's care.

5. Help the parents express their fears and concerns about their infant's welfare. Assure them that their response is normal.

6. Inform the parents that a caregiver will be present whenever needed for support and information.

7. Refer the parents to community resources for assistance.

8. Additional individualized interventions: _____

_____

4. Parental participation promotes contact and bonding.

5. Expressing fears decreases anxiety by externalizing feelings.

6. This communicates caring, acceptance, and support.

7. These resources provide the parents with continued support, guidance, and follow-up.

8. Rationales: _____

_____

Documentation checklist

During the hospital stay, document:
- ❏ patient status and assessment findings, especially maternal history, Apgar scores, neurologic status, and ICP level
- ❏ changes in patient status
- ❏ pertinent laboratory and diagnostic findings, especially CSF results, HCT, ABG levels, maternal or infant toxicology screen (if done), and results of CT scan, cranial ultrasound, and transillumination
- ❏ patient's response to treatment
- ❏ family's reaction to the diagnosis and possible long-term effects
- ❏ parent-infant interaction
- ❏ family teaching guidelines
- ❏ discharge planning guidelines.

Associated plans
- ❏ Drug addiction and withdrawal
- ❏ Hyperbilirubinemia
- ❏ Hypocalcemia
- ❏ Hypoglycemia
- ❏ Postoperative care
- ❏ Pregnancy-induced hypertension
- ❏ Preoperative care

Additional nursing diagnoses
- ❏ Anticipatory grieving (parental) related to potential loss of infant experiencing severe hemorrhage or potential loss of normal infant functioning
- ❏ Ineffective breathing pattern related to apnea or irregular breathing
- ❏ Ineffective family coping: compromised related to situational crisis of sick infant
- ❏ Knowledge deficit (parental) related to limited exposure to information regarding infant care
- ❏ Risk for caregiver role strain related to infant's condition

- ❏ Risk for infection related to lumbar puncture that may introduce microorganisms
- ❏ Risk for injury related to neurologic dysfunction

Meconium aspiration syndrome

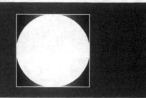

Definition

Meconium aspiration syndrome occurs when an infant aspirates meconium that has entered the amniotic fluid before, during, or after delivery. This syndrome usually occurs in full-term infants. Meconium is found in the amniotic fluid of 10% of all neonates, indicating some degree of in utero asphyxia. The asphyxia causes an increase in intestinal peristalsis because the diminished oxygenated blood flow relaxes the anal sphincter, allowing the meconium to be released. The sickest, most severely distressed fetuses, while making gasping attempts to save themselves in utero, suck meconium so deeply into their airways that the meconium cannot be retrieved with normal suctioning after delivery. Aspiration of the meconium causes partial or complete airway obstruction and pulmonary vasospasm. Bile salts in the meconium act as detergents, producing chemical burns on lung tissue. As the condition progresses, atelectasis, pneumothorax, persistent pulmonary hypertension, and bacterial pneumonia may develop.

With intervention, this disorder usually subsides in a few days, but death occurs in at least 28% of those affected. The prognosis depends on the amount of meconium aspirated, the degree of lung infiltration, and how quickly and effectively suctioning is implemented. Suctioning should include aspiration of the nasopharynx as the infant's head appears during birth and, if thick meconium is present, direct suctioning of the trachea through an endotracheal tube immediately after birth.

This plan focuses on caring for the infant who has aspirated meconium and is at risk for pulmonary complications.

Etiology and precipitating factors
• Fetal asphyxia
• Prolonged labor

Physical findings
Maternal antenatal history
• Intrauterine stress
Infant status at birth
• Full term, preterm, or small for gestational age
• Apgar score below 5
• Meconium in amniotic fluid
• Suctioning, resuscitative measures, or oxygen administration
Pulmonary
• Respiratory distress with gasping, tachypnea (more than 60 breaths/minute), grunting, retractions, and nasal flaring
• Possibly increased breath sounds with crackles, depending on meconium spread to lungs
• Cyanosis if severe
• Barrel chest with increased anteroposterior (AP) diameter
• Rhonchi

Behavioral findings
• Diminished activity

Diagnostic studies
• Chest X-ray to reveal patches of density representing atelectasis, increased AP diameter, hyperinflation, flattened diaphragm and, possibly, pneumothorax
• Arterial blood gas (ABG) studies to identify respiratory or metabolic acidosis with decreased partial pressure of oxygen (PO_2) and increased partial pressure of carbon dioxide (PO_2) levels

COLLABORATIVE PROBLEM

Risk for respiratory insufficiency related to meconium aspiration (two expected outcomes)

Expected outcome 1

The patient will exhibit no signs of meconium aspiration.

Interventions

1. Observe for immediate need to suction the nasopharynx when the infant's head appears during birth (performed by the doctor or nurse practitioner).

Rationales

1. Meconium in the amniotic fluid is an indication for suctioning before the infant takes a breath.

2. If thick meconium is present, suction the infant's trachea through an endotracheal tube immediately after birth.

3. Continue to suction the infant's mouth to remove larger meconium particles.

4. If an endotracheal tube is inserted, continue mouth suctioning as the tube is withdrawn.

5. Provide rest and quiet for the infant.

6. Additional individualized interventions: _____

2. This procedure should be performed before stimulating the infant to prevent further aspiration of thick meconium.

3. The infant who aspirates meconium needs resuscitation, especially if the infant is in respiratory distress.

4. Continued suctioning retrieves meconium that clings to the tube's tip.

5. Crying or agitation may increase intrathoracic pressure, causing pneumothorax.

6. Rationales: _____

Expected outcome 2

The patient will exhibit no respiratory compromise.

Interventions

1. Assess for indications of meconium aspiration, including:
• tachypnea (rate more than 60 breaths/minute), increased depth, and decreased ease of breathing
• grunting

• nasal flaring

• retractions with accessory muscle use

• cyanosis
• ABG levels showing increased Pco_2 and decreased Po_2
• serial lung X-ray results indicating atelectasis, hyperinflation, or pneumothorax.

2. Administer oxygen therapy, using an oxygen hood with humidification, nasal or oral continuous positive airway pressure (CPAP) at pressures of 4 to 6 cm H_2O, or mechanical ventilation, as ordered.

3. Set the mechanical ventilator to provide higher distending pressures with short inspiratory rates (60 to 70 breaths/minute).

4. Maintain hyperoxygenation and pH levels at 7.45 to 7.55 and Pco_2 at 22 to 30 mm Hg.

5. Provide physiotherapy with percussion and vibration every 1 to 2 hours. Use a percussor or fine vibrator if the infant can tolerate treatments.

Rationales

1. All are indications that meconium was aspirated and that the infant needs immediate treatment.
• Respiratory rate increases to enhance the oxygen level.

• The sound results from the glottis closing to stop exhalation of air by forcing air against the vocal cords.
• Narrowing of the nostrils produces resistance to respirations; flaring is an attempt to reduce this.
• Retractions indicate inadequate distention of lungs during inspiration.
• Cyanosis results as oxygen levels decrease.
• These values indicate impending acidosis.
• Atelectasis, hyperinflation, and pneumothorax indicate meconium aspiration.

2. Mechanical ventilation may or may not be needed. If the infant's condition is mild, an oxygen hood improves oxygenation without undue pressure; nasal or oral CPAP also improves oxygenation with minimal pressure. If the infant does need mechanical ventilation, many hospitals give surfactant to decrease surface tension and increase oxygenation or use high-frequency ventilation to reduce the risk or barotrauma or both. Positive pressure is administered after bronchoscopy or laryngotracheal therapy to prevent pushing meconium down into smaller airways (see the "Respiratory distress syndrome" plan, page 297, for oxygen therapy and mechanical ventilation procedures).

3. These settings are needed to ventilate distal alveoli in infants with severe meconium aspiration.

4. Hyperoxygenation prevents persistent fetal circulation. Respiratory alkalosis helps reduce pulmonary vasoconstriction in infants with meconium aspiration.

5. Percussion and vibration help remove secretions, but the infant's condition determines which procedure and equipment are used.

Extracorporeal membrane oxygenation

In major neonatal care facilities, extracorporeal membrane oxygenation (ECMO) may be used to maintain gas exchange and perfusion during preoperative management of diaphragmatic hernia and for selected neonates with refractory respiratory failure or meconium aspiration syndrome. ECMO maintains ventilation and oxygenation by oxygenating the neonate's blood outside the body through an arterial shunt. This permits cardiopulmonary recovery at low fractions of inspired oxygen and reduced mechanical ventilator settings.

In the neonate, ECMO usually involves venoarterial bypass. A cannula is inserted into the right atrium by way of the right internal jugular vein; the aortic arch is cannulated by way of the right common carotid artery. After circulating through the tubing by means of a pumping device, blood circulates through a membrane oxygenator. The oxygenated blood then flows through a heating device and into the carotid cannula. The neonate remains on mechanical ventilation during ECMO, with ventilator settings reduced to the lowest level required.

---

6. Prevent infection (pneumonitis) by administering I.V. antibiotics such as ampicillin, if ordered.

6. Antibiotics destroy bacteria by binding to the bacterial cell wall, resulting in cell death.

7. Slowly administer I.V. aminoglycosides, such as kanamycin, if ordered. Monitor serum peak and trough levels.

7. Aminoglycosides destroy bacteria by prohibiting protein synthesis, resulting in cell death. Slow administration prevents renal toxicity and ototoxicity. Monitoring peak and trough levels maximizes the effectiveness of drug therapy.

8. If ordered, administer steroids to reduce an inflammatory response to meconium.

8. Although hydrocortisone is the drug of choice, its use is controversial.

9. Prepare the infant for transfer to an agency for surgery and for attachment to an extracorporeal membrane oxygenation (ECMO) pump if the infant has severe aspiration and lung involvement. If ECMO is used:

9. ECMO maintains gas exchange and perfusion. This technology is available in selected hospitals. Surgery is performed to implant two thick tubes in the neck. These tubes are attached to an ECMO machine that pumps blood through an artificial lung. This procedure keeps the infant alive until the lungs can be supported with mechanical ventilation.

• Assess the infant's fluid intake and output.

• Maintaining fluid balance is essential to preventing fluid overload.

• Monitor transcutaneous blood oxygen tension or pulse oximetry values.
• Assess the infant's neurologic status.

• These readings evaluate tissue oxygenation and alert caregivers to changes in the infant's status.
• Neurologic signs may reflect changes in the infant's oxygenation status.

• Suction the endotracheal tube, as ordered.

• Suctioning maintains airway patency, aiding treatment. (For details on ECMO, see *Extracorporeal membrane oxygenation*.)

10. Additional individualized interventions: _____

10. Rationales: _____

NURSING DIAGNOSIS

Ineffective family coping: compromised related to anxiety, guilt and, possibly, long-term care

Expected outcome

The parents will express minimal anxiety and guilt.

Interventions

1. Assess the parents' verbal and nonverbal expressions of feelings and use of coping mechanisms.

Rationales

1. Assessment helps the caregiver and parents identify and develop constructive coping strategies.

2. Help the parents to verbalize their concerns about their sick infant, the prolonged care, and the procedures and equipment used in that care.

3. Provide consistent and accurate information concerning the infant's condition and progress, future care, and potential for pulmonary problems.

4. Encourage the parents to visit, give care if appropriate, and telephone for information.

5. Inform the parents of care needed after discharge and, if they will be providing specific procedures after discharge, teach them how to perform these procedures.

6. Refer the parents to community agencies, and inform them of available home care resources.

7. Additional individualized interventions: _____
_____

2. Verbalization helps to maintain a trusting, secure environment and acceptance of parents' concerns and fears.

3. Information reduces anxiety about the course of the disease and the rate at which the infant is improving.

4. Visitation, communication, and participation in the infant's care promote the bonding process.

5. Some infants need ventilatory assistance after discharge to home.

6. Referrals provide the family with additional support and follow-up. Equipment and supplies needed for home care are available to buy or rent.

7. Rationales: _____
_____

Documentation checklist
During the hospital stay, document:
❑ patient status and assessment findings, especially intrapartal history, including whether the infant received perineal suctioning before taking its first breath, character of secretions suctioned, Apgar scores, respiratory status, and presence of murmurs
❑ changes in patient status
❑ pertinent laboratory and diagnostic findings, especially ABG levels and chest X-rays
❑ types of therapies used, such as high-frequency ventilation or ECMO
❑ patient's response to treatment, especially if given surfactant or steroids or placed on ECMO
❑ family's reaction to the diagnosis
❑ parent-infant interaction
❑ family teaching guidelines
❑ discharge planning guidelines.

Associated plan
❑ Respiratory distress syndrome

Additional nursing diagnoses
❑ Altered nutrition: less than body requirements related to increased caloric needs
❑ Fear (parental) related to possible death of infant, responsibility of long-term care, and providing ventilatory assistance at home
❑ Impaired gas exchange related to chemical pneumonitis and respiratory compromise resulting from meconium aspiration
❑ Ineffective airway clearance related to meconium aspiration

❑ Ineffective infant feeding pattern related to respiratory compromise
❑ Knowledge deficit (parental) related to infant's long-term care needs after discharge
❑ Risk for fluid volume deficit related to insensible water losses from increased respirations
❑ Risk for infection related to pneumonia as result of meconium in lungs
❑ Risk for injury related to complications of pneumothorax, atelectasis

Necrotizing enterocolitis

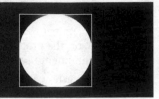

Definition

Necrotizing enterocolitis (NEC), also called inflammatory bowel disease, primarily affects preterm and low-birth-weight (LBW) infants. Its development seems to be linked to ischemia and bacterial invasion, along with certain conditions created by infant feeding.

NEC is characterized by ischemia of the gut, mucosal damage, edema, ulceration, and perforation. Hypoxemic, hypothermic, or shock states cause blood to be shunted to vital organs, decreasing mesenteric circulation, which damages the mucus-producing cells that protect the bowel wall. This allows bacteria to invade areas in the intestinal wall and proliferate in the poorly functioning bowel. If the infant has been fed, the milk also sits in the gut and provides a perfect medium for bacterial growth. Free gas accumulates in the intestine, causing pneumatosis intestinalis and necrosis. Disease onset usually occurs within 72 hours of the first feeding.

NEC is associated with such disorders as respiratory distress syndrome (RDS), asphyxia, patent ductus arteriosus, sepsis, and polycythemia and with such procedures as catheterization of the umbilical artery or vein and exchange transfusions. If medical management does not contain the infection or if severe acidosis persists and perforation occurs, the perforated area is surgically resected and ileostomy or colostomy is performed. The survival rate has dramatically increased with improved medical and surgical care and the use of total parenteral nutrition (TPN). Overall mortality is 33%, but this varies with treatment. The long-term prognosis is good; the survival rate depends on how much of the bowel is resected. If the small intestine or a significant portion of it (including the ileocecal valve) is lost, severe feeding problems develop.

This plan focuses on care of the infant with or at risk for NEC, with emphasis on preventing progression or complications of the disease.

Etiology and precipitating factors

• Uncertain; may result from ischemic insult to the bowel and the effect of microorganisms on this vascular insult
• Possibly reestablishment of circulation
• Certain types of feeding (hyperosmolar formula), volume of feeding, and effect of microorganisms on formula
• Infection with *Escherichia coli, Klebsiella, Clostridium, Salmonella,* or other bacteria
• Viral infection

Physical findings
Maternal history
• Such conditions as placenta previa, abruptio placentae, sepsis, pregnancy-induced hypertension, drug abuse, and diabetes mellitus
• Prolonged rupture of membranes
Infant status at birth
• Prematurity and LBW
• Low Apgar score, asphyxia, and respiratory distress
• Breech or cesarean birth
Cardiovascular
• Murmur
• Delayed capillary filling time
• Heart failure
Gastrointestinal
• Bile-colored (bilious) vomitus
• Possibly retention of feedings from poor absorption
• Abdominal distention
• Blood in stools
• Decreased or absent bowel sounds (ileus)
Integumentary
• Possibly jaundice
Neurologic
• Temperature instability
Pulmonary
• Apnea with bradycardic episodes

Behavioral findings
• Lethargy
• Irritability

Diagnostic studies
• X-ray (left lateral decubitus, upright) studies to detect bubbles or gas in the wall of the bowel, portal venous gas, or pneumatosis intestinalis (free air in peritoneum may mean perforation of the bowel)
• Clinitest to detect glucose (reducing substances)
• Hematest or guaiac test to identify occult blood in emesis, nasogastric (NG) tube aspirate, or stool
• Platelet count to indicate severe infection and deterioration if decreased to 100,000/mm³ or below
• Complete blood count (CBC) to detect white blood cell (WBC) count less than 5,000/mm³ or greater than 25,000/mm³; absolute neutrophil count less than 5,000; and immature to total neutrophil ratio as follows: 0.25:0.49 is suspicious, 0.50:0.79 indicates sepsis, and 0.8 or above indicates fulminating NEC.

• Clotting profile of prothrombin time (PT), partial thromboplastin time (PTT), and fibrinogen to indicate coagulation complication
• Typing and crossmatching of blood to prepare for exchange transfusion if needed

• Electrolyte levels to determine need for correction (with vomiting and gastric decompression)
• Cultures of blood, urine, stool, cerebrospinal fluid, and peritoneal fluid to determine causative organism

COLLABORATIVE PROBLEM

Risk for extension of bowel injury related to continued or further bowel infection and to necrosis (two expected outcomes)

Expected outcome 1

The patient will exhibit no signs of progressive bowel involvement.

Interventions

1. Assess the infant at risk, and monitor for early symptoms of NEC, as follows:
• Review maternal history.
• Watch for signs of NEC if the infant has asphyxia, RDS, sepsis, or other illness or is undergoing exchange transfusions.
• Note onset of vomiting, lethargy, change in feeding pattern, jaundice, apnea, or temperature instability within 72 hours of first formula feeding.
• Review stool Hematest and Clinitest results.

2. Assess for later signs, including:
• abdominal distention
• bile-colored vomitus
• decreased or absent bowel sounds and bowel movements.

3. Review X-rays, cultures of body fluids and stools, platelet count, WBC count, segmented cell count, and electrolyte levels.

4. Additional individualized interventions: _____

Rationales

1. Early recognition of the disease increases the survival rate, and nursing observations of subtle changes are essential for early intervention or preventive therapy. Early, nonspecific signs are similar to those of other conditions.

2. Later signs usually appear 12 to 24 hours after retained gastric contents are noted because of poor absorption.

3. These studies identify infection and infectious agents. The platelet count decreases in infection, the WBC count may increase or decrease, and the neutrophil count decreases.

4. Rationales: _____

Expected outcome 2

The patient will exhibit no further signs of infection.

Interventions

1. Discontinue oral feedings for 7 to 14 days.

2. Insert an NG tube and attach it to low intermittent suction, or aspirate by hand at frequent intervals. Measure abdominal girth every 4 to 8 hours.

Rationales

1. This allows the injured bowel to rest.

2. These actions maintain gastric decompression to eliminate vomiting and distention. Abdominal girth measurements provide information about changes in distention.

3. Start an I.V. infusion of dextrose 10% in water ($D_{10}W$) at 150 ml/kg/24 hours.

3. An infant 3 to 4 days old needs volume expansion to reperfuse. An I.V. infusion of $D_{10}W$ at 60 ml/kg/24 hours may be given initially for the first 24 hours. An electrolyte replacement of minerals and sodium may also be considered.

4. Prepare and administer I.V. antibiotic therapy, such as ampicillin or aminoglycosides, as prescribed.

4. These broad-spectrum antibiotics inhibit protein biosynthesis of the bacterial cell wall.

5. Additional individualized interventions: _____

5. Rationales: _____

_____

COLLABORATIVE PROBLEM

Nutritional deficiency related to infant's inability to ingest and absorb nutrients because of bowel infection

Expected outcome

The patient will maintain adequate nutritional intake.

Interventions

1. Maintain I.V. parenteral nutritional support for 2 weeks as follows:
• Start with $D_{10}W$, using an infusion-control device.
• Add amino acid mixture to $D_{10}W$ infusion.
• Add a supplement of fat administered by way of another setup and device.

2. Administer TPN after sepsis is controlled.

3. Resume feedings slowly and in small amounts by gastric gavage.

4. Aspirate gastric contents before each feeding.

5. Measure abdominal girth before feedings and note increases. Note the presence or absence of bowel sounds, tone of stomach, and abdominal musculature.

6. Weigh the infant every 8 hours. Record and report losses.

7. Calculate the infant's calorie needs to be given intermittently or continuously by NG tube.

8. Additional individualized interventions: _____

Rationales

1. Parenteral nutrition supplies nutritional needs while allowing the bowel to rest. Poor absorption of feedings and the need to rest the injured bowel make withholding of food and water necessary. Formula feedings also contribute to the production of hydrogen gas, which increases gas-forming bacteria.

2. Parenteral nutrition is continued to maintain nutritional intake until the infant can take oral feedings (see the "Tracheoesophageal fistula or esophageal atresia" plan, page 326, for the correct TPN procedure).

3. This prevents exacerbation of GI symptoms caused by retained gastric contents.

4. Increasing gastric residual contents may indicate poor absorption, which could result in distention and vomiting if the feeding is given.

5. Girth measurement helps detect increasing distention. Normal bowel sounds indicate an adequately functioning bowel.

6. Weight measurements help determine whether growth and fluid status are adequate.

7. Identifying calorie needs ensures appropriate nutrient administration. Formula or breast milk (preferred) is given in the amounts needed for growth and in progressive amounts as tolerated.

8. Rationales: _____

NURSING DIAGNOSIS

Risk for fluid volume deficit related to fluid loss through gastric decompression and to withholding of food and water

Expected outcome

The patient will exhibit no fluid and electrolyte imbalance.

Interventions

1. Monitor fluid intake by I.V. infusion, by feedings through an NG tube or other route, or by TPN, and compare with output.

2. Monitor fluid output, including:
• weight of diapers (1 g = 1 ml) and oliguria
• weight loss
• gastric aspirate and emesis
• insensible water loss.

3. Review serum electrolyte levels and osmolality, and urine specific gravity and osmolality.

4. Assess for dehydration, including:
• hot, dry skin and poor skin turgor
• depressed fontanels
• elevated temperature
• increased urine specific gravity
• dry mucous membranes.

5. Additional individualized interventions: _____

Rationales

1. Comparison of fluid intake and output helps prevent imbalance, dehydration, and overhydration.

2. Urine output should be at least 1 ml/kg/hour, with a low specific gravity of 1.005 to 1.010. Weight is the best indication of fluid loss in the infant.

3. Assessment reveals imbalance in sodium, potassium, and urine concentration, indicating dehydration. Specific gravity and sodium and potassium levels increase with dehydration.

4. Signs of dehydration are related to third-space fluid shifting associated with NEC.

5. Rationales: _____

COLLABORATIVE PROBLEM

Physiologic injury and infection related to failure of disease to resolve (two expected outcomes)

Expected outcome 1

The patient will exhibit no actual or potential complications of NEC.

Interventions

1. Assess for signs of disseminated intravascular coagulation (DIC), including:
• bleeding or oozing from any site (such as incision and I.V. puncture) or in stools, urine, and vomitus
• pallor, petechiae, ecchymoses, and poor capillary filling time
• frank bleeding from the intestine.

2. Review serial laboratory results for decreased hemoglobin (Hb) and fibrinogen levels and platelet count in the CBC, WBC count, and differential and increased PT, activated partial thromboplastin time (APTT), and thrombin time.

Rationales

1. DIC can develop in infants with NEC because infections are the most common stimuli that activate the clotting process; the damaged bowel releases thromboplastin.

2. A decreased Hb level indicates blood loss from bleeding. A platelet count below 100,000/mm^3 increases the risk of DIC. A reduced fibrinogen level slows the clotting process. Increases in PT, APTT, and thrombin time indicate a clotting abnormality and potential bleeding.

3. Assess for signs of septic shock, including:
• decreased blood pressure with wide pulse pressure
• tachycardia
• warm arms and legs.

4. Assess for signs of peritonitis, including:
• listlessness and "rag-doll" limpness
• apnea
• bradycardia
• hypothermia
• abdominal rigidity and distention; shiny red abdomen.

5. Additional individualized interventions: _____

3. The infectious process may eventually result in severe systemic involvement.

4. Continued inflammation and damage to the intestinal mucosa may cause perforation and peritonitis.

5. Rationales: _____

Expected outcome 2

The patient will exhibit minimal effects from complications of NEC.

Interventions

1. Treat DIC as follows:

• Record the amounts of blood taken for frequent testing.
• Avoid I.M. injections; monitor heelstick and I.V. sites.

• Administer I.V. phytonadione (vitamin K).

• Administer antithrombin III (AT-III) at a concentration of 50 IU/kg, low-dose heparin at 10 units/kg/hour, and fresh frozen plasma and platelets at concentrations of 10 ml/kg, if ordered.

• Apply pressure to bleeding sites.
• Prepare and assist with transfusion of volume expanders, such as plasma protein fraction (Plasmanate).
• Prepare and assist with transfusion of packed red blood cells (RBCs).
• Prepare and assist with transfusion of platelets and crystalloids.

2. Treat for septic shock as follows:
• Prepare and administer hydrocortisone sodium succinate (Solu-Cortef). (This is not always used because it may mask infection.)
• Monitor the infant's blood pressure and heart rate electronically and continuously.
• Prepare and assist with administration of the transfusion.

Rationales

1. Therapy for coagulopathy may prevent life-threatening hemorrhage.
• Frequent testing may result in significant additional blood loss.
• Puncture wounds may predispose the infant to blood loss.
• Vitamin K is given in an emergency to aid liver synthesis of clotting factors.
• AT-III replaces regulatory proteins; low-dose heparin may be ordered if infused fibrinogen and platelet survival time is less than 12 hours, and plasma and platelet concentrations are administered to maintain levels of fibrinogen above 100 mg/dl and platelets at 100,000/mm^3.
• Pressure helps control bleeding.
• A volume expander is given if clotting factors are the problem.
• Packed RBCs are given if bleeding is a problem and hematocrit is decreased.
• Platelets and crystalloids are given if PTT and WBC count are low.

2. Septic shock may complicate NEC.
• A corticosteroid is given to increase cardiac output and peripheral perfusion.

• Increased heart rate and decreased blood pressure indicate shock.
• Whole blood, plasma, or crystalloid infusion may be given to maintain blood pressure and urine output.

3. Treat perforation and peritonitis as follows:
• Remove the umbilical artery catheter (UAC), if present and if possible.

• Limit palpation of the abdomen.
• Handle the infant as little as possible.
• Measure abdominal girth for increases every 2 hours.
• Assist with paracentesis, and collect a specimen for culture.
• If the culture is positive for gram-negative or gram-positive rods, give additional I.V. antibiotics. The usual drugs of choice are ampicillin and gentamicin, oxacillin, and methicillin.
• Prepare the infant for surgery.

4. Additional individualized interventions: _____
_____

3. Perforation may complicate uncontrolled NEC.
• Removal of the UAC prevents further injury, but this is not possible if the infant is critically ill and the UAC is needed for monitoring.
• Palpation may cause further trauma to the abdomen.
• Unnecessary handling may cause injury.
• Increases in girth indicate distention.
• Paracentesis relieves distention by removing fluid; culture identifies infection in peritoneal cavity.
• An antibiotic specific to these organisms is given to inhibit protein biosynthesis of the bacterial cell wall.

• Perforation and peritonitis may require surgical intervention (see the "Preoperative care" plan, page 284).

4. Rationales: _____
_____

NURSING DIAGNOSIS

Anxiety (parental) related to the uncertain outcome of surgical intervention

Expected outcome

The parents will express minimal anxiety.

Interventions

1. Maintain a calm and accepting manner.

2. Encourage the parents to ask questions, and give honest and accurate answers or obtain needed information about:
• surgery involving resection of affected parts and reconnection of the bowel
• possibility of ileostomy or colostomy (usually temporary) and accompanying short-bowel syndrome
• care being given before and after surgery and its rationale. (See the "Postoperative care" plan, page 277, and the "Preoperative care" plan, page 284, for details on knowledge deficit.)

3. Spend as much time as possible with the parents, keeping them informed of the infant's care and progress.

4. Help the parents to appraise the crisis in terms of their needs and the needs of their infant.

5. Refer the parents to community agencies for follow-up.

6. Additional individualized interventions: _____

Rationales

1. This allows the parents to feel comfortable in expressing their feelings.

2. An open discussion with honest information promotes trust and decreases anxiety.

3. This involvement shows caring and support.

4. This appraisal identifies changes in needs brought on by the crisis.

5. These agencies can provide the family with support and guidance.

6. Rationales: _____

Documentation checklist

During the hospital stay, document:

❒ patient status and assessment findings, especially intrapartal history of any hypoxic episodes, Apgar scores, abdominal girth, presence of bowel loops, tenderness on palpation (which should be limited), stool color and presence of blood in stool, feeding tolerance (if receiving oral feedings), color of any vomitus, cardiopulmonary status (including peripheral perfusion), and pulmonary sounds indicating heart failure

❒ changes in patient status

❒ pertinent laboratory and diagnostic findings, especially Clinitest results, results of Hematest or guaiac tests of any excretions, CBC with differential, serum electrolyte levels, and any culture results

❒ patient's reaction to surgery (if performed), including tolerance of procedure, thermal stability, and appearance of suture line

❒ patient's response to treatment, especially gastric decompression or stopping of feedings

❒ family's reaction to the diagnosis and surgery (if performed)

❒ parent-infant interaction

❒ family teaching guidelines, especially care of suture line (if present), feeding schedule and type of feeding, and care of ostomy (if present)

❒ discharge planning guidelines.

Associated plans

❒ Abruptio placentae
❒ Cesarean section birth
❒ Hyperbilirubinemia
❒ Hypothermia and hyperthermia
❒ Placenta previa
❒ Postoperative care
❒ Pregnancy-induced hypertension
❒ Premature rupture of membranes
❒ Preoperative care
❒ Preterm infant
❒ Sepsis neonatorum and infectious disorders
❒ Tracheoesophageal fistula or esophageal atresia

Additional nursing diagnoses

❒ Altered nutrition: less than body requirements related to short-bowel syndrome

❒ Altered parenting related to compromised bonding process, misunderstanding, or lack of information

❒ Altered body temperature related to infection affecting regulation

❒ Impaired skin integrity related to injury, irritation caused by the NG tube

❒ Impaired tissue integrity related to surgery

❒ Ineffective family coping related to guilt, anxiety about sick infant

❒ Ineffective infant feeding pattern related to bowel infection

❒ Knowledge deficit (parental) related to care of infant after surgery

Postoperative care

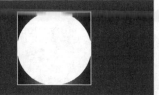

Definition

Postoperative care in this plan consists of the care given to infants after surgical interventions for palliative or corrective procedures. The potential for altering each infant's physiologic status depends on the type of surgical procedure, the organs involved, and the system most severely affected by the surgery.

This plan presents general information on infant care after surgery and focuses on preventing complications related to surgery. Postoperative care for specific surgical procedures is also included, but each infant has individual needs based on the infant's status and the disorder's severity. Specific nursing diagnoses and interventions may need to be modified to fit a specific infant.

Etiology and precipitating factors

• Congenital defect that produces a life-threatening situation in the infant and requires immediate correction (some surgeries require more extensive follow-up procedures when the infant is older and in better condition to undergo permanent correction)
• Conditions such as gastroschisis, myelomeningocele, and patent ductus arteriosus (PDA) ligation that require immediate surgery but no further surgical procedures

• Conditions that develop later and require surgical procedures, such as gastrostomy tube insertion, shunting when intraventricular hemorrhage results in hydrocephalus, and retinopathy

Physical findings
Infant status at birth
• Congenital anomalies that threaten any system functions
• Conditions that develop soon after birth because of abnormalities
Body systems
• Signs and symptoms included in the assessment of each system noted in the plan

Behavioral findings
• Depend on condition necessitating surgery (see specific plan for more information)

Diagnostic studies
See the "Preoperative care" plan, page 284, for appropriate tests; postoperative tests are included in this plan as they relate to the system affected by surgery.

COLLABORATIVE PROBLEM

Respiratory compromise related to inadequate spontaneous respirations, with decreased lung expansion and increased tracheobronchial secretions from trauma or surgical anesthesia

Expected outcome

The patient will exhibit optimal respiratory effort and oxygenation after surgery

---

Interventions

1. Assess the infant's respiratory status hourly, noting:
• rate, depth, and ease of respirations
• return of respiratory effort
• vital signs, including hourly blood pressure
• apneic episodes
• chest retractions and movements
• decreased or absent breath sounds with crackles or rhonchi
• central or peripheral cyanosis
• abdominal distention.

Rationales

1. An infant going to surgery usually receives pancuronium bromide (Pavulon), a skeletal muscle relaxant; this drug, combined with an anesthetic, affects respiratory status. Continual assessment can identify problems before they become serious. Infants usually are intubated preoperatively and not extubated until respiratory status is controlled.

2. Have ventilatory support ready for the infant's return from surgery.

2. Having ventilation support on hand allows for prompt treatment if a problem should arise. Information from surgery ensures proper ventilation.

3. Monitor the fraction of inspired oxygen (FIO_2) hourly.

3. FIO_2 identifies oxygen levels, ensuring proper oxygenation and preventing hypoxia.

4. Provide suction, if needed.

4. Suction removes excess secretions that interfere with breathing by obstructing airways.

5. Avoid restraining the infant, and minimize handling.

5. Minimizing movement helps stabilize the infant.

6. Maintain a neutral thermal environment by using an incubator or a radiant warmer, which should be warm and ready for use when the infant returns from surgery.

6. A neutral thermal environment reduces metabolic expenditure of energy and oxygen demands. A hypothermic infant may develop disseminated intravascular coagulation if it gets cold in the operating room (OR).

7. Monitor arterial blood gas (ABG) values after establishing a patent airway and ventilation.

7. Monitoring ABG levels helps identify the adjustments needed in oxygen administration and helps prevent acid-base imbalances.

8. Review complete blood count (CBC) results, electrolyte analyses, chest X-ray, and reagent strip test results for glucose level.

8. Test results establish a baseline for comparison. Deviations may indicate improvement or abnormalities.

9. Check if a chest tube was inserted in the OR. If it was, monitor its patency.

9. Specific interventions ensure tube patency if surgery was performed in the chest area.

10. Perform chest physiotherapy, unless the infant had chest surgery or is still intubated.

10. Chest physiotherapy may help loosen secretions. This procedure may be considered 2 to 3 days postoperatively; small percussors with cup may be used.

11. Assess for signs of pain, including restlessness, changes in baseline vital signs, and crying when touched (indicating tenderness); give pain medications as ordered.

11. Adequate pain management may allow the infant to breathe more deeply and easily, helping the infant to heal faster.

12. Allow the parents to see the infant as soon as possible after surgery.

12. Seeing the infant alive reassures the parents and helps relieve their anxiety.

13. Additional individualized interventions: _____

13. Rationales: _____

COLLABORATIVE PROBLEM

Decreased cardiac output related to anesthesia, an inadequate shunt, or PDA ligation

Expected outcome

The patient will maintain optimal cardiac output after surgery.

Interventions

1. Monitor cardiovascular status every 1 to 2 hours, assessing for:
- irregular apical pulse
- blood pressure changes and narrowing pulse pressure
- capillary refill time greater than 5 seconds
- diminishing peripheral pulses and cool arms and legs
- distant heart sounds
- skin mottling
- oliguria.

Rationales

1. Monitoring allows for prompt intervention to return the infant to the optimal cardiac function needed to deliver oxygen and nutrients to body tissues and enhance recovery.

2. Monitor ABG measurements, hematocrit (HCT), X-ray results, and serum calcium and potassium levels.

3. Provide calcium or other electrolyte replacement as indicated.

4. Prepare and administer digoxin or other medications, as ordered.

5. Prepare and administer prostaglandin E and titrate to the lowest dose.

6. Attach a cardiopulmonary monitor, turn on the alarm, and observe the infant's status as appropriate.

7. Additional individualized interventions: _____

2. Monitoring laboratory results helps to identify changes quickly. Abnormal results may indicate complications.

3. Reduced electrolyte levels may cause arrhythmias.

4. Digoxin improves cardiac output and is given to treat heart failure that results from cardiac dysfunction.

5. This drug is given if the shunt is functioning improperly.

6. Continuous monitoring allows prompt assessment and intervention if changes should occur. An alarm warns of inappropriate oxygenation and cardiac changes

7. Rationales: _____

NURSING DIAGNOSIS

Risk for infection related to surgical incision

Expected outcome

The patient exhibits optimal wound healing and an intact suture line without infection.

Interventions

1. Assess the surgical site for infection; note:
• redness, breaks, irritation, or edema of the skin
• color, type, amount, and odor of any wound drainage
• inflammation at chest tube insertion site (if infant has a chest tube).

2. Perform proper hand washing before approaching the infant, using an antiseptic.

3. Change your gown before caring for the infant. Follow hospital protocol for reverse isolation if indicated.

4. Take the infant's axillary temperature hourly or monitor temperature electronically until it stabilizes. Be alert for readings over 96.8° F (36° C) and poor temperature control.

5. Review results of cultures from wound exudate and results of white blood cell count and differential.

6. Maintain sterile technique when caring for the wound or performing dressing changes, irrigation, and other procedures.

7. Additional individualized interventions: _____

Rationales

1. An infant is more susceptible to infection because of deficient phagocytic action and an immature immune system, which decrease the inflammatory response. Postoperatively, decreased resistance further compromises the infant's status.

2. Hand washing removes transient bacteria and prevents the transmission of contaminants.

3. These measures protect the infant from infection and cross-contamination.

4. Temperature elevations may indicate infection.

5. When infection is suspected, cultures identify the infecting organism and blood tests confirm the presence of an infectious process.

6. Sterile technique helps prevent contamination that predisposes the infant to infection.

7. Rationales: _____

COLLABORATIVE PROBLEM

Altered nutrition: Less than less than body requirements, related to withholding food and fluid and to inadequate nutritional intake from parenteral infusion

Expected outcome

The patient will maintain optimal nutritional intake after surgery.

Interventions

1. Assess for changes in nutritional status and intervene as appropriate:
• Weigh the infant daily to determine loss or gain.
• Note vomiting.
• Determine how long the infant has gone without food or water.
• Note lethargy and irritability.
• Monitor glucose levels using reagent and glucose reagent strip testing; monitor serum calcium levels.
• Begin I.V. infusion of dextrose and electrolytes, gavage feedings, or total parenteral nutrition (TPN), as ordered.

2. Maintain nutritional requirements as follows:
• Calculate the infant's calorie needs, and document the infant's fluid intake and output hourly.
• Weigh the infant daily unless its condition prohibits weighing.
• Administer and monitor I.V. glucose, gavage feedings, or TPN as ordered.

3. Additional individualized interventions: _____

Rationales

1. An infant has the potential for developing hypoglycemia and hypocalcemia because it has limited glucose and calcium reserves. The caregiver must be alert for signs of a developing disorder and intervene promptly to restore balance.

2. The most appropriate route for nutrition depends on the infant's condition and the type of surgery. Initially, the infant may receive an I.V. infusion, followed by other methods as tolerated (see the "Tracheoesophageal fistula or esophageal atresia" plan, page 326, for procedures).

3. Rationales: _____

COLLABORATIVE PROBLEM

Fluid imbalance related to withholding food and fluid or to blood or fluid loss

Expected outcome

The patient will maintain a stable fluid and electrolyte balance.

Interventions

1. Document the infant's fluid intake every 1 to 2 hours, recording:
• parenteral fluids
• fluids received in the OR
• volume expanders or blood products given
• medications given I.V. or by mouth
• oral feedings, including breast, bottle, or gavage feedings.

Rationales

1. These records help predict the infant's potential for imbalances before they occur, allowing for appropriate replacement therapy.

2. Document the infant's fluid output every 1 to 2 hours, recording:
• urine output, including urine output in the OR
• liquid or loose stools
• nasogastric or thoracic drainage or drainage from other routes
• blood loss in surgery, from blood tests, or from other bleeding sites.

2. These records help predict the potential for excess losses.

3. Compare fluid intake and output for positive or negative fluid balance.

3. The ratio of fluid intake to output identifies or predicts fluid imbalances.

4. Monitor HCT; CBC; ABG, blood urea nitrogen (BUN), creatinine, and electrolyte levels; and urine specific gravity. Report results and intervene as appropriate.

4. These tests indicate changes in cardiac output and renal function as well as fluid and electrolyte losses.

5. Monitor heart rate, blood pressure, and central venous pressure every 1 to 2 hours.

5. These parameters indicate changes in cardiac and renal functions.

6. Ensure hydration:
• Administer I.V. fluids as ordered.
• Provide electrolyte replacement as needed and ordered.
• Administer blood or volume expanders as ordered.
• Monitor urine output; output should be at least 2 ml/kg/hour.
• Monitor urine specific gravity; values should range from 1.005 to 1.015, indicating normal urine concentration.

6. Proper fluid replacement is essential to prevent or minimize fluid losses. See appendix G, Fluid and nutritional needs in infancy, for fluid requirements.

7. Additional individualized interventions: _____

7. Rationales: _____

NURSING DIAGNOSIS

Altered parenting related to separation from infant because of surgery

Expected outcome

The parents will exhibit positive bonding behavior.

Interventions

1. Frequently and accurately inform the parents of their infant's condition and progress after surgery. Permit parental visits as soon as possible.

2. Allow the parents to express their feelings and fears, and show acceptance of these feelings.

3. Allow the parents to visit frequently, to participate in infant care, and to telephone around the clock.

4. Reassure the parents that they will be able to care for the infant after discharge; teach them how to provide appropriate care.

5. If appropriate, reinforce information from the doctor that the surgical outcome may be temporary and that the child may need hospitalization for further procedures in the future.

Rationales

1. Informing the parents helps decrease their anxiety and increase their comfort level with the infant.

2. This establishes a trusting relationship.

3. Visiting, participating in care, and being able to call as needed promote bonding.

4. Proper infant care instructions and reassurance help the parents feel confident in their ability to provide care.

5. Adequate information enhances compliance and alleviates further stress. Some procedures are temporary until the infant is old enough for permanent corrective surgery.

6. Additional individualized interventions: _____
_____

6. Rationales: _____
_____

Nursing diagnosis

Knowledge deficit (parental) related to postoperative care of infant at home

Expected outcome

The parents will receive information about their infant's condition and necessary follow-up care and will express understanding of that information.

Interventions

1. Teach the parents about:
• infant's disease and surgery
• treatments and procedures
• signs and symptoms of complications
• follow-up care and therapy.
Reinforce teaching as needed.

2. Teach the parents about ordered treatments and infant care, which may include:
• home oxygen therapy and chest physiotherapy
• drug, nutritional, and fluid therapy
• incisional care and dressing changes
• skin care.

3. Encourage the family to participate in the infant's care.

4. Teach the parents and other family members about signs of infection, such as:
• fever
• redness, warmth, and inflammation at the surgical site
• foul-smelling, purulent drainage from the incision.

5. Have the parents perform return demonstrations of all required procedures.

6. Teach the parents and other family members how to balance activities with rest and how to evaluate the infant's tolerance for activities.

7. Arrange for home health care follow-up.

8. Additional individualized interventions: _____
_____

Rationales

1. Providing information alleviates the parents' anxiety and helps them prepare adequately for the infant's discharge.

2. Proper instruction promotes compliance and helps dispel the parents' fears about equipment and procedures.

3. Participation in care helps relieve feelings of inadequacy and prepares the family to care for the infant at home.

4. Early identification of signs of infection allows prompt intervention.

5. Return demonstrations foster parental feelings of adequacy and independence in caring for the infant and may signal the need for more instruction.

6. Stimulation of activity is crucial for normal infant growth and development; prolonged hospitalization may delay development. Activity tolerance varies from one infant to the next.

7. A home health care referral provides the family with continued support outside the hospital.

8. Rationales: _____
_____

Documentation checklist

During the hospital stay, document:

❏ patient status and assessment findings, especially the patient's tolerance of the surgery, any signs of pain, cardiorespiratory status, fluid balance (including intake and output), appearance of suture line (if applicable) and any secretions from the surgical site, and neurologic status
❏ changes in patient status
❏ pertinent laboratory and diagnostic findings, especially CBC with differential; HCT; hemoglobin, electrolyte, glucose, BUN, creatinine, calcium, and ABG levels; reagent and glucose reagent strip results; urine specific gravity; appropriate X-rays; and daily weight
❏ patient's response to treatment and surgery
❏ family's reaction to the diagnosis and surgical procedure
❏ parent-infant interaction
❏ family teaching guidelines, especially any wound care or specialized treatments secondary to the surgery that must be carried out in the home
❏ discharge planning guidelines.

Associated plans

❏ Bowel obstruction
❏ Cleft lip and cleft palate
❏ Congenital heart disease
❏ Intracranial hemorrhage
❏ Necrotizing enterocolitis
❏ Preoperative care
❏ Spinal cord defects and hydrocephalus
❏ Tracheoesophageal fistula or esophageal atresia

Additional nursing diagnoses

❏ Anticipatory grieving (parental) related to possible loss of infant during or as a result of surgery or loss of the anticipated perfect child
❏ Fear (parental) related to separation from infant
❏ Impaired adjustment (parental) related to infant requiring surgery
❏ Impaired gas exchange related to anesthesia
❏ Impaired skin integrity related to drainage from colostomy, ileostomy
❏ Ineffective breathing pattern related to anesthesia
❏ Ineffective family coping: disabled related to guilt, anxiety
❏ Knowledge deficit (parental) related to lack of exposure to information or care of infant after surgery
❏ Pain related to surgical tissue trauma
❏ Risk for altered body temperature related to extremes in age and weight
❏ Risk for aspiration related to anesthesia
❏ Risk for fluid deficit related to withholding of fluids postoperatively

Preoperative care

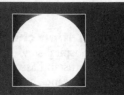

Definition

Preoperative care is given to an infant before surgical intervention for palliative or corrective procedures. Preparatory procedures depend on the infant's chronologic and gestational age and the defect or abnormal condition to be corrected. In most cases, the decision to intervene surgically is based on the infant's condition, the disorder's acuity (or life-threatening potential), the surgeon's and neonatologist's diagnoses and evaluations of the infant, and parental desires.

This plan focuses on the preoperative needs of most infants undergoing surgery for congenital defects, obstructions, relief of intracranial pressure, and other abnormalities. Because each infant's needs vary according to health status and severity of the disorder to be corrected, the following plan is general rather than specific to any disease or condition.

Etiology and precipitating factors

• Cardiac defects, such as tetralogy of Fallot, truncus arteriosus, coarctation of the aorta, hypoplastic heart syndrome, and any of the ductal-dependent lesions
• GI defects, such as gastroschisis, omphalocele, imperforate anus, strangulated inguinal hernia, volvulus, intestinal atresia or stenosis, necrotizing enterocolitis, tracheoesophageal fistula or esophageal atresia, and cleft lip or cleft palate
• Musculoskeletal defects, such as talipes deformity
• Neurologic defects, such as meningocele and hydrocephalus (shunt placement)
• Pulmonary defects, such as choanal atresia and diaphragmatic hernia

Physical findings
Infant status at birth

• Immaturity, low birth weight and height or, possibly, full-term infant with cardiac defects not identified at birth
• Visible congenital anomalies, such as umbilical cord with only two vessels, cleft lip or cleft palate
• Low Apgar score, asphyxia

Behavioral findings

• Depend on condition necessitating surgery (see specific plan for more information)

Diagnostic studies

• X-ray to determine presence and extent of abnormality and area dependent on assessment
• Computed tomography scan or magnetic resonance imaging to detect abnormalities
• Cardiac catheterization to determine the nature and extent of cardiac defects
• Serum glucose levels to identify hypoglycemia
• Electrolyte studies to identify hypocalcemia and hypernatremia
• Prothrombin time (PT), partial thromboplastin time (PTT), and blood typing and crossmatching to prepare for blood replacement if needed
• Complete blood count (CBC) to identify changes indicating blood loss or infection
• Screening for sexually transmitted infections to identify possible viral infections
• Arterial blood gas (ABG) studies to identify changes indicating altered gas exchange
• Chromosomal studies to identify genetic abnormalities

NURSING DIAGNOSIS

Anxiety (parental) related to uncertain outcome of surgery

Expected outcome

The parents will express minimal anxiety.

Interventions

1. Maintain a calm and accepting manner.

2. Encourage the parents to ask questions; give honest and accurate answers and obtain necessary information, as needed.

Rationales

1. This allows the parents to feel comfortable expressing feelings and asking questions.

2. This promotes trust by decreasing parental anxiety and fear of the unknown.

3. Use pamphlets and drawings to reinforce the doctor's information about the infant's surgical procedure, prognosis, and postsurgical care.

4. Stay with the parents or spend as much time as possible with them.

5. Inform the parents if the infant must be moved to another hospital, and explain the methods of safe transfer. The father or other family members may be allowed to accompany the infant and visit if the mother is still hospitalized.

6. Keep the parents informed of the infant's care and progress. Allow them unlimited time with the infant as its condition permits.

7. Additional individualized interventions: _____

_____

3. Reinforcing the doctor's information ensures that the parents learn information they may have been too anxious to comprehend earlier. It also ensures that the parents can give their fully informed consent before surgery.

4. The caregiver's presence shows support and caring.

5. Some hospitals do not have intensive care nursery (ICN) facilities. Although transferring the infant to a hospital with an ICN will benefit the infant, the move may cause additional parental anxiety because of separation.

6. Providing reports about the infant's condition and care alleviates parental anxiety. Allowing time with the infant promotes bonding.

7. Rationales: _____

_____

NURSING DIAGNOSIS

Risk for infection related to a break in skin integrity from surgery or from a defect in which a sac protrudes from the skin surface

Expected outcome

The patient will exhibit no signs of infection.

Interventions

1. Before approaching the infant, wash your hands properly with an antiseptic.

2. Take the infant's axillary temperature every 2 to 4 hours. Note readings over 96.8° F (36° C) and poor temperature control.

3. Monitor skin cultures.

4. Note changes such as lethargy, irritability, dyspnea, and cyanosis.

5. Maintain sterile technique when caring for infants with such defects as gastroschisis or myelomeningocele. Clean the equipment and supplies used on the infant daily or as hospital policy dictates. Cover the sac with a moist sterile saline dressing.

6. Position the infant with a lumbosacral myelomeningocele on its abdomen with its legs in a froglike position.

7. Additional individualized interventions: _____

_____

Rationales

1. Hand washing removes transient bacteria and prevents transmission of contaminants.

2. Temperature elevation indicates possible infection.

3. Culture results identify infectious organisms.

4. Early identification of these signs may reveal that the infant has an infection and allow for prompt treatment.

5. These actions prevent contamination, which predisposes the infant to infection.

6. This position minimizes tension on the sac.

7. Rationales: _____

_____

NURSING DIAGNOSIS

Knowledge deficit (parental) related to lack of familiarity with hospital procedures and perioperative routines

Expected outcome

The parents will express appropriate understanding of the surgical procedure their infant will undergo.

Interventions

1. Determine the parents' readiness to learn.

2. Assess the effect of the infant's medical problem on the parents and on the family's lifestyle.

3. Determine each parent's stage of adaptation to the infant's condition (such as shock and disbelief, developing awareness, and resolution and reorganization). Base your teaching approach on that stage.

4. Assess the parents' knowledge of the infant's disorder, including its implications and potential complications.

5. Determine the parents' learning needs.

6. Set realistic goals, and work with the family to ensure mutually acceptable goals.

7. Set priorities and divide teaching content into information to teach now and information to teach later.

8. Determine the best time for teaching sessions.

9. Use various teaching strategies and tools, including:
• printed materials, such as booklets, at the appropriate reading level
• discussions
• demonstrations
• films and videotapes
• models or dolls.

10. Teach the family about the infant's perioperative care, such as:
• food and fluid restrictions
• time of surgery
• type of anesthesia
• insertion of I.V. or intra-arterial lines
• operating room and postanesthesia care unit personnel and environments
• equipment and procedures, such as monitors, tubes, drains, dressing changes, and respiratory therapy.

Rationales

1. This helps you plan your teaching method and the type and amount of material to present.

2. This helps determine the extent of teaching required; teaching should be structured according to the areas most affected.

3. Teaching focus and issues differ with the stage of adaptation, requiring a different teaching approach.

4. Teaching works best when it is based on the learner's previous experience and knowledge.

5. The parents' needs determine the appropriate content. Responding to these needs conveys sensitivity to the family's concerns.

6. Goals affect teaching content. Family participation in goal setting improves the chance of success.

7. Setting priorities and dividing teaching content into these categories ensure coverage of important information without overwhelming the family.

8. Choosing appropriate times for teaching sessions enhances the parents' attention and receptivity, improving their retention of information.

9. Parents are more likely to retain information when learning engages multiple senses.

10. Such teaching reduces the parents' fears and anxieties by helping them understand what to expect. Also, parents are more likely to remember and comply with perioperative care if they understand the rationales for using equipment and performing procedures.

11. Evaluate the parents' response to teaching.

11. This determines whether goals have been met and may reveal the need for further teaching.

12. Additional individualized interventions: _____

12. Rationales: _____

Documentation checklist
During the hospital stay, document:
❏ patient status and assessment findings, especially cardiorespiratory status, temperature stability, description of the situation or condition that requires surgery, and neurologic status before surgery
❏ changes in patient status
❏ pertinent laboratory and diagnostic findings, especially serum glucose and electrolyte levels, ABG studies, PT and PTT, platelet count, CBC with differential, screening for sexually transmitted infection (if done), chromosomal studies (if done), urine specific gravity, and any culture results
❏ patient's response to treatment before surgery
❏ family's reaction to the diagnosis and the need for surgery
❏ parent-infant interaction
❏ family teaching guidelines about the condition requiring surgery.

Associated plans
❏ Bowel obstruction
❏ Cleft lip and cleft palate
❏ Congenital heart disease
❏ Hypothermia and hyperthermia
❏ Intracranial hemorrhage
❏ Necrotizing enterocolitis
❏ Spinal cord defects and hydrocephalus
❏ Tracheoesophageal fistula or esophageal atresia

Additional nursing diagnoses
❏ Altered growth and development related to environmental and stimulation deficiencies
❏ Altered nutrition: less than body requirements related to withholding food and water
❏ Fear (parental) related to possible separation from infant or death of infant as result of surgery
❏ Ineffective family coping related to guilt and anxiety
❏ Ineffective infant feeding pattern related to withholding of food and fluids
❏ Risk for altered body temperature related to extremes in age and weight
❏ Risk for fluid volume deficit related to withholding food and water or to gastric decompression

Preterm infant

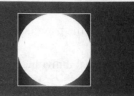

Definition

An infant whose gestational age is 37 weeks or less at birth is called preterm. Although small, a preterm infant may be appropriately sized for its gestational age, but poor intrauterine growth may complicate the postnatal period of the already compromised infant.

An infant whose birth weight is about 5 lb, 8 oz (2,500 g) or less and whose gestational age is more than 37 weeks is considered small for gestational age (SGA) rather than preterm, although about 75% of neonates who weigh less than 2,500 g are born prematurely. Preterm births constitute 8% to 10% all live births in the United States.

Clinical problems occur more often in a preterm infant than in a full-term infant. Prematurity results in immaturely developed and functioning systems, limiting the infant's ability to cope with problems and illnesses.

Common problems include respiratory distress syndrome (RDS), necrotizing enterocolitis, hyperbilirubinemia, hypoglycemia, poor thermoregulation, patent ductus arteriosus (PDA), pulmonary edema, and intraventricular hemorrhage. Additional stressors for the infant and parents include separation and prolonged hospitalization for the high-risk or critically ill infant. Parental responses and coping mechanisms may interfere with the parent-infant relationship; special allowances and planning may be needed to support the bonding process.

The preterm infant's survival depends on weight, gestational age, and illnesses or abnormalities. Preterm delivery accounts for 75% to 80% of neonatal morbidity and mortality. This plan focuses on caring for the preterm infant and preventing potential complications in specific systems.

Etiology and precipitating factors
• Maternal factors, including:
  – disorders, such as hypertensive disease, pregnancy-induced hypertension (PIH), placenta previa, abruptio placentae, cervical incompetence, multiple gestation, malnutrition, and diabetes mellitus
  – low socioeconomic status and little or no prenatal care
  – history of preterm deliveries or induced abortion
  – maternal use of any or all of the following: prescribed, over-the-counter, or illegal drugs; alcohol; cigarettes; or caffeine

Physical findings
Maternal history
• Age under 16 years and poor educational background
• Multiple gestation
• Low socioeconomic status, little or no prenatal care, and poor nutrition
• Possibly genetic counseling
• Previous preterm births and closely spaced pregnancies
• Infections, such as sexually transmitted infections
• Conditions, such as PIH, premature rupture of membranes, abruptio placentae, placenta previa, and prolapsed umbilical cord
• Use of caffeine, cigarettes, alcohol, or prescribed, over-the-counter, or illegal drugs
• Blood type, Rh factor, amniocentesis for lung profile, alpha fetoprotein with history of previous infants with neurologic defects
• Antenatal steroids received

Infant status at birth
• Gestational age usually 23 to 37 weeks, low birth weight, SGA, or large for gestational age
• Weight usually less than 5 lb, 8 oz (2,500 g)
• Thin, minimal subcutaneous fat deposits
• Large head in proportion to body: circumference about 1¼" (3 cm) larger than chest circumference
• Possibly visible physical anomalies
• Apgar score at 1 and 5 minutes: 0 to 3 indicates severe distress; 4 to 6, moderate distress; and 7 to 10, normal adjustment probable
• Surfactant received

Cardiovascular
• Heart rate 110 to 160 beats/minute at apical site with regular rhythm
• At birth, possible murmur auscultated over base of heart or at third or fourth intercostal space at left sternal edge, indicating right-to-left shunt from pulmonary hypertension or atelectasis

Gastrointestinal
• Protruding abdomen
• Meconium passage usually within 12 hours
• Weak sucking and diminished swallowing reflexes
• Patent anus unless congenital abnormality present

Integumentary
• Pallid, cyanotic, jaundiced, mottled, red, or bright pink skin
• Little vernix caseosa, with lanugo over entire body
• Thin, transparent appearance, both smooth and shiny

- Generalized edema or localized edema in presenting part at delivery
- Short nails; fine, fuzzy, scant, or no head hair
- Possibly petechiae or ecchymoses
- Minimally creased soles and palms

Musculoskeletal
- Ear cartilage poorly developed but soft and pliable
- Fontanels and separation at suture lines present
- Soft skull and rib bones
- Relaxed state, inactive, or lethargic

Neurologic
- Reflexes and movement to neurologic test meet with no resistance; reflex activity is only partly developed
- Sucking, swallowing, gag reflex, and coughing may be weak or ineffectual
- Absent or diminished neurologic signs
- Eyes may be closed or fused before 25 to 26 gestational weeks
- Unstable body temperature; usually hypothermic, adjusting to various environmental temperatures
- Possibly tremors, twitching, and eye rolling; usually transient but may indicate neurologic abnormalities

Pulmonary
- Respiratory rate ranging from 40 to 60 breaths/minute with short periods of apnea
- Possibly irregular respirations, with nasal flaring, grunting, and retractions (intercostal, suprasternal, or substernal)
- Possibly audible fine crackles

Renal
- Voiding occurring within 8 hours after birth
- Possibly inability to excrete solutes in urine

Reproductive
- Girls: prominent clitoris with poorly developed labia majora
- Boys: underdeveloped scrotum with minimal rugae and testes not down in scrotum, with inguinal hernia

Behavioral findings
- Possibly weak cry
- Jitteriness
- Inactivity

Diagnostic studies
- X-ray studies of chest or other organs to confirm or rule out suspected abnormalities
- Ultrasonography to detect organ abnormalities
- Heelstick blood glucose levels (reagent or glucose reagent strip testing) to identify blood glucose decreases, followed by serum glucose test if values are less than 40 mg/dl, with second test for verification
- Serum calcium level to identify decreases that may lead to hypocalcemia
- Bilirubin levels to identify increases (because a preterm infant is more vulnerable to hyperbilirubinemia than a full-term infant); umbilical cord blood is tested
- Complete blood count (CBC) for hematocrit and hemoglobin decreases, red blood cell count decreases, platelet count decreases, and white blood cell (WBC) count and differential abnormalities
- Electrolyte levels to determine potassium, sodium, and magnesium levels
- Arterial blood gas (ABG) studies to identify changes in oxygen, carbon dioxide, bicarbonate, or pH, indicating acidosis
- Blood type, Rh factor, and Coombs' test to identify potential incompatibilities
- Culture of blood, other body fluids, or drainage to identify infectious agents, if any
- Urinalysis for specific gravity and culture to identify infection
- Stool analysis to identify occult blood (first stool usually is positive from blood swallowed during delivery)
- Additional tests as appropriate, depending on presenting signs

COLLABORATIVE PROBLEM

Risk for respiratory distress related to pulmonary immaturity with decreased surfactant production causing hypoxemia and acidosis

Expected outcome

The patient will maintain optimal pulmonary function.

Interventions	**Rationales**
1. Compile assessment data focusing on possible respiratory distress, including:	**1.** Assessment data provide baseline information, permitting early interventions and a better prognosis if the infant should display respiratory distress signs (see the "Respiratory distress syndrome" plan, page 297, for care of respiratory distress in the preterm infant).
• maternal history of drug use or abnormal conditions during pregnancy or labor and delivery	• Maternal conditions may predispose the infant to respiratory distress.

• infant's condition at birth, including Apgar score and need for resuscitation
• respiratory rate, depth, and ease; note tachypnea with a rate over 60 breaths/minute
• expiratory grunting, nasal flaring, or retractions with the use of accessory muscles (intercostal, suprasternal, or substernal)
• cyanosis when breathing room air and decreased breath sounds.

2. Assess for apneic episodes lasting longer than 20 seconds, noting:
• bradycardia
• lethargy, position (side-lying, prone, or supine), and activity (for example, while sleeping or feeding) before, during, and after apneic episode; airway obstruction caused by mask (Bilimask) over nose
• abdominal distention
• skin temperature and mottling
• spontaneous return of breathing
• need for stimulation, including type and amount
• episode's duration
• cause of apnea, such as cold stress, sepsis, respiratory failure, or preterm birth
• results of CBC with differential, blood culture, chest X-ray, and ABG studies, if performed.

3. Provide and monitor respiratory support:

• Administer warm and humidified oxygen, with a pulse oximeter or transcutaneous blood oxygen tension monitor in place. Check oxygen hourly. Reposition the probe every 3 hours.
• Carefully suction the infant's nostrils and mouth for no longer than 5 seconds.
• Maintain a neutral thermal environment.

• Position the infant on its abdomen in the supine position with a small pad beneath the shoulders or on its side with its head supported.
• Stimulate the infant by stroking its feet, hands, and back and then its trunk, face, arms, and legs. Start with gentle motions, making them more vigorous if needed.

4. Monitor serial ABG studies to identify respiratory or metabolic acidosis.

5. Prepare and administer methylxanthine pharmacologic therapy, such as caffeine, theophylline, or aminophylline. Monitor blood levels every 1 to 2 days for toxicity.

6. Additional individualized interventions: _____

_____

• This provides data indicating respiratory distress at birth.
• Respiratory rate increases with respiratory distress as the infant's need for oxygen increases.
• Respiratory distress signs appear as the infant attempts to increase oxygen intake. They may also result from meconium aspiration or diaphragmatic hernia.
• These signs appear as respiratory distress worsens.

2. Apneic episodes may occur because of hypoxia and carbon dioxide retention and decreased pH. Breathing cessation that lasts less than 20 seconds is known as periodic breathing; breathing cessation that lasts for 20 to 30 seconds is apnea. Apnea may be a sign of sepsis, intracranial hemorrhage, RDS, cold stress, hypoglycemia, pneumonia, PDA, maternal oversedation, or other problems. An infant with apneic pauses that last 15 seconds or more should be placed on an apnea monitor with alarms set to detect apneic episodes of 15 seconds (see the "Sepsis neonatorum and infectious disorders" plan, page 306, for procedure).

3. Respiratory support provides the infant with needed oxygen. Monitoring prevents oxygen toxicity.
• Oxygen administration supplements the infant's oxygen supply. Monitoring ensures the optimal oxygen level necessary for respiratory support. Changing the position of the probe prevents burns.
• Suctioning may be needed to maintain a patent airway if the infant is receiving mechanical ventilation.
• Temperature changes may contribute to apnea and increased oxygen consumption, which leads to decreased surfactant production.
• These positions make breathing easier and promote chest expansion.

• Stimulating the central nervous system promotes spontaneous resumption of breathing during apneic episodes.

4. ABG studies signal respiratory depression; for example, partial pressure of oxygen less than 50 mm Hg indicates hypoxia; partial pressure of carbon dioxide more than 55 mm Hg indicates hypercapnia; and pH less than 7.3 indicates acidosis.

5. Methylxanthines are given for apnea. They increase ventilation through central stimulation, which causes bronchodilation. Monitoring ensures that therapeutic drug levels are maintained without toxicity.

6. Rationales: _____

_____

COLLABORATIVE PROBLEM

Risk for hypothermia or hyperthermia related to prematurity or changes in environmental temperatures

Expected outcome

The patient will maintain a stable temperature in a neutral thermal environment.

Interventions	Rationales
1. Maintain an ambient nursery temperature of 77° F (25° C).	**1.** An optimal room temperature minimizes heat loss.
2. Assess the infant's temperature every 2 hours or as needed.	**2.** A preterm infant is susceptible to cold stress or temperature fluctuations because of decreased subcutaneous fat deposits, low metabolic reserves of substances needed for heat and energy, inability to shiver, and smaller ratio of body mass to surface area (see the "Hypothermia and hyperthermia" plan, page 247).
3. Carry out appropriate warming procedure after the infant's delivery.	**3.** Warming conserves the infant's body heat and helps prevent temperature changes.
4. Place the infant under a radiant warmer or in an incubator, if indicated.	**4.** A radiant warmer or an incubator ensures a neutral thermal environment, which helps the infant maintain its body temperature and reduce oxygen consumption.
5. Apply the temperature control (Servo-Control) probe over the abdomen, set the heater output for 98.6° to 99.5° F (37° to 37.5° C), and maintain a skin temperature of 96° to 97° F (35.6° to 36.5° C).	**5.** The device controls the infant's body temperature by turning on or off when the infant's temperature varies from a set point. The temperature setting depends on the infant's age and weight.
6. Protect the infant from external contact with sources of cold or heat and exposure to cold or hot air. Take steps to conserve the infant's body heat, such as keeping it dry and covering its head.	**6.** These steps help prevent potential hypothermic or hyperthermic responses by minimizing heat loss through radiation, conduction, convection, and evaporation and preventing cold stress.
7. Assess the infant for status changes that may indicate cold stress.	**7.** Cold stress increases oxygen and caloric needs, which may lead to hypoxia and acidosis (see the "Hypothermia and hyperthermia" plan, page 247).

COLLABORATIVE PROBLEM

Altered nutrition: less than body requirements, related to inadequate stores of glycogen, iron, and calcium and to the depletion of these stores by the infant's higher metabolic rate and increased requirements, inadequate calorie intake, and loss of calories

Expected outcome

The patient will maintain adequate calorie intake and optimal nutritional status.

Interventions	Rationales
1. Assess the infant's sucking and gag reflexes and swallowing ability. Begin oral feedings when the infant is stable and its respirations are controlled.	**1.** Immature reflexes, lethargy, or weakness may postpone oral feedings.
2. Assess and calculate the infant's calorie requirements.	**2.** For optimal weight gain, the preterm infant requires about 120 to 150 cal/kg/24 hours once oral feedings begin.

3. Initiate breast-feeding or bottle-feeding 2 to 6 hours after birth. Begin with 3 to 5 ml per feeding every 3 hours and increase as tolerated. Breast-feeding may need to be postponed until the infant demonstrates that it can feed by nipple and gain weight; if so, the mother can pump milk to be bottle-fed to the infant.

4. Weigh the infant daily, comparing weight with calorie intake, to determine if the infant needs to increase its intake.

5. Provide dextrose 10% in water ($D_{10}W$) I.V. if the infant does not feed orally.

6. Provide gavage feedings as appropriate.

7. Provide total parenteral nutrition (TPN) and intralipids as appropriate.

8. Monitor heelstick blood glucose levels with reagent or glucose reagent strip testing; monitor serum for calcium, iron, and glucose levels.

9. Additional individualized interventions: _____

3. Feedings should begin as soon as possible because the immature infant has not had the opportunity to build up stores of iron and glucose. The stable preterm infant may be able to tolerate oral feedings.

4. Daily weighing determines whether the infant is taking in enough calories for adequate weight gain (see appendix G, Fluid and nutritional needs in infancy).

5. I.V. $D_{10}W$ meets the preterm infant's immediate fluid and glucose requirements, preventing hypoglycemia that can result from depleted glucose stores.

6. This alternate route ensures nutritional intake if the infant's condition prevents oral feeding (see the "Respiratory distress syndrome" plan, page 297, for gavage procedure and care).

7. TPN meets the infant's nutritional requirements during a prolonged illness or after surgery (see the "Tracheoesophageal fistula or esophageal atresia" plan, page 326, for TPN procedure and care).

8. Monitoring identifies low glucose, calcium, or iron levels that signal the need for replacement to prevent complications.

9. Rationales: _____

COLLABORATIVE PROBLEM

Fluid imbalance related to losses from immaturity, use of a radiant warmer, phototherapy, or through skin or lungs

Expected outcome

The patient will maintain a stable fluid and electrolyte balance.

Interventions

1. Carefully assess and calculate the infant's fluid requirements.

2. Provide from 150 to 180 ml/kg of fluids, up to 200 ml/kg if necessary. Fluids should not be withheld for very long.

3. Weigh the infant daily.

4. Monitor and record the infant's fluid intake and output hourly. Compare amounts to identify imbalances. Include all sources of intake and output.

5. Test the infant's urine for specific gravity and glycosuria.

Rationales

1. This allows accurate fluid administration. An infant's immature renal system affects its ability to concentrate urine and conserve fluid. A preterm infant loses more fluid through the skin than a full-term infant during treatments (as much as 190%). (See the "Postoperative care" plan, page 277, for input-output procedure.)

2. This fulfills the infant's fluid requirement; the specific amount depends on the infant's needs and fluid loss.

3. A daily weight record reflects the infant's growth progress as well as fluid losses or gains.

4. Comparing fluid intake and output allows the detection of excess fluid losses.

5. The urine test provides information about potential dehydration or glycosuria.

6. Maintain a neutral thermal environment, and dress the infant in proper clothing to help prevent fluid loss.

7. Assess the infant for indications of increased fluid needs, such as:
- increased body temperature
- hypovolemic shock with decreased blood pressure and increased heart rate, diminished peripheral pulses, cool hands and feet, and skin mottling
- sepsis
- asphyxia and hypoxia.

8. Monitor potassium, sodium, and chloride levels; replace electrolytes and fluids (with $D_{10}W$ I.V.), if needed.

9. Additional individualized interventions: _____

6. A preterm infant lacks insulating fat. Its thin skin, with blood vessels close to the body surface, increases the potential for fluid and heat loss through the skin.

7. A sick preterm infant needs careful hemodynamic monitoring because it is prone to arrhythmias from immature cardiac conduction tissue and autonomic nervous system or from susceptibility to congenital heart defects other than PDA; these arrhythmias might occur secondary to prolonged exposure to decreased oxygen level.

8. Electrolyte and fluid replacement maintains fluid and electrolyte balance (see appendix G, Fluid and nutritional needs in infancy, for requirements).

9. Rationales: _____

COLLABORATIVE PROBLEM

Risk for infection related to infant's immunologic immaturity and possible infection transmission from mother or health care personnel

Expected outcome

The patient will remain free from infection.

Interventions

1. Assess for temperature fluctuations, lethargy, apnea, poor feeding, irritability, and jaundice.

2. Review maternal history, the infant's condition at birth, and infection epidemics in the nursery.

3. Obtain samples of blood and drainage from any source.

4. Review laboratory data, including CBC with WBC count and differential and platelet count. Note immunoglobulins with WBC count less than 5,000 or greater than 25,000/mm³; absolute neutrophils less than 5,000; immature to total neutrophil ratios of 0.25:0.49; platelets less than 80,000/mm³; and immunoglobulin M increases.

5. Provide an environment that protects the infant from infection.
- Follow protocol for gown changes and hand washing before and between infant care.
- Follow protocol for isolating infants or excluding them from the nursery.
- Follow meticulous sterile technique when caring for the infant and performing procedures.
- Follow protocol to protect the infant from contact with people who might transmit infection.
- Institute standard precautions as indicated.
- Instruct the parents how to prevent cross-contamination of the infant and transmission of microorganisms.

Rationales

1. Identifying early signs of infection allows prompt treatment.

2. Infections may be transmitted perinatally by the mother or by hospital personnel.

3. Cultures identify microorganisms responsible for infection, making treatment choices possible.

4. The infant's immature defense systems at birth (with a deficiency in phagocytic and immune system activity and decreased inflammatory response) increase the potential for acquiring infection. This is a special concern for the compromised preterm infant. Reviewing laboratory data identifies actual or potential infection.

5. These actions prevent the transmission of infection to the infant (see the "Sepsis neonatorum and infectious disorders" plan, page 306, for complete care of infection in the preterm infant).

6. Additional individualized interventions: _____ | **6.** Rationales: _____

_____ | _____

NURSING DIAGNOSIS

Risk for impaired skin integrity related to fragile, transparent, immature skin

Expected outcome

The patient will maintain optimal skin integrity.

Interventions	**Rationales**
1. Assess the infant's skin for redness, irritation, rashes, and lesions and for breakdown in all pressure areas.	**1.** The preterm infant has thinner, more fragile skin, with capillaries near the surface and minimal subcutaneous fat to protect bony pressure areas.
2. Assess I.V., electrode, and catheter sites or other insertion sites for signs of infection, skin breakdown, and extravasation of fluid.	**2.** A preterm infant is more likely to undergo invasive therapeutic procedures, further exposing the skin to breakdown.
3. Provide appropriate daily skin care but, as much as possible, protect the infant's skin from contact with cleaning agents, other solutions, and tapes.	**3.** This protects the skin by maintaining cleanliness and preventing loss of the protective bactericidal barrier or skin layer.
4. Additional individualized interventions: _____	**4.** Rationales: _____

NURSING DIAGNOSIS

Sensory/perceptual alteration: visual, auditory, kinesthetic, gustatory, tactile, and olfactory related to decreased or excessive stimulation of intensive care environment

Expected outcome

The patient will receive sensory stimulation without sensory overload.

Interventions	**Rationales**
1. Assess the infant's ability to respond to stimuli. Observe for: • neurologic deficits • alertness or inattention • inappropriate response to noise, eye contact, or feeding and absent normal reflexes • effects of medications on behavior.	**1.** Assessment results suggest the types and amounts of sensory stimulation to provide or reduce.
2. Provide visual stimulation: • Dim bright lights. • Suspend a black-and-white mobile with geometric shapes 7″ to 9″ [17.8 to 22.9 cm] from the infant's eyes. • Hold the infant at eye level for eye contact; hold the infant upright on your shoulder if possible.	**2.** The infant should be able to look at and respond to an object; too much visual stimulation may cause the infant to look away or sigh or cause respiratory changes.

3. Provide auditory stimulation:
• Talk to the infant, speaking in a quiet, gentle voice.
• Call the infant by name and talk to the infant while giving care.
• Sing, play tapes, or turn on a radio.
• Avoid excessive noises and conversations around the infant.
• Reduce monitor noises if possible.

4. Provide tactile stimulation as follows:
• With warmed hands, stroke the infant gently from head to toe as well as all other parts of the infant's body.
• Hold and caress the infant, if appropriate.
• Give the infant a pacifier for sucking satisfaction.
• Touch the infant with articles of differing textures, such as cotton balls or smooth and napped cloth.
• Change the infant's position every other hour, if appropriate.
• Carry the infant in a strap-on carrier, if appropriate.
• Flex the infant's knees, hips, and elbows and cover its flexed body with your hand.

5. Provide gustatory stimulation by offering a pacifier or feeding the infant breast milk or formula as indicated.

6. Provide uninterrupted rest and sleep periods.

7. Additional individualized interventions: _____

3. Auditory responses, such as the infant turning its head toward the sounds, should occur; overstimulation may cause apnea, bradycardia, or minimal body response.

4. Tactile responses, such as motor activity, should occur based on the infant's condition; overstimulation may cause hyperactivity or hypoactivity. Tactile deficiency may cause inappropriate crying spells or response only during procedures. The flexed position decreases stress in the preterm infant.

5. Gustatory responses, such as hand-to-mouth activity, feeding, and sucking pacifier, should occur.

6. Rest periods prevent overstimulation.

7. Rationales: _____

NURSING DIAGNOSIS

Knowledge deficit related to care of sick infant at home

Expected outcome

The parents will express appropriate understanding about the infant's condition and follow-up care.

Interventions

1. Inform the parents and family about:
• disease process
• care procedures
• signs of respiratory problems
• follow-up care and therapy.

2. Teach the parents and family about ordered treatments, such as:
• home oxygen therapy
• mechanical ventilation
• chest physiotherapy
• drug therapy
• nutritional and fluid therapy
• specialized monitoring, such as apnea or blood glucose monitoring.

Rationales

1. Learning about the infant's condition and treatment relieves family members' anxiety and allows them to prepare for the infant's discharge.

2. Such teaching promotes family compliance and helps dispel their fears about equipment and procedures.

3. Have the parents and family give return demonstrations of all required procedures.

4. Encourage the parents and family to participate in the infant's care.

5. Teach the parents and family how to balance the infant's activities with rest and how to evaluate the infant's tolerance for activities. Provide them with appropriate written information they can use for reference at home.

6. Arrange for home health care follow-up.

7. Additional individualized interventions: _____

_____

3. Return demonstrations boost family members' feelings of adequacy and independence and may alert the nurse to the need for more instruction.

4. Participation helps alleviate feelings of inadequacy and prepares family members to care for the infant at home.

5. Stimulation of activity is crucial for normal infant growth and development, which may be delayed from prolonged hospitalization. Activity tolerance varies from one infant to the next. Written information gives the parents a resource they can refer to at home.

6. Home health care provides the parents and family with continued support outside the hospital.

7. Rationales: _____

_____

Documentation checklist

During the hospital stay, document:
❒ patient status and assessment findings, especially whether mother received antenatal steroids, Apgar scores, gestational age by examination, presence of any murmurs, respiratory effort, tolerance of enteral feedings (if infant received enteral feedings), skin integrity, daily weight, head circumference, and skin and core temperature variations (axillary, aural, and infrared)
❒ changes in patient status, especially changes in respiratory status
❒ pertinent laboratory and diagnostic findings, especially serum calcium, phosphorus, total protein, potassium, sodium, magnesium, bilirubin, and glucose levels; CBC with differential; ABG results (oxygen, carbon dioxide, bicarbonate, and pH); type and crossmatch; Coombs' test; Rh factor; culture results; urine specific gravity; occult blood in stools; and chest X-rays
❒ patient's response to treatment, especially to surfactant (if given)
❒ family's reaction to the diagnosis
❒ parent-infant interaction
❒ family teaching guidelines, especially any special care required and guidelines for stability and stress cues
❒ discharge planning guidelines.

Associated plans

All plans for the full-term infant have applications relevant to the preterm infant, whose condition usually is compromised and who usually is vulnerable to the conditions discussed in this section. See the plan appropriate to the individual infant.

Additional nursing diagnoses

❒ Altered family processes related to birth of high-risk infant
❒ Altered growth and development related to functional immaturity and prolonged environmental stress
❒ Altered parenting related to infant's need for intensive care nursery
❒ Anxiety (parental) related to vulnerability of small infant to illnesses
❒ Caregiver role strain related to infant's status and need for intensive care
❒ Impaired gas exchange related to pulmonary immaturity
❒ Ineffective breathing pattern related to respiratory and neurologic immaturity
❒ Ineffective individual coping (parental) related to stress of preterm birth
❒ Powerlessness (parental) related to health care environment and limited infant interaction
❒ Risk for injury related to lack of cushioning from inadequate subcutaneous fat

Respiratory distress syndrome

Definition

Respiratory distress syndrome (RDS), also known as hyaline membrane disease, is an acute disorder found primarily in preterm infants at birth or shortly after birth. It occurs most often in infants under 32 weeks' gestation who weigh less than 3 lb, 4 oz (1,500 g). Roughly 60% of infants born before 29 weeks' gestation develop RDS.

Normal respiratory function depends on adequate lung development and surfactant production. A lipoprotein that lines the alveoli, surfactant decreases surface tension, preventing alveolar collapse and decreasing the work of breathing. Preterm infants are born before they can produce sufficient surfactant on their own. As a result, surface tension increases, causing alveolar collapse and decreased lung compliance. This reduces alveolar ventilation, leading to a poor ventilation-perfusion ratio in pulmonary circulation and resulting in hypoxemia and hypercapnia with respiratory acidosis. Tissue hypoxia, metabolic acidosis, and atelectasis occur as respiratory failure progresses.

To prevent such complications, the mother can receive steroids to stimulate fetal lung maturation if premature birth is imminent. Ideally, she should receive the steroids 48 to 72 hours before the birth. Once the infant is born, it receives surfactant to decrease the chances of such long-term complications of RDS as oxygen toxicity, retinopathy of prematurity, bronchopulmonary dysplasia, and ventilator dependence. Despite such preventive treatments, RDS remains the leading cause of morbidity and mortality in preterm infants.

This plan focuses on caring for the infant at risk for or with RDS and on the associated respiratory support the infant may need.

Etiology and precipitating factors

• Prematurity with immature lungs (ranges from 32 to 35 weeks' gestation) and absence, alteration, or deficiency of pulmonary surfactants
• Cesarean delivery of preterm infant
• Decreased oxygen in fetus or at birth in full-term or preterm infant

Physical findings
Maternal history
• Disorder such as diabetes mellitus
• Condition such as placental bleeding
• Type and length of delivery
• Fetal or intrapartal stress
Infant status at birth
• Prematurity, small for gestational age (large if mother is diabetic)
• Apgar score indicating asphyxia
• Cesarean delivery of preterm infant
Cardiovascular
• Bradycardia (less than 100 beats/minute) with severe hypoxemia
Integumentary
• Pallor caused by peripheral vasoconstriction
• Pitting edema in hands and feet within 24 hours
• Mottling
Neurologic
• Immobility, motionlessness; flaccidity
• Decreased body temperature
Cardiovascular
• Systolic murmur
• Heart rate within normal limits
Pulmonary
• Tachypnea (more than 60 breaths/minute; may be as high as 100 breaths/minute)
• Expiratory grunting or whining
• Nasal flaring
• Intercostal, suprasternal, or substernal retractions
• Cyanosis (circumoral followed by central) related to percentage of desaturated hemoglobin
• Decreased breath sounds, crackles, apneic episodes
Behavioral findings
• Lethargy

Diagnostic studies

• Serial chest X-rays reveal clouded appearance with grainy look, areas of density or atelectasis, and elevated diaphragm with overdistended alveolar ducts.
• Air bronchograms reveal ventilation of the airway, not the alveoli.
• A fetus predisposed to RDS should have a lung profile performed on amniotic fluid to determine lung maturity. Specific tests include the automated fluorescence polarized assay (TDx instrument) for rapid testing of lecithin-

sphingomyelin (L/S) ratio and the Amino-Stat-FLM test for determining phosphatidyglycerol (PG) levels; these two tests together produce highly reliable results:
 – Normal L/S ratio is 2:1 or more, indicating pulmonary maturity; ratio must be 3:1 if mother is diabetic.
 – PG should appear in amniotic fluid by 35 weeks' gestation.
 – Phosphatidylinositol level should decrease.

• Arterial blood gas (ABG) levels, which include a partial pressure of arterial oxygen (PaO_2) less than 50 mm Hg while on 100% oxygen, partial pressure of arterial carbon dioxide ($PaCO_2$) less than 60 mm Hg, oxygen saturation 92% to 94%, and pH 7.31 to 7.45.
• Potassium levels in RDS increase as potassium is released from injured alveolar cells.

COLLABORATIVE PROBLEM

Respiratory insufficiency related to reduced lung volume and compliance, lung perfusion, and alveolar ventilation (two expected outcomes)

Expected outcome 1

The infant at risk for respiratory distress will be identified early to prevent complications of RDS.

Interventions

1. Assess for infant at risk for RDS, including:
• history of mother with diabetes or placental bleeding
• prematurity of infant
• fetal hypoxia
• cesarean birth.

2. Assess for changes in respiratory status, including:

• tachypnea (more than 60 breaths/minute and possibly as high as 100 breaths/minute)
• expiratory grunting

• nasal flaring

• intercostal, suprasternal, or substernal retractions with the use of accessory muscles
• cyanosis (circumoral followed by central) on room air

• apneic episodes, decreased breath sounds, and crepitant crackles.

3. Assess for associated signs of RDS, including:
• pallor and pitting edema in hands and feet within 24 hours
• flaccid muscles, motionlessness, or lying in a froglike position with the head to the side
• heart rate less than 100 beats/minute in late-stage RDS
• serial ABG levels that show PaO_2 level less than 40 mm Hg, $PaCO_2$ level greater than 65 mm Hg, and pH less than 7.15
• grainy appearance and ground-glass appearance on air bronchograms.

Rationales

1. Assessment permits early interventions if an infant displays signs of respiratory distress and, consequently, results in a better prognosis.

2. These changes indicate RDS, calling for immediate treatment.
• The infant's respiratory rate increases in an attempt to increase oxygen levels.
• This is the sound of the glottis closing to stop exhalation of air by forcing it against the vocal cords.
• Flaring is an attempt to widen nostrils to reduce resistance to respirations.
• Retractions indicate inadequate lung expansion during inspiration.
• Cyanosis becomes apparent as a later sign of RDS, with partial pressure of oxygen (PO_2) as low as 40 mm Hg.
• Apneic episodes and decreased breath sounds occur as respiratory distress becomes more severe.

3. These signs indicate RDS.
• Pallor and pitting edema result from peripheral vasoconstriction and altered vascular permeability.
• These signs result from exhaustion caused by energy expenditure during difficult breathing.
• Bradycardia results from severe hypoxemia.
• These ABG levels indicate respiratory acidosis and metabolic acidosis if the infant is hypoxic.

• This is diagnostic of RDS.

4. Monitor transcutaneous Po_2 or pulse oximetry values continuously or every hour.

4. Transcutaneous Po_2 and noninvasive pulse oximetry devices measure oxygen percentage in inspired air. Monitoring these values ensures proper forced inspiratory oxygen (Fio_2) concentration and accuracy of readings.

5. Additional individualized interventions: _____
_____

5. Rationales: _____
_____

Expected outcome 2

The patient will maintain optimal pulmonary function.

Interventions

1. Administer warm and humidified oxygen as follows, according to hospital policy.

- Warm oxygen to 89° to 93° F (31.7° to 33.9° C).
- Humidify oxygen to 40% to 60%.
- Use a small oxygen hood (Oxyhood) for an infant weighing 2 lb, 8 oz (1,134 g) or less and a medium hood for an infant weighing from 2 lb, 9 oz to 8 lb (1,135 to 3,629 g).
- Provide continuous positive airway pressure (CPAP) or continuous distending pressure by endotracheal tube (using mechanical ventilation) to achieve intermittent buildup of positive pressure in the airway. Nasal prongs, nasopharyngeal prongs, face mask, nasal mask, and head box are methods used for respiratory distress conditions and may be used for RDS, but they are more commonly used for other conditions.
- Provide positive end-expiratory pressure (PEEP) or continuous negative pressure using the same techniques to achieve intermittent negative pressure around the chest wall.
- Provide intermittent positive-pressure ventilation (IPPV) by endotracheal intubation (mechanical ventilation).
- Provide high-frequency or conventional mechanical ventilation.

2. Assist with surfactant administration.

3. Prepare and administer pancuronium bromide (Pavulon).

4. Place the infant in a neutral thermal environment, and monitor axillary temperature every hour.

Rationales

1. Methods vary, depending on oxygen needs, infant acuity, and the need for ventilatory assistance; these methods can also be used for other respiratory distress conditions.
- Warmed oxygen prevents hypothermia.
- Humidified oxygen prevents mucosal dryness.
- An oxygen hood delivers prescribed concentrations of oxygen for the infant who can breathe spontaneously.

- CPAP is used for the infant with recurrent apnea and RDS who requires more than 70% oxygen to maintain a Pao_2 of more than 60 mm Hg and to maintain breathing with positive pressure throughout the respiratory cycle. An infant weighing 1,500 g may be mechanically ventilated, depending on other factors, such as gestational age.

- Like CPAP, PEEP prevents the collapse of alveoli by exerting positive pressure at the end-expiratory phase, forcing the alveoli to retain air.

- IPPV is the best way of assuring effective ventilation; it is used when Pao_2 is not corrected by CPAP of 6 cm H_2O and 80% oxygen.
- High-frequency ventilation requires less pressure; it decreases the risk of barotrauma but increases the risk of intravascular bleeding. Conventional mechanical ventilation carries less risk of intravascular bleeding but may cause barotrauma, such as air leak or bronchopulmonary dysplasia.

2. Surfactant increases pulmonary function.

3. This drug may be ordered as a muscle relaxant to prevent the infant from working against the ventilator and causing injury.

4. A neutral thermal environment reduces oxygen requirements and carbon dioxide production by stabilizing the infant's temperature. This may prevent a life-threatening situation from developing (see the "Hypothermia and hyperthermia" plan, page 247).

5. Continually monitor vital signs electronically for changes in heart rate, respiratory rate, and blood pressure, and auscultate for breath sounds every hour.

5. Electronic monitoring allows the detection of changes without disturbing the infant. Blood pressure is monitored for indications of hypovolemia; respiratory rate is monitored to detect periods of apnea.

6. Observe for changes in skin color, movement, and activity.

6. Changes in skin color, movement, and activity may indicate increased metabolism of oxygen and glucose. They indicate the need to assess the infant further for changing fluid, calorie, and oxygen requirements.

7. Conserve the infant's energy by clustering procedures and handling the infant as little as possible.

7. Handling the infant and performing procedures require the infant to use energy, increasing its need for oxygen and, possibly, causing a drop in PaO_2 level.

8. Monitor serial ABG studies for PaO_2, $PaCO_2$, bicarbonate, and pH levels at least hourly and every hour after any change; continuous monitoring of PaO_2 is ideal.

8. A PaO_2 level in the abdominal aorta of 60 to 80 mm Hg and a pH above 7.25 are normal values; changes indicate the potential for respiratory or metabolic acidosis.

9. If appropriate, perform a heelstick to obtain capillary blood for blood gas measurements (warm heel for 5 to 10 minutes).

9. Oxygen levels of 35 to 55 mm Hg in capillary blood are equal to oxygen levels of 40 to 65 mm Hg in arterial blood.

10. Start and maintain an I.V. infusion of dextrose 10% in water ($D_{10}W$), depending on the infant's age and additional fluid requirements.

10. An infusion is given immediately to meet fluid and caloric requirements, based on calculations per kilogram of body weight, because poor gastric motility prevents oral feeding.

11. Additional individualized interventions: _____
_____

11. Rationales: _____
_____

COLLABORATIVE PROBLEM

Risk for complications related to medical therapy and treatments

Expected outcome

The patient will exhibit no complications of therapy.

Interventions

1. Maintain safe use of the oxygen hood and head box as follows:
• Do not plug holes or seal the space between the hood and the neck.
• Ensure that the hood does not touch the infant and that air does not blow directly into the infant's face.

• Adjust the flow rate as ordered, and measure the amount the infant receives with an oxygen analyzer, placing the probe near the infant's nose.

2. Maintain safe administration of oxygen by nasal or nasopharyngeal prongs, as follows:

• Select prongs of an appropriate size.

• Check for kinks in tubing when using nasopharyngeal prongs.

Rationales

1. The oxygen hood has the advantage of being noninvasive, although the neck seal is difficult to achieve.
• Holes allow carbon dioxide to escape.

• Stimulation of facial nerves from the hood touching the infant could cause apnea; air in the infant's face could cause cold stress.
• Proper adjustment ensures correct concentration of oxygen and prevents administration of higher amounts.

2. Prongs may injure the turbinates and septum, causing excessive crying from discomfort. The infant may need sedation with chloral hydrate I.V.; if so, the infant should be switched to assisted ventilation.
• Using the appropriate-sized prongs prevents irritation and leaks.
• Straight tubing ensures patency.

• Apply a small amount of water-soluble lubricant to the outside of the prongs and insert them into the infant's nostrils.

• Secure the prongs in the infant's nostrils.
• Remove the prongs every 4 hours to check for redness and exudate, and clean and dry nostrils and prongs.

3. Maintain safe administration of oxygen by face mask, as follows:
• Secure the mask to the face snugly.
• Check for skin trauma every 2 to 4 hours.

4. Maintain safe administration of oxygen by endotracheal tube, as follows:
• Monitor the infant's pulse and respiratory rates during intubation and use a handheld resuscitation bag for ventilation with 100% FiO_2.
• Based on the infant's weight, select the proper tube size:
−less than 1,000 g = 2.5-mm inner diameter
−1,000 to 2,000 g = 3-mm inner diameter
−2,000 to 3,000 g = 3.5-mm inner diameter
−greater than 3,000 g = 4-mm inner diameter.
• Have an extra endotracheal tube, resuscitation bag, and mask at hand.
• Place the infant on a flat surface with its head tilted backward slightly and shoulders elevated slightly with a folded towel.
• After intubation by appropriate personnel, secure the tube in the proper position after placement is verified by X-ray or auscultation of air entering the lungs.

• Connect the tube to the oxygen source or mechanical ventilator.
• Set alarms and maintain them in the ON position; monitor and record all settings hourly, including changes made and who made them.
• Monitor both endotracheal and ventilator tubes to make sure they are patent, free of moisture, and not displaced.

5. Administer the prescribed amount of CPAP or PEEP safely. One possible schedule is the following:

• Start with 3 to 4 cm H_2O.

• Monitor ABG measurements with each change of pressure or oxygen.
• Increase inspired oxygen in 5% to 10% increments if PaO_2 level remains below 50 mm Hg at pressures of 12 to 15 cm H_2O.

• Lubricant permits easier application and decreases mucosal excoriation. An infant with nasal prongs who needs CPAP in addition to oxygen may have difficulty maintaining constant pressure.
• A proper fit prevents air leak.
• Cleaning the infant's nostrils prevents the breakdown of nasal mucosa from pressure; cleaning the prongs ensures patency.

3. A face mask is a simple method of oxygen administration, but fixation is difficult.
• A proper fit prevents air leak.
• Pressure from the mask on the face may cause injury or skin breakdown.

4. Safety measures prevent complications.

• Monitoring ensures proper ventilation until the tube is in place and oxygenation begins.

• Proper fit helps prevent injury to the trachea. Tube size can also be determined by equating the width of the infant's little finger with the diameter of the trachea.

• An extra tube can be used in the event of extubation or failure of the ventilator.
• This position maintains an open airway for intubation; hyperextension may close the airway.

• Verifying placement ensures that the tube is not in the esophagus or positioned too far into the trachea. Once placement is verified, securing the tube prevents displacement.
• Connection to the oxygen source permits oxygen flow.
• Alarms provide a warning that the ventilator is not functioning or needs adjustment.

• This ensures patency for proper functioning and prevents suffocation from overhumidification or infection (moisture in the tubing provides a growth medium for bacteria).

5. CPAP or PEEP prevents the collapse of alveoli by exerting positive pressure at the end-expiratory phase. Procedures vary with hospitals and policy.
• Starting at a lower pressure and increasing pressure, as appropriate, is a safety measure.
• This helps determine whether the pressure needs to be adjusted; however, continuous monitoring is ideal.
• Oxygen increases must be made cautiously and according to protocol to prevent complications.

6. Maintain safe use of the ventilator and document hourly as follows:

- Check that the circuit to be used is leakproof.
- Check that the heated nebulizer is working and that nebulization of inspired gas is correct.
- Check the tubing for condensation and accumulated moisture.
- Check for tube kinking.
- Check ventilator settings for concentration and volume, and maintain as prescribed; levels vary according to the type of ventilator used and the infant's needs.
- Set alarms and maintain them in the ON position.

- Check the manometer to maintain pressure and the in-line thermometer for correct temperature.

7. Using sterile technique, provide safe suctioning every 4 hours for copious secretions to prevent occluding the endotracheal tube. Suctioning should be performed by one pass through the tube with a 5F or 6F suction catheter. If the infant is on a closed system, administer 6 to 8 hyperinflated breaths with the ventilator; do not use a handheld resuscitation bag. If the infant is on an open system and is taken off the ventilator during suctioning, use a handheld resuscitation bag to give 6 to 8 hyperinflated breaths before returning the infant to the ventilator.

8. If an oxygen hood or incubator is used or needed in other methods, place an oxygen analyzer with probe in the area to be measured, such as near the infant's nose.

9. If transcutaneous PO_2 monitoring or pulse oximetry is used, monitor continuously or assess hourly and record your findings. Calibrate the sensor each shift, and rotate the sensor position every 3 to 4 hours.

10. Additional individualized interventions: _____

6. Ventilators used for infants are time-cycled or volume-cycled to ensure an adequate volume of gas to ventilate the lungs and oxygenate and remove carbon dioxide from the blood. A respiratory therapist performs checks and documents findings on the chart.
- A leakproof circuit ensures safe functioning.
- This is necessary for safe ventilator function.

- Moisture in the tubing provides a medium for bacterial growth.
- This ensures patency.
- This ensures safe functioning.

- An active alarm system indicates problems with the ventilator.
- These ensure safe ventilator functioning.

7. If performed incorrectly, suctioning may produce atelectasis or lesions by removing gas from small airways or may cause trauma from the catheter tip. Infection may occur from introduction of contaminants. Hypoxia may also result. Hyperinflated breaths help inflate the lungs and promote oxygenation.

8. An analyzer measures oxygen concentrations administered in a confined environment. An alarm sounds if oxygen deviates from the desired concentrations.

9. Monitoring ensures appropriate FIO_2 concentrations and accurate readings. Rotating the sensor prevents skin burns. Electrode sites include the chest, abdomen, and inner thigh. The oxygen diffusing through the skin from capillaries directly beneath the skin is measured. The oximeter is preferred because it doesn't produce heat.

10. Rationales: _____

NURSING DIAGNOSIS

Altered nutrition: less than body requirements related to inability to ingest feedings, decreased gastric motility, and withholding of food and water

Expected outcome

The patient will maintain optimal nutritional intake.

Interventions

1. Establish an I.V. infusion of $D_{10}W$ at a rate ranging from 65 to 80 ml/kg/day.

Rationales:

1. This rate is for initial calorie intake rather than for oral feedings.

2. Insert a nasogastric or an orogastric tube (5F to 8F) to provide gavage feedings if indicated, to evaluate stomach contents, or to assist with placement of a naso-duodenal or nasojejunal tube for feedings if prescribed.

3. Verify placement of the tube as follows:
• Aspirate gastric contents.
• Inject a minimal amount of air and auscultate for entry into the stomach.
• Place the tip in water; if no bubbles appear, the tip is in the stomach.

4. For a premature infant who weighs more than 1,000 g, provide gavage feedings as follows:
• Elevate the infant's head slightly.
• Allow breast milk or formula to flow into the tube by low gravity from a height of 6″ to 8″ [15 to 20 cm] above the infant's head.
• Make sure the breast milk or formula is at room temperature.
• Give 2 to 4 ml/minute as tolerated, and then flush the tube with sterile water. Use just enough water to clear the tube.

• Place the infant on its side for 1 hour after feeding.

• Follow your institution's feeding schedule. A suggested schedule follows:
−Start with about 4 ml of formula or breast milk every feeding for the 1st day.
−Advance the feedings 2 to 4 ml each day, depending on how well the infant tolerated the previous feeding.
−If the infant is preterm, advance the feedings slowly. This helps prevent necrotizing enterocolitis. Reduce the feeding at the first indication of trouble. As an alternative to intermittent feedings, provide continuous feedings at a rate of 1 to 2 ml/hour through an indwelling feeding tube attached to a kangaroo pump.
−Check residuals before feedings, and report remainders of more than 2 ml to the doctor. Subtract the residual amount from the amount to be given, provided it is a minimal amount. Residuals higher than 30% of the previous feedings might mean that the next feeding will be omitted. If large residuals occur persistently, discontinue feedings.

5. Provide TPN when indicated.

6. Additional individualized interventions: _____

2. This provides a choice of routes for feedings when feedings are allowed, although feedings are withheld when an umbilical arterial catheter is in place. The tube for gavage feedings must be placed cautiously; the infant usually is too sick for feedings.

3. Verification prevents feedings from entering the trachea.

4. Gavage feedings provide nutritional requirements with minimal energy expenditure.
• This position usually is used for feedings.
• This flow rate minimizes metabolic activity and prevents distention, reducing pressure on the diaphragm.

• Room-temperature breast milk or formula are better tolerated and prevent body temperature changes.
• Small feeding amounts accommodate the infant's small stomach capacity. Flushing maintains tube patency; using too much water could overload the infant with fluid.
• This position promotes gastric emptying and prevents regurgitation.
• Feeding by gavage should include 20 kcal/30 ml, increasing to 120 to 144 ml/kg/day. Continuous feedings are better tolerated and help maintain stable serum glucose levels without the peaks and troughs that result from intermittent feedings.

5. TPN is an alternative method for maintaining nutrition if bowel sounds are not present and the infant remains in an acute stage (see the "Tracheoesophageal fistula or esophageal atresia" plan, page 326, for information on TPN). They are considered if feedings cannot be achieved in 4 to 5 days.

6. Rationales: _____

NURSING DIAGNOSIS

Risk for fluid volume deficit related to sensible and insensible fluid losses

Expected outcome

The patient will maintain fluid and electrolyte balance.

Interventions

1. Maintain an I.V. infusion of $D_{10}W$ at a rate of 60 to 100 ml/kg/day.

2. Increase the infusion by 10 ml/kg/day, depending on urine output, radiant heater use, and the amount of enteral feedings.

3. Maintain the I.V. at the prescribed rate, using an infusion pump.

4. Monitor fluid intake and output by:
• weighing the infant every 8 hours
• weighing diapers to determine urine output
• keeping track of the number and amount of stools
• monitoring the amount of fluid infused hourly.

5. Review electrolyte levels for sodium and potassium increases every 12 to 24 hours.

6. Additional individualized interventions: _____

Rationales

1. Initial fluid replacement prevents imbalance.

2. Maintain fluids based on the patient's needs. Tachypnea and the use of a radiant warmer increase fluid loss.

3. Administering too much fluid or infusing it too rapidly can cause fatal circulatory overload.

4. Fluid intake and output indicate potential imbalances and serve as a basis for fluid replacement.

5. Changes in electrolyte levels indicate dehydration and potential electrolyte imbalance.

6. Rationales: _____

NURSING DIAGNOSIS

Ineffective family coping: compromised related to anxiety, guilt, and separation from the infant as result of situational crisis

Expected outcome

The parents will express their concerns about their infant and demonstrate positive parent-infant interaction.

Interventions

1. Assess the parents' verbal and nonverbal expression of anxiety and their use of coping mechanisms.

2. Help the parents verbalize their feelings about the sick infant, prolonged care in the neonatal intensive care unit, and procedures and equipment used in infant care.

3. Provide consistent and accurate information about the infant's condition and progress.

4. As appropriate, encourage the parents to visit, stroke, and care for the infant.

Rationales

1. This helps identify and develop constructive coping strategies.

2. Encouraging the parents to express their feelings helps maintain a trusting, secure environment and shows acceptance of parents' concerns and fears.

3. Information reduces anxiety about the course of the disease and whether the infant is improving.

4. Touching promotes bonding.

5. Refer the parents to social services and community agencies.

5. These resources offer additional support, information, and assistance to the parents during the acute illness and after discharge.

6. Additional individualized interventions: _____

6. Rationales: _____

Documentation checklist

During the hospital stay, document:
- ❏ patient status and assessment findings, especially respiratory effort, murmurs, tissue perfusion, cyanosis, use of ventilatory supports, and characteristics of any mucus suctioned
- ❏ changes in patient status
- ❏ pertinent laboratory and diagnostic findings, especially ABG levels, chest X-rays, pulse oximeter readings, and serum glucose and electrolyte levels
- ❏ patient's response to treatment
- ❏ family's reaction to diagnosis
- ❏ parent-infant interaction
- ❏ family teaching guidelines
- ❏ discharge planning guidelines.

Associated plans and appendices
- ❏ Abruptio placentae
- ❏ Cesarean section birth
- ❏ Hypoglycemia
- ❏ Hypothermia and hyperthermia
- ❏ Meconium aspiration syndrome
- ❏ Pregnancy complicated by diabetes mellitus
- ❏ Preterm infant
- ❏ Tracheoesophageal fistula or esophageal atresia
- ❏ Aspects of psychological care — maternal (appendix D)
- ❏ Assessing vital signs in the infant (appendix H)
- ❏ Normal laboratory values for the newborn infant (appendix I)

Additional nursing diagnoses
- ❏ Altered cardiopulmonary tissue perfusion related to disease process
- ❏ Altered family processes related to critically ill infant
- ❏ Altered parenting related to interruption in bonding process and unrealistic expectations for self, infant
- ❏ Anticipatory grieving (parental) related to perceived potential loss of child
- ❏ Anxiety (parental) related to threat of infant's death
- ❏ Dysfunctional ventilatory weaning response related to lung immaturity and prolonged use of mechanical ventilation
- ❏ Inability to sustain spontaneous ventilation related to respiratory distress

- ❏ Knowledge deficit (parental) related to lack of exposure to information regarding care of infant
- ❏ Risk for altered body temperature related to immaturity
- ❏ Risk for infection related to inadequate primary defenses, skin, mucous membranes, and invasive procedures

Sepsis neonatorum and infectious disorders

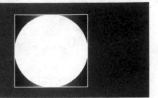

Definition

Infectious diseases may occur in the infant before, during, and after birth. They may be acquired in the ascending genital tract, by intrauterine infection, or by transplacental inoculation. Postnatally, they may be acquired from nursery personnel or from equipment used during the infant's treatment and care. Nosocomial infections are hospital-acquired. Viral and protozoan infections include toxoplasmosis, rubella, cytomegalovirus, and herpes simplex virus Type 1 or 2; other sexually transmitted infections include syphilis, varicella, chlamydia, hepatitis B, group B streptococcus, and gonorrhea (see *Etiology of infection* for mode of transmission to the fetus or infant). The most common neonatal infections are pneumonia and septicemia; the most severe cases result from group B beta-hemolytic streptococci, with onset a few days after delivery. Infections caused by this organism are acquired in utero, by the ascending route, or by contact with infected tissue during birth.

The incidence of infection is higher in a preterm infant than in a full-term infant, indicating an association between the immature immune system, the infection, and the predisposing factors leading to infection. Like an adult, an infant defends itself against invasion by infectious agents with its intact skin and mucous membranes, by phagocytosis, by the inflammatory response, and by producing antibodies that act against a specific microorganism. Because of immaturity, the preterm infant's defenses are deficient, limited, or reduced in their actions, leaving the infant more susceptible to infection.

This plan focuses on identifying potential or existing infectious states and caring for the infant with an infection.

Physical findings
Maternal history
• Little or no prenatal care, low socioeconomic status
• Premature rupture of membranes (PROM), dilation of cervix 24 hours or more before delivery, or precipitous delivery
• Birth outside of delivery or operating room
• Previous or current sexually transmitted infections, such as syphilis, herpes, *Chlamydia,* and gonorrhea
• Infectious diseases, such as toxoplasmosis, rubella, cytomegalovirus, tuberculosis, hepatitis, and acquired immunodeficiency syndrome, during pregnancy or at delivery

• Amnionitis, maternal bleeding, or pregnancy-induced hypertension
• Positive for group B streptococcus; no antibiotics given before delivery
• Positive for hepatitis B; may or may not have received treatment during the antenatal and intrapartal periods
Infant status at birth
• Prematurity
• Hypothermia or hypoglycemia from sepsis
• Low Apgar score or use of resuscitation or invasive procedures
Cardiovascular
• Pallor; mottling; cold, clammy skin with septic shock or delayed perfusion or refilling of nail beds
• Hypotension
• Tachycardia
Gastrointestinal
• Feeding difficulty
• Vomiting, diarrhea, or abdominal distention with sepsis or meningitis
• Splenomegaly, hepatomegaly with toxoplasmosis or hepatitis
Integumentary
• Jaundice with meningitis, hepatitis, cytomegalovirus, toxoplasmosis, or sepsis neonatorum
• Petechiae with cytomegalovirus
• Pustules or lesions with herpes
• Erythema with omphalitis (periumbilical)
• Pustules, abscesses, or furuncles with streptococcal or staphylococcal septicemia
• Maculopapular rash with toxoplasmosis
Neurologic
• Temperature instability (usually hypothermia with sepsis)
• Hypertonia or hypotonia with sepsis
• Abnormal eye movements
• Seizure activity
Pulmonary
• Apnea, tachypnea, cyanosis with group B streptococcal disease, causing sepsis, pneumonia, or meningitis

Behavioral findings
• Lethargy
• Irritability
• Shrill cry

Etiology of infection

Infection	Causative agent	Means of transmission
Viral		
Acquired immunodeficiency syndrome	Human immunodeficiency virus	In utero by way of transplacental passage of virus, during labor and delivery through exposure to infected blood or vaginal secretions, and through breast milk
Cytomegalovirus	Cytomegalovirus	In utero, during birth, from contact with infected maternal cervical secretions, and in breast milk
Hepatitis	Hepatitis B virus	During birth and in breast milk
Herpes simplex	Herpes simplex virus Type 2	Genital tract during birth and in utero
Rubella	Rubella virus	In utero
Protozoal		
Toxoplasmosis	*Toxoplasma gondii*	In utero
Bacterial		
Conjunctivitis	*Neisseria gonorrhoeae, Chlamydia trachomatis,* and *Staphylococcus* sp.	During birth (*N. gonorrhoeae* and *C. trachomatis*) or acquired postpartum (*Staphylococcus* sp.)
Diarrhea	*Escherichia coli, Salmonella* sp., *Shigella* sp., and *Staphylococcus* sp.	Acquired postpartum
Listeriosis	*Listeria monocytogenes*	In utero and during birth
Meningitis	Group B streptococci and *L. monocytogenes*	Acquired postpartum
Pneumonia	Group B streptococci, *E. coli, Pseudomonas aeruginosa,* and penicillin-resistant staphylococci	In utero (B streptococci and *E. coli*) or acquired postpartum (*P. aeruginosa* and penicillin-resistant staphylococci)
Septicemia	Group A or B streptococci (most often B), *E. coli,* and *P. aeruginosa*	In utero, during birth, or acquired postpartum
Syphilis	*Treponema pallidum*	In utero
Tuberculosis	*Mycobacterium tuberculosis*	In utero or acquired postpartum

Diagnostic studies

• Chest X-ray to show pulmonary changes or involvement
• Skull X-ray and long bone and joint X-ray to screen for sexually transmitted infections
• Complete blood count (CBC) to identify white blood cell (WBC) count less than 3,000/mm³ or greater than 25,000/mm³; absolute neutrophils less than 5,000; and ratio of immature to total neutrophils as follows: 0.25:0.49 is suspicious of infection, 0.50:0.79 indicates sepsis, and 0.8 or above indicates fulminating infection

• Peripheral blood smear to identify platelet count less than 80,000/mm³, Döhle's inclusion bodies, and toxic granulation
• Gram stain of buffy coat of bacteria in association with blood culture positive for sepsis to confirm sepsis
• Gastric aspirate smear to indicate intrauterine contamination by examining for WBC count and bacteria
• C-reactive protein levels to indicate sepsis
• Serum immunoglobulin studies to identify increase of immunoglobulin M (IgM)

- Presence of bands in WBC differential
- Radioimmunoassay to detect hepatitis B surface antigen (even though results are usually negative for the first 4 weeks)
- Enzyme-linked immunosorbent assay, Western blot, and CD4 levels to identify presence of human immunodeficiency virus antibody and immune function (for more information, see the "Acquired immunodeficiency syndrome—infant" plan, page 162)
- Serum glucose, calcium, and bilirubin studies to detect abnormal increases or decreases

- Blood culture from peripheral vein sample (two different sites) to identify type of microorganism
- Urine culture of specimen secured by suprapubic bladder aspiration to identify type of microorganism
- Cultures of fluid from ear, lesions, stool, drainage from umbilical stump, suction aspirate, conjunctiva, or from around central line if one is present, to identify microorganism
- Cerebrospinal fluid (CSF) studies (culture, protein, glucose, and cell count) to identify abnormal levels or microorganisms

COLLABORATIVE PROBLEM

Infection related to transmission of infectious agent to infant before, during, or after birth (two expected outcomes)

Expected outcome 1

The patient will exhibit no signs of infection.

Interventions

1. Assess the infant for the risk of infection, including:
- prematurity, being small or large for gestational age
- low Apgar score
- surgery performed on the infant
- epidemics of *Escherichia coli* or streptococcal infections in the nursery
- invasive or resuscitative procedures.

Note: Review maternal history, noting ethnic group, socioeconomic status, vaginal flora, PROM, illness, and infections; note if the mother is positive for group B *Streptococcus* on culture taken from vagina or rectum at 36 weeks' gestation.

2. Assess for early signs of infection, including:
- temperature instability (usually hypothermia)
- apnea
- jaundice
- poor feeding and sucking or abdominal distention
- lethargy or irritability.

3. Assess for system-related signs of infection, including:
- respiratory distress; apnea; tachypnea; cyanosis; and pallor, hypotension, and tachycardia (indicating shock) with group B streptococcal sepsis, pneumonia, or systemic infections from *Staphylococcus, E. coli, Klebsiella, Candida,* or others
- hypothermia, lethargy, hypertonia, hypotonia, jitteriness, bulging fontanels, abnormal eye movements, or seizures with sepsis or meningitis
- jaundice, petechiae, pustules, lesions, rash, or abscesses with sexually transmitted infections
- difficulty feeding, vomiting, diarrhea, or weight loss with sepsis.

Rationales

1. The infant's immature defense system at birth, with a deficiency in phagocytic responses and in the immune system, decreases the inflammatory response and increases the infant's susceptibility to infection. The preterm infant is further compromised. Maternal involvement (both antepartum and intrapartum) always precedes infection.

2. Many early signs of infection are similar to those of other conditions. Unless early subtle signs are identified while the infant still seems generally healthy, infection might become difficult to manage.

3. Signs may or may not be related to a specific system but result from the infection's effect on a system or an organ. Similar signs may present themselves in infections that involve different systems.

4. Review CBC with WBC count and differential; platelet studies; immunoglobulin analysis; results of Gram stain of buffy coat; glucose, calcium, and bilirubin levels; and screening results for sexually transmitted infections.

4. Blood study results help determine the cause of infection.

5. Obtain samples, as needed, for cultures, including blood, ear fluid, lesions, stool, drainage (such as from the eye), and gastric aspirate. Assist with obtaining a urine specimen by suprapubic bladder aspiration and CSF by lumbar puncture. Send samples to the laboratory for examination. Repeat as appropriate.

5. Cultures identify microorganisms and their sensitivity to antibiotics.

6. Review chest, skull, long bone, and joint X-rays.

6. Results reveal changes caused by infection in these areas.

7. Additional individualized interventions: _____

7. Rationales: _____

Expected outcome 2

The patient will exhibit minimal or no signs of infection or its complications.

Interventions

1. Provide a neutral thermal environment.

2. Provide for the infant's fluid and nutritional needs by I.V. infusion, according to the infant's weight, age, and condition.

3. Monitor vital signs continuously by transducer and other mechanical means.

4. Prepare and administer antibiotic and aminoglycoside therapy as follows:
• Calculate the amount of drug needed per kilogram of body weight.
• Administer I.V. drugs at the appropriate rate regulated by an infusion pump.
• Administer such antibiotics as penicillin G, ampicillin, or methicillin.
• Administer such aminoglycosides as gentamicin, kanamycin, or chloramphenicol.
• Monitor peak and trough levels for antibiotics and aminoglycosides as ordered.

5. Prepare and administer fresh frozen plasma I.V. as ordered.

6. Prepare and administer glucose, calcium, and electrolyte replacement therapy, as ordered.

7. Prepare for exchange transfusion with packed red blood cells, if indicated for sepsis.

8. Additional individualized interventions: _____

Rationales

1. This environment prevents temperature instability that further compromises the infant.

2. This action supports fluid and electrolyte balance and nutritional status.

3. Continuous monitoring allows for early detection of changes and prompt intervention.

4. The infant receives prophylactic anti-infective therapy until culture results can identify the infectious microorganism and its sensitivity. Antibiotics destroy bacteria by binding to the cell wall, killing the cell; aminoglycosides destroy bacteria by inhibiting protein synthesis. Antimicrobial therapy dosage depends on drug absorption, metabolism, and excretion, all of which vary with the infant's weight, gestational age, chronological age, and condition. Therapy is administered for up to 10 days (longer in meningitis) or until cultures are normal for 72 hours.

5. Fresh frozen plasma may be given for severe infection.

6. This action corrects abnormally low electrolyte levels associated with sepsis.

7. Transfusion may be needed for blood replacement in sepsis.

8. Rationales: _____

COLLABORATIVE PROBLEM

Altered nutrition: less than body requirements related to poor feeding or feeding intolerance

Expected outcome

The patient will maintain an optimal nutritional state.

Interventions

1. Assess for feeding intolerance, noting:
• weight loss (weigh daily on the same scale)
• vomiting or diarrhea
• abdominal distention or residual gastric contents before feeding with gavage
• poor sucking ability and poor swallowing reflex.

2. If the infant cannot tolerate oral feedings, initiate appropriate measures to meet nutritional needs:
• Discontinue oral feedings and insert a gastric tube; attach the tube to a suctioning device or suction by hand.
• Provide dextrose 10% in water I.V. initially, and follow with total parenteral nutrition (TPN) as appropriate or provide gavage feedings, if appropriate and needed.
• As the infant's condition improves, initiate oral feedings with breast milk, if possible, or formula.

• Continue increasing calorie intake until daily weight gain, as calculated according to gestational age and expected weight gain, is achieved.

3. Additional individualized interventions: _____

Rationales

1. Poor feeding and absorption as well as vomiting and diarrhea cause caloric loss and nutritional deficit.

2. Maintaining optimal nutritional status enhances the infant's ability to withstand infection.
• Gastric distention and mucus production occur with sepsis; decompression prevents aspiration.
• These measures provide nutritional needs during acute sepsis.

• Small quantities of formula or breast milk, with advancement as tolerated, provide essential nutrients; breast milk also provides IgA and IgC as well as additional phagocytic cells needed to fight infection.
• Increasing daily calorie intake ensures adequate nutrition.

3. Rationales: _____

COLLABORATIVE PROBLEM

Irregular respiratory effort related to apnea or periodic breathing

Expected outcome

The patient will exhibit optimal pulmonary function and oxygenation.

Interventions

1. Assess for respiratory changes, including tachypnea, nasal flaring, retractions, grunting, cyanosis, periodic breathing with apneic periods of more than 10 seconds, and crackles.

Rationales

1. Early detection of changes ensures prompt treatment. These respiratory changes occur with pneumonia and other pulmonary infections.

2. Electronically monitor heart rate for tachycardia or bradycardia and blood pressure for changes. Monitor apnea with a thoracic impedance monitor as follows:
• Apply electrode jelly to electrodes and place them on the infant's chest.
• Plug in the monitor and attach leadwires to the electrodes.
• Adjust the system and set the alarms.
• Turn on the monitor, and adjust it so that the lights blink with each breath and heartbeat.
• If the alarm sounds, check the infant and confirm apnea by assessing color and breathing.
• If the infant is breathing and pink, readjust the controls and electrodes. If the infant is not breathing but pink, stimulate gently by stroking the sole or more vigorously by flicking the sole with your finger.
• If apnea continues, begin resuscitation.

2. Close monitoring allows detection of changes in the infant's condition as well as apneic periods that may cause brain damage. The thoracic impedance monitor detects changes caused by respiratory alterations and has an alarm to signal bradycardia.

3. Provide warm, humidified oxygen therapy at the minimal fraction of inspired oxygen concentration necessary to maintain energy expenditure and color.

3. Supplemental oxygen support may be needed with respiratory distress and decreased partial pressure of oxygen (PO_2).

4. Provide assistive or mechanical ventilation as appropriate.

4. The infant may need respiratory support to sustain breathing.

5. Suction the airway carefully, if appropriate.

5. Suctioning removes mucus from the nasopharynx or endotracheal tube.

6. Review arterial blood gas (ABG) studies as available or draw blood and monitor ABG levels as needed.

6. ABG levels indicate acid-base balance and may suggest acidosis if PO_2 is low, partial pressure of carbon dioxide (PCO_2) is high, and pH is low.

7. Cluster infant care to prevent excessive handling.

7. Handling increases the infant's energy expenditure and need for oxygen.

8. Additional individualized interventions: _____

8. Rationales: _____

Nursing diagnosis

Risk for injury related to transmission of infection to infant by personnel

Expected outcome

The patient will not develop a nosocomial infection.

Interventions

1. Institute standard precautions; follow institutional policy for excluding or removing from the nursery infants with diarrhea, draining infections, or viral infections.

Rationales

1. Standard precautions minimize the risk of infection transmission. Disease may be transmitted to and from healthy and sick infants if they are exposed to or cared for by the same personnel.

2. Follow the hospital's protocol for hand washing or take the following steps:
• Before entering the nursery, wash your hands to above the elbows for 2 minutes, using an antiseptic iodophor preparation or chlorhexidine (Hibiclens).
• Wash your hands for 15 seconds before caring for another infant.
• A doctor, a relative, or any other person who enters the nursery briefly should wash hands and, if hospital policy dictates, cover clothing with a clean gown.
• All nursing staff should wear short-sleeved gowns in the nursery.
• No caregiver should wear artificial fingernails.

3. Use an incubator to isolate infants coming from outside the nursery until their blood, skin, and urine cultures are negative.

4. If an infant's mother has an infection or a communicable disease, exclude the infant from the nursery or place it in an isolation nursery.

5. Ensure that all personnel, relatives, and other caregivers are free of fever; respiratory or GI disorders; open, draining lesions or skin breaks; and any communicable disease before allowing them to enter the nursery or care for an infant.

6. Sterilize all equipment before use. Change all tubing, lines, and humidifiers or sterilize daily or according to hospital protocol.

7. Wash all cribs, incubators, and other apparatus with an antiseptic solution once a week and after each use.

8. Clean and sterilize daily any equipment or sinks that become wet.

9. Use meticulous sterile technique for cord care, for all procedures, and when caring for catheters (umbilical or vein), I.V. lines, and dressings.

10. Take samples for culture from equipment, supplies, and any possibly contaminated items in the nursery.

11. Tell visiting parents that they should:
• touch only their own infant
• wash hands properly and put on a gown according to hospital protocol
• not handle another infant's equipment or supplies or move things from one crib to another.

12. Additional individualized interventions: _____
_____

2. Hands are the principal mode of infection transmission and spread to infants.
• This is a general hand-washing procedure. Individual hospital protocols may vary.

• Hands are considered contaminated after touching an infant or any materials in the nursery.
• Anyone can be a potential carrier of infection and should follow infection-preventing protocols.

• Wearing short sleeves allows for washing above the elbows.
• Studies indicate that artificial fingernails harbor infection.

3. This prevents cross-contamination with unknown microorganisms to other infants in the nursery.

4. An infant may have a disease at birth that was transmitted in utero or during delivery.

5. Contact with sick people creates a health hazard and encourages possible transmission of infections that might endanger all infants in the nursery.

6. Sterilization and frequent changes of equipment lines prevent the spread of bacteria from the objects to infants.

7. Washing maintains cleanliness and provides bacteriostatic action to reduce contaminants.

8. Dampness provides a good medium for microorganisms to thrive.

9. Any break in the first line of defense offers microorganisms an opportunity to enter and cause infection.

10. Culturing identifies the infection potential.

11. These steps help protect infants in the nursery from infection.

12. Rationales: _____
_____

Documentation checklist

During the hospital stay, document:

❒ patient status and assessment findings, especially color, feeding difficulties, level of activity and alertness, Apgar scores, capillary refill, jaundice, skin and core temperature (axillary, aural, or infrared), seizure activity, characteristic of cry, apneic or bradycardic episodes, irritability, rashes, and respiratory effort

❒ changes in patient status

❒ pertinent laboratory and diagnostic findings, especially serum calcium, phosphorus, total protein, potassium, sodium, magnesium, bilirubin, glucose, and C-reactive protein levels; CBC with differential; gram stains; culture and sensitivity results; ABG results (including PO_2, PCO_2, and bicarbonate levels and pH); type and crossmatch, Coombs' test, Rh factor; urine specific gravity, guaiac stools; and chest X-rays. If the patient is on TPN, note weekly blood urea nitrogen, creatinine, aspartate aminotransferase, alanine aminotransferase, triglyceride, ammonia, and electrolyte levels; clotting studies; and hematocrit.

❒ patient's response to treatment, especially antibiotic therapy

❒ family's reaction to the diagnosis

❒ parent-infant interaction

❒ family teaching guidelines, especially any specialized care required and stability and stress cues

❒ discharge planning guidelines.

Associated plans

❒ Acquired immunodeficiency syndrome — infant

❒ Acquired immunodeficiency syndrome — maternal

❒ Anemia

❒ Hyperbilirubinemia

❒ Hypocalcemia

❒ Hypoglycemia

❒ Hypothermia and hyperthermia

❒ Intracranial hemorrhage

❒ Necrotizing enterocolitis

❒ Sexually transmitted diseases

Additional nursing diagnoses

❒ Altered growth and development related to illness and hospitalization

❒ Hyperthermia related to infectious process

❒ Hypothermia related to infectious process

❒ Ineffective airway clearance related to infection

❒ Ineffective individual coping related to guilt and anxiety from transmitting infection to infant and possible serious consequences of the infection

❒ Knowledge deficit (parental) related to infection control

❒ Risk for altered parenting related to separation from infant as result of severe infection

❒ Risk for fluid volume deficit related to losses from vomiting and diarrhea

Infant

Spinal cord defects and hydrocephalus

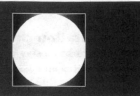

Definition

Spinal cord defects include congenital neurologic abnormalities that involve defective embryonic neural tube closure during the first trimester. The defects may be found in the cervical, thoracic, or sacral area but commonly occur in the lumbosacral area. Hydrocephalus, an excessive accumulation of cerebrospinal fluid (CSF) in the ventricles, often accompanies spinal cord defects, affecting about 90% of infants with myelomeningocele.

Spina bifida occulta, the incomplete closure of one or more vertebrae without protrusion of the cord or meninges, is the most common and least severe of the defects. Other forms of spina bifida, in which spinal contents protrude into an external sac through the incomplete closure, are considered more severe.

Meningocele is the protrusion of an external sac containing meninges and CSF with the spinal cord and nerve roots in their normal positions; myelocele is the protrusion of an external sac containing the spinal cord. Myelomeningocele is the protrusion of an external sac containing meninges, CSF, and a portion of the spinal cord or nerve roots; it is the most severe of the spinal cord defects and the one with the most serious long-term neurologic consequences.

Surgery may be performed early to close the protruding sac in meningocele, but repair of the sac in myelomeningocele may not reverse the neurologic deficit. Hydrocephalus may be surgically treated with a shunt to relieve pressure caused by fluid accumulation. The method of treatment depends on the type and extent of the defect, the infant's condition, associated defects, the family's desires, and the availability of and potential for rehabilitation. A multidisciplinary approach to the care of these infants is carried out by a team composed of nurses, a neurologist, a neurosurgeon, a pediatrician, an orthopedist, a urologist, and a physical therapist. The prognosis depends on the number and severity of abnormalities; infants who are totally paralyzed below the defect have the poorest prognosis.

This plan focuses on care of the infant with a spinal cord defect, hydrocephalus, and other abnormalities and the prevention of associated complications before surgery.

Etiology and precipitating factors
Spinal cord defects
• Genetic predisposition
• Possibility of viruses, radiation, or other environmental factors

Hydrocephalus
• Excessive production, inadequate reabsorption, or obstruction of circulating CSF through ventricles, preventing reabsorption

Physical findings
Maternal and family history
• Other children with similar defect
• Amniocentesis that shows an increase in alpha-fetoprotein (AFP) levels in open neural tube defects; in closed defects (about 10% of cases), results are negative
• Possibly one or both parents of Irish descent (incidence higher in families of Irish descent)

Infant status at birth
• Depression or dimple over defect area
• Tuft of hair and soft fatty deposits over defect area
• Port wine nevus over defect area
• Sac protruding from spine
• Other defects, such as hydrocephalus, talipes, hip dislocation, curvature of spine, and Arnold-Chiari syndrome (a form of hydrocephalus)

Gastrointestinal
• Poor feeding if lethargic
• Projectile vomiting with increasing intracranial pressure (ICP)

Integumentary
• Thin, shiny, fragile scalp skin; bulging fontanels; prominent scalp veins; possibly enlarged head in hydrocephalus
• Palpable depression over spinal defect area

Neurologic
• Vary with level of defect
• Flaccid or spastic paralysis of legs and trunk, fixed downward gaze in hydrocephalus, and setting-sun sign
• Fever and nuchal rigidity with meningitis

Behavioral findings
• Irritability
• Lethargy

Diagnostic studies
• Analysis of AFP levels from amniocentesis to reveal increase, possibly indicating neural tube defect
• Maternal serum AFP levels to detect increase, possibly indicating neural tube defect
• X-rays of spine, skull, hips, arms, and legs to reveal bone defects, with separating fontanels in hydrocephalus
• Cranial ultrasonography to differentiate hydrocephalus from other conditions associated with increasing head size

• Computed tomography (CT) scan to reveal ventricular distention and intracranial lesions
• Magnetic resonance imaging (MRI) to differentiate hydrocephalus from other conditions associated with increasing head size

• Ventriculography in hydrocephalus with possible culture of CSF to detect suspected infection
• Transillumination to reveal meningocele, but not myelomeningocele (may be performed during surgery), and to differentiate hydrocephalus from other conditions associated with increasing head size

NURSING DIAGNOSIS

Risk for infection related to breakdown or rupture of protruding sac

Expected outcome

The patient will show no signs of infection.

Interventions

1. Assess the infant for signs of infection, including:
• restlessness and irritability
• excessive crying
• temperature increase
• changes in white blood cell count, differential, and platelet count
• increased sensitivity to light and noise
• breaks or abrasion of sac and leakage from sac.

2. Prevent exposure of sac to contaminants by:
• cleaning the area gently with warm, sterile normal saline solution
• covering the defect with sterile dressings moistened with sterile saline solution and changing the dressings every 2 hours
• covering the dressings with plastic wrap and placing a "myelo" apron between the anus and the defect
• positioning the infant in the prone position to avoid contact with urine or feces; do not position the infant on its back until the defect is repaired and has healed.

3. Be prepared to administer prophylactic antibiotics, such as penicillin G, ampicillin, or methicillin, or aminoglycosides, such as kanamycin or gentamicin, if ordered.

4. Additional individualized interventions: _____

Rationales

1. Early identification of infection allows for early treatment. These signs indicate possible infection. Sac rupture increases the infant's risk of contracting meningitis.

2. These actions maintain cleanliness and prevent the defect from coming into contact with microorganisms, urine, or feces.

3. Anti-infectives are administered to prevent central nervous system infection; they kill bacteria by inhibiting protein biosynthesis of the bacterial cell wall.

4. Rationales: _____

NURSING DIAGNOSIS

Impaired skin integrity related to irritation or abrasions

Expected outcome

The patient will maintain skin integrity and will exhibit minimal trauma to the sac.

Interventions

1. Assess the skin for irritation, redness, and breaks.

2. Keep the skin clean and dry. Wash sensitive and pressure areas gently, using warm water.

3. Place sheepskin and foam pad under the infant.

4. Apply cream or emollient to knees, elbows, and other pressure areas, massaging gently.

5. Handle the infant carefully without putting pressure on the defect or on the thin, fragile skin of the head.

6. Place the infant in a prone position supported by small pillows and sandbags or in a side-lying position, if allowed. Change position every 2 hours or as needed. Place a roll between the legs at hip level.

7. Support the enlarged head when moving or feeding the hydrocephalic infant.

8. Position the infant with a spinal cord defect on the abdomen when holding the infant on your lap.

9. Dress the infant lightly, omitting a diaper and shirt if they would cover the defect, and place the infant in an Isolette to maintain a neutral thermal environment.

10. Additional individualized interventions: _____

Rationales

1. Assessment helps prevent continued deterioration by promoting immediate preventive treatment.

2. This prevents mechanical injury and promotes cleanliness.

3. Sheepskin and foam pad decrease pressure on skin.

4. Cream and emollients protect these areas from rubbing against linens, and the massaging action promotes circulation.

5. Careful handling prevents the possibility of rupturing the sac or injuring the skin on the head.

6. These positions prevent pressure on the sac or head. Raising the foot of the bed decreases pressure on the sac. Placing a roll at hip level maintains abduction of the legs.

7. Supporting the head avoids straining the infant's neck.

8. This position avoids pressure on the sac.

9. Dressing the infant lightly reduces pressure on the defect; the Isolette maintains the infant's warmth with little or no clothing.

10. Rationales: _____

COLLABORATIVE PROBLEM

Risk for neurologic, musculoskeletal, or elimination impairment related to complications of spinal cord defect or hydrocephalus (two expected outcomes)

Expected outcome 1

The patient will exhibit no signs of infection from spinal cord defect or hydrocephalus.

Interventions

1. Assess the infant for signs of neurologic complications, including:
• increasing head circumference measurements; bulging, full, or tense fontanels; lethargy and feeding difficulty; and projectile or other vomiting
• irritability or nuchal rigidity
• variations in vital signs and temperature (taken every 2 hours)

• pupillary changes (assessed every 2 hours), including inequality and sluggish response to light.

Rationales

1. Assessment data identify the infant at risk.

• These are signs of hydrocephalus; because of developments in ultrasonography, few infants are born with gross hydrocephalus.
• These indicate meningeal irritation.
• Increased temperature indicates infection. Blood pressure with widening pulse pressure changes indicates increased ICP.
• Pupillary changes indicate neurologic involvement and, possibly, increased ICP.

2. Assess for musculoskeletal complications, such as:

• reduced movement of arms and legs, reduced response to stimulation, and muscle weakness
• talipes or hip displacement abnormalities.

3. Assess for urinary and bowel elimination complications, such as:
• continuous passage of stool and urine retention

• urinary tract infection (by culture).

4. Additional individualized interventions: _____

2. Assessment data identify the infant at risk for paralysis and congenital deformity.
• These signs indicate potential paralysis with motor or sensory involvement.
• These are common congenital defects associated with spina bifida.

3. These complications are associated with spinal cord defects.
• These signs indicate lack of control, not diarrhea, and lack of innervation to the bladder and bowel.
• Culture identifies urinary tract infection.

4. Rationales: _____

Expected outcome 2

The patient will exhibit minimal signs of the effects of complications from spinal cord defect.

Interventions

1. Perform passive range-of-motion exercises every 4 hours or as needed as well as muscle-stretching exercises.

2. Perform exercises carefully while supporting the arms and legs properly.

3. Position the hips in slight to moderate abduction.

4. Perform the procedures for hip dislocation or talipes if present.

5. Help the infant empty its bladder every 2 hours by applying slight pressure to the suprapubic area (Credé's maneuver) from the umbilicus to the symphysis pubis.

6. After bowel elimination, gently clean and apply petroleum jelly to the infant's perianal area.

7. Arrange a comfortable position for feeding, facing the infant when possible.

8. Caress, fondle, and speak to the infant.

9. Additional individualized interventions: _____

Rationales

1. These exercises prevent contractures and muscle weakness.

2. Support prevents injury to fragile bones.

3. This position prevents hip dislocation.

4. Immediate serial casting, splinting, or another intervention may be needed (see the "Developmental dysplasia of the hip" plan, page 193, or the "Talipes deformity" plan, page 321).

5. Assistance prevents urine retention by releasing residual urine retained in the neurogenic bladder; this technique may also help the infant pass stool.

6. These actions prevent excoriation of the perianal area and skin breakdown.

7. Facing the infant while feeding provides both adequate intake and stimulation by eye contact.

8. Stroking and talking to the infant provide stimulation by touch and sound.

9. Rationales: _____

NURSING DIAGNOSIS

Anxiety (parental) related to defect in infant and potential defects in future children

Expected outcome

The parents will express minimal anxiety.

Interventions

1. Offer information and referral to genetic counseling. Explain that tests can be performed early in pregnancy to detect neural tube defects, allowing more options.

2. Review the family history. Answer questions honestly and accurately or refer parents to the doctor for information.

3. Help the parents adjust to the shock related to their infant's defect, and help them grieve over having an infant with an anomaly.

4. Refer the parents and other family members to local associations and support groups.

5. Additional individualized interventions: _____

Rationales

1. Information may reduce the parents' fear of the unknown.

2. Open discussion increases the parents' knowledge about the condition and reduces the potential for recurrence.

3. Adjustment to the physical and emotional aspects of the infant's condition promotes parent-infant interaction.

4. Such referrals allow family members to share their feelings with others in similar situations, which helps them work through anxieties and fears.

5. Rationales: _____

NURSING DIAGNOSIS

Ineffective family coping related to guilt, emotional conflict, and fear about the infant's immediate and long-term care

Expected outcome

The parents will demonstrate appropriate coping skills.

Interventions

1. Encourage and allow the parents to express feelings and fears about infant care, about what others might say, and about the loss of the "perfect child."

2. Allow the parents to see and hold the infant as soon after birth as possible, after the obstetrician has informed them of the defect.

3. Reinforce the normal and healthy aspects of the infant when interacting with the parents.

4. Handle the infant in a caring manner, and instruct the parents how to hold and cuddle the infant, being careful to avoid placing pressure on the sac and supporting the infant on the side or abdomen.

5. Allow the parents to visit the infant when desired, and encourage them to participate in the infant's care.

6. Encourage the parents to participate in support groups, such as the Spina Bifida Association of America.

7. Additional individualized interventions: _____

Rationales

1. The birth of a child with a congenital defect precipitates a major family crisis, and the parents and family must mourn the loss of the "perfect child" that they had expected.

2. Delay in seeing the infant may heighten parental anxiety and sadness, causing unrealistic expectations. Important bonding takes place as soon after birth as possible and is reinforced by continued close contact between the infant and its parents.

3. This reinforcement helps reduce the parents' chronic sorrow and anger.

4. These actions promote bonding and the infant's normal social and emotional development.

5. Open visitation promotes a flexible, secure environment for the development of a parent-infant relationship.

6. Group involvement offers the parents a support system and a positive view of the treatment outcome.

7. Rationales: _____

NURSING DIAGNOSIS

Knowledge deficit (parental) related to long-term care of child

Expected outcome

The parents will express appropriate understanding of their infants' condition and care needs.

Interventions

1. Assess the family's understanding of spina bifida, hydrocephalus, or other deformity if present.

2. Provide information about:

• infant's condition

• defect's cause, occurrence, and type

• infant's immediate needs and care

• surgery to insert a shunt, if the infant is hydrocephalic, or to correct myelomeningocele, if the infant has spina bifida
• infant's potential and long-term problems with myelomeningocele, such as paralysis with motor and sensory deficits, renal disorders, bowel and bladder training, mental retardation, and pulmonary infections.

3. Teach parents about ordered procedures and treatments, such as range-of-motion exercises, shunt care, skin care, positioning, handling, and feeding.

4. Allow the parents to ask as many questions as they like; answer them honestly and patiently. Encourage family participation in care.

5. Arrange for home health care follow-up.

6. Additional individualized interventions: _____

Rationales

1. Assessment reveals what the family needs to learn, their readiness for learning, and what misinformation needs to be corrected.

2. Information maximizes the parents' understanding of the defect and the care their infant will need.
• This information addresses the parents' anxiety about the seriousness of the infant's condition.
• This helps resolve the parents' guilt feelings about the infant's abnormality.
• This clarifies the reasons for the infant's treatment regimen while in the hospital.
• The parents need to understand the surgery their infant may need and its potential for success so that they can participate in medical decisions.
• This helps the parents understand the long-term care and resources their child will need.

3. Proper instruction aids compliance and helps dispel the parents' fears.

4. Questions may indicate that adaptation is taking place and that the parents' interest in caring for the infant is increasing. Participation helps to alleviate feelings of inadequacy and prepares for home care.

5. Home health care follow-up provides continued support outside the hospital.

6. Rationales: _____

NURSING DIAGNOSIS

Risk for altered parenting related to lack of attachment and bonding opportunities because of intensive care and surgery performed in another hospital

Expected outcome

The parents will exhibit appropriate bonding behavior with their infant.

Interventions

1. Encourage the parents to visit, provide care, and touch the infant.

Rationales

1. Visitation and infant contact promote bonding.

2. Provide time for the parents to be alone with the infant.

3. Provide support when the parents hold the infant.

4. Accept parental reactions without showing anger or shock or withdrawing from the situation.

5. Explain the need to transfer the infant to a different facility for special procedures if this is indicated. Allow the father to accompany the infant if the mother is still hospitalized.

6. Give anticipatory guidance in caring for the infant. Explain that the family may feel chronic sorrow if the infant has severe anomalies.

7. Additional individualized interventions: _____
_____

2. Time spent with the infant enhances bonding.

3. The parents may be afraid of injuring the infant.

4. Parents need time to overcome probable shock.

5. Understanding the need for the transfer and having the opportunity to accompany the infant prevent parental feelings of abandoning the infant and not knowing where and when they can be with their infant.

6. This adds to parental understanding that sorrow is a normal feeling that may persist.

7. Rationales: _____
_____

Documentation checklist
During the hospital stay, document:
- ❏ patient status and assessment findings, especially family history of spinal cord defects, Apgar scores, gestational age by examination, appearance and location of spinal cord lesion, any movements of the extremities, necessity of using Credé's maneuver to empty bladder, lethargy or irritability, head circumference, feeding difficulties, and vomiting
- ❏ changes in patient status, especially size and appearance of head, level of alertness, or movement of extremities
- ❏ pertinent laboratory and diagnostic findings, especially serum calcium, phosphorus, total protein, and glucose levels; complete blood count with differential; spinal, skull, hip, arm, and leg X-rays; cranial ultrasound; CT and (if performed) MRI scan results; transillumination results (if performed); and results of any cultures; note weekly blood urea nitrogen, creatinine, aspartate aminotransferase, alanine aminotransferase, triglyceride, ammonia, and electrolyte levels; clotting studies; and hematocrit
- ❏ patient's response to treatment, especially to any surgery for spinal cord defect (including movement of extremities and whether bladder is emptying) or hydrocephalus (including if shunt is working, head circumference, and level of alertness)
- ❏ family's reaction to the diagnosis and possible need for surgery
- ❏ parent-infant interaction
- ❏ family teaching guidelines, including care of an infant with limited movement and, possibly, impaired bladder and bowel function; signs of shunt malfunctioning; and types of follow-up care needed
- ❏ discharge planning guidelines.

Associated plans
- ❏ Developmental dysplasia of the hip
- ❏ Talipes deformity

Additional nursing diagnoses
- ❏ Altered growth and development related to neurologic impairment
- ❏ Dysfunctional grieving (parental) related to loss of perfect child
- ❏ Impaired home maintenance management (parental) related to care of infant with defect and cost of long-term habilitation
- ❏ Impaired tissue integrity related to spinal cord defect
- ❏ Knowledge deficit (parental) related to prevention and care of complications associated with defect
- ❏ Risk for injury related to protruding sac
- ❏ Total incontinence related to bladder and bowel involvement from spinal cord defect

Talipes deformity

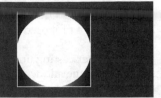

Definition
Talipes deformity, also known as clubfoot, is a congenital deformity of the muscles and bones of one or both feet. Common types of talipes include:
• talipes varus, in which the foot is bent inward (inversion)
• talipes valgus, in which the foot is bent outward (eversion)
• talipes calcaneus, in which the toes are higher than the heel (dorsiflexion)
• talipes equinus, in which the toes are lower than the heel (plantar flexion).

Combinations of these malformations also may occur; the most common is talipes equinovarus, in which the foot is abducted and turned inward and downward, with a shortened Achilles tendon. Some deformities can be manipulated into a correct position; true clubfoot cannot.

Treatment begins shortly after birth. It varies from serial casting to splinting to corrective shoes, depending on the severity and type of the deformity. Surgical correction may be needed at a later date. The prognosis is based on early detection and initiation and consistent application of corrective measures.

Found in 1 in 1,000 live births, this abnormality commonly occurs with other congenital defects. It is thought to result from familial tendencies; it is twice as common in boys as in girls. When unilateral, talipes usually occurs on the right side.

This plan focuses on the care of the infant at the beginning of the first stage of treatment, immediately after birth.

Etiology and precipitating factors
• Cause unknown
• May be genetic (familial tendency exists)
• May result from position of fetus in utero or from lack of movement or activity in utero
• May result from arrested development during early fetal stage

Physical findings
Family history
• Other members of family with clubfoot
Infant status at birth
• Exaggerated attitudes or positioning of feet
• Other congenital abnormalities, especially spinal cord defects
• Obvious deformity of feet with or without a decrease in the degree of manipulation allowed

Diagnostic studies
• X-rays to reveal abnormality of talus and calcaneus and ladderlike appearance of metatarsals

COLLABORATIVE PROBLEM
Physiologic injury related to failure to provide appropriate care, leading to complications (two expected outcomes)

Expected outcome 1
The patient will receive treatment for talipes deformity.

Interventions
1. Assess the infant's feet as follows:
• Check position, turning, and flexion of foot and toes.
• Note how easily each foot moves.

Rationales
1. Early recognition and treatment produce the best results because cartilage and muscles are supple and the feet are more malleable at birth.

2. Be aware of proposed medical treatment, including:

• serial plaster casting until the defect is corrected, starting with the adduction deformity (most common therapy)
• splint in an infant less than 1 year old

• Denis Browne splint where shoes are fixed to a metal crossbar.

3. Prepare and assist in the application of a cast or splint, holding the feet in the correct position.

4. Additional individualized interventions: _____
_____

2. Medical treatment varies with the type and severity of the deformity.
• In first-stage correction, plaster casting accommodates the infant's rapid growth; the second stage focuses on inversion, and the third stage focuses on plantar flexion.
• The infant's feet are fastened to two padded metal plates with tape and then connected to a metal crossbar that can be adjusted to permit rotation, eversion, and dorsiflexion of the feet.
• This device fixes shoes to allow adjustment of the feet to a desired position.

3. For good result, the feet must be correctly positioned during cast application.

4. Rationales: _____
_____

Expected outcome 2

The patient will show no signs of circulatory impairment to the legs.

Interventions

1. Assess for signs of circulatory impairment in the legs, including:
• tightness of the cast or splint
• coolness, duskiness, and lack of motion of toes if the leg is in a cast (assess every 1 to 2 hours)
• edema of toes
• decreased capillary refill of toes.

2. Elevate casted feet on pillows.

3. Additional individualized interventions: _____

Rationales

1. Assessment provides for interventions to prevent complications.
• Pressure impairs circulation to tissues.
• The space between the cast and skin should be wide enough so that a finger can be inserted.
• Edema is a sign of decreased circulation.
• Decreased capillary refill indicates impaired circulation.

2. Elevation promotes venous return and reduces edema.

3. Rationales: _____

NURSING DIAGNOSIS

Risk for impaired skin integrity related to casting or splinting

Expected outcome

The patient will maintain skin integrity

Interventions

1. Assess the infant's skin, noting:
• level of cleanliness and dryness under and around cast or splint
• redness, excoriation, abrasions, pallor, paresthesias, lack of pulse, and pinprick sensitivity
• cast-related irritation from rough edges touching skin.

Rationales

1. Assessment data suggest measures to prevent skin irritation and breakdown.

2. Protect the skin with foam rubber padding and petal the cast edges.

3. Turn the infant every 2 hours during the day and every 4 hours at night.

4. Wash the skin under the splint and around the cast and dry it thoroughly.

5. Additional individualized interventions: _____

2. Foam rubber padding and petaling prevent rough edges from irritating the skin.

3. Change of position relieves pressure on the area.

4. These actions maintain cleanliness and dryness. Oils and powders are not advised.

5. Rationales: _____

NURSING DIAGNOSIS

Ineffective family coping: compromised related to situational crisis of infant with congenital deformity and probability of long-term therapy

Expected outcome

The parents will exhibit appropriate coping skills.

Interventions

1. Encourage and allow the parents to express fears about caring for the infant, the need for long-term care and rehabilitation, and possible future surgical correction.

2. Inform the family about the abnormality, and allow them to see and hold the infant as soon as possible after birth. Encourage them to hold and cuddle the infant, regardless of the cast.

3. Help the parents identify necessary coping skills and available support systems.

4. Assess the family's understanding of the talipes deformity.

5. Assure the family that the abnormality can be corrected with appropriate treatment.

6. Provide information about:

• infant's condition

• cause, prevalence, and nature of the abnormality

• infant's long-term needs, such as serial casting with the foot held in position for several days or weeks, followed by maintaining the alignment of the feet with night splints as well as exercise and orthopedic shoes

• possible surgery to correct the deformity

• importance of immediate and ongoing therapy and orthopedic supervision until the child's growth is completed.

Rationales

1. Parents may feel disappointment because of the abnormality and future effects on the child's appearance and function.

2. Parental involvement with the child promotes bonding and a normal parent-child relationship.

3. This enables parents to determine the need for assistance in adapting to the new situation.

4. Assessment reveals what the family needs to learn and what misinformation needs to be corrected.

5. This should reassure the family and help them cope with the crisis.

6. Increased knowledge enhances the family's understanding of the defect.
• Information about the infant's condition allays potential anxiety.
• Information helps the parents resolve guilt feelings about the abnormality.
• Information prepares the family for long-term correctional care (usually for 3 months but longer in certain cases). The cast may be completely changed or wedged (Kite method) to change its shape when needed. The Denis Browne splint may be used to promote correction and strengthen the foot muscles.
• Resistant clubfoot, which usually is the result of recurrent neglected deformities, may need surgical correction.
• Long-term therapy is needed to ensure correction of the abnormality, and permanent correction requires time and patience.

7. Additional individualized interventions: _____

7. Rationales: _____

Nursing diagnosis

Knowledge deficit (parental) related to care of infant with cast or splint device

Expected outcome

The parents will receive appropriate information about infant care and will express understanding of that information.

Interventions

1. Identify the parents' knowledge and their interest, readiness, and ability to learn.

2. Inform the parents that the treatment may be long and requires patience.

3. Encourage the parents to fondle, hold, and cuddle the infant, regardless of the cast.

4. Provide instruction on caring for the splint device or cast. Cast care instructions include the following:
• Elevate the infant's feet on pillows after casts are reapplied.
• Check the infant's toes every 1 to 2 hours after each new cast application; report coolness, pallor, lack of movement and sensation, and edema to the doctor.
• Protect skin by petaling cast edges or padding them with adhesive tape or foam rubber; check for irritation every 2 to 4 hours.
• Protect the cast from urine and wetness during bathing by covering the cast with a plastic bag and securing the bag with rubber bands.

5. Inform the parents of the importance of keeping appointments with the orthopedist for cast changes and evaluations.

6. Allow time for questions, clarifications, and demonstrations of cast care techniques, as needed.

7. Refer the parents to community agencies and home health care.

8. Additional individualized interventions: _____

Rationales

1. Assessment provides the basis for developing a teaching plan appropriate to the parents' needs and abilities.

2. Restrictive movement may make the infant irritable at first, but the infant eventually will adjust.

3. Fondling, holding, and cuddling the infant provide stimulation and promote development.

4. Teaching ensures safe infant care and prevents skin or circulatory complications.
• Elevating the feet promotes venous return and prevents edema.
• These are indications of circulatory impairment.

• These measures prevent skin irritation or breakdown from the cast's rough edges.

• Wetness softens cast, impairing its corrective effect.

5. Ongoing therapy is necessary for successful correction.

6. Discussions and demonstrations reinforce parents' learning and reduce their anxiety.

7. These referrals provide continued support and enhance compliance with follow-up care.

8. Rationales: _____

Documentation checklist

During the hospital stay, document:

❒ patient status and assessment findings, especially other congenital anomalies and any family history of talipes deformity

❒ changes in patient status

❒ pertinent laboratory and diagnostic findings, especially X-rays of legs and feet

❒ patient's response to treatment

❒ family's reaction to the diagnosis

❒ parent-infant interaction

❒ family teaching guidelines, especially any specialized treatment or exercises required

❒ discharge planning guidelines.

Associated plans

❒ Developmental dysplasia of the hip

❒ Preoperative care

❒ Spinal cord defects and hydrocephalus

Additional nursing diagnoses

❒ Altered growth and development related to effects of long-term therapy, stimulation deficiencies

❒ Impaired physical mobility related to casting and splinting

❒ Risk for altered parenting related to lack of knowledge, lack of support from significant other, or unrealistic expectations for infant

❒ Risk for peripheral neurovascular dysfunction related to ill-fitting cast or splint device

Tracheoesophageal fistula or esophageal atresia

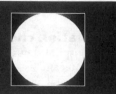

Definition
Tracheoesophageal fistula (TEF) is an abnormal congenital opening between the trachea and the esophagus with or without an associated esophageal interruption. The most common of the abnormalities is atresia of a segment of the esophagus involving an upper blind pouch and the lower portion connected to the stomach. A fistula connects the trachea to the lower portion of the esophagus.

An esophageal atresia without tracheal involvement or a fistula that connects an otherwise normal trachea and esophagus (H-type fistula) may also occur. At birth, this defect may be associated with congenital heart disease, GI disorders, skeletal defects, or neurologic disorders.

All these defects are repaired surgically by transthoracic extrapleural fistula ligation and end-to-end esophageal anastomosis, depending on the length of the proximal and distal ends of the esophagus and whether the infant can tolerate the surgery. If the infant cannot yet tolerate surgery, a gastrostomy tube is inserted under local anesthesia to perform GI decompression. Feeding by total parenteral nutrition (TPN) may be indicated until surgery is performed. The survival rate is about 97% for full-term infants and about 50% for preterm infants; pneumonia, septicemia, and other anomalies are the usual cause of death.

This plan focuses on care of the infant before surgery and preventing complications while maintaining pulmonary and nutritional status.

Etiology and precipitating factors
• Defective separation of the trachea and esophagus and incomplete fusing of the trachea after this separation; occurs during the 4th and 5th weeks of gestation.

Physical findings
Maternal history
• Polyhydramnios or hydramnios
Infant status at birth
• Prematurity and small size for gestational age
• Low Apgar score and cyanosis
• Inability to pass catheter into stomach
• Congenital anomalies
Gastrointestinal
• Pooling of secretions with excessive drooling from mouth
• Difficulty feeding with regurgitation of feedings

• Excessive gastric air and gastric distention caused by air from lungs traveling to stomach by way of the fistula
Pulmonary
• Respiratory distress and tachypnea if secretions are aspirated
• Coughing, choking, sneezing, or cyanosis during feeding

Diagnostic studies
• Chest X-ray to reveal pneumonia, atelectasis in upper lobe of right lung, blind pouch filled with air, and excessive gastric air; after attempt to pass radiopaque catheter from nares through esophagus into stomach, X-ray may show tube ending or coiling in upper esophageal pouch
• Contrast studies with bronchoscopy or barium X-ray to detect TEF (performed with caution because aspiration of contrast medium can cause chemical pneumonia)
• Upper GI series
• White blood cell count and differential for neutrophils and platelets to determine whether pneumonitis is present
• Serum glucose level to ensure adequate glucose level
• Arterial blood gas (ABG) values to determine pH, oxygen, and carbon dioxide levels with respiratory distress
• Cultures to identify infectious organisms

COLLABORATIVE PROBLEM

Risk for respiratory distress related to excessive secretions in mouth and blind pouch or aspiration of secretions and feedings (three expected outcomes)

Expected outcome 1

The patient will maintain a patent airway with no signs of aspiration.

Interventions

1. Assess for respiratory distress, noting:
• increased respiratory rate and distress, use of accessory muscles, nasal flaring, retractions, and grunting
• cyanosis, mottling, or pallor
• choking and coughing
• regurgitation of feedings through mouth and nose
• increased secretions.

2. Additional individualized interventions: _____

Rationales

1. Assessment determines the presence of the anomaly. The signs noted indicate respiratory problems and, possibly, aspiration (swallowed secretions or feedings entering the esophageal pouch and then being aspirated into the trachea). The normal respiratory rate for a neonate ranges from 40 to 60 breaths/minute.

2. Rationales: _____

Expected outcome 2

The patient will maintain a patent airway and optimal pulmonary function.

Interventions

1. Have suctioning and intubation equipment, oxygen, and a resuscitation bag on hand at all times.

2. Perform oral, nasal, and endotracheal suctioning every 1 to 2 hours or more frequently if needed.

3. Withhold oral food and fluids.

4. Insert a #10 Replogle tube into the blind pouch; then attach it to low intermittent suction according to the doctor's order, and monitor output.

5. Position the infant on its abdomen or side, as tolerated, with the head elevated 20 to 40 degrees. Reposition the infant every 2 hours if feasible. Position the infant with its head down if the defect involves a blind pouch at each end only or a fistula from the trachea to the upper esophageal segment.

6. If a gastrostomy tube is inserted for decompression, attach it to straight drainage to check patency.

7. Institute comfort measures to prevent crying.

8. Additional individualized interventions: _____

Rationales

1. Emergency apparatus should be on hand in case aspiration causes respiratory difficulty.

2. Suctioning clears secretions from the oropharynx and maintains a patent airway.

3. This prevents aspiration of feedings.

4. The tube provides continuous removal of secretions from the pouch if the infant has an esophageal atresia.

5. The abdominal or side-lying position prevents aspiration of mucus or stomach contents and reduces gastric reflux. It also allows for better lung expansion and breathing pattern. The head-down position in an infant with a blind pouch at each end only or a fistula from the trachea to the upper esophageal segment reduces the risk of aspiration.

6. Gastrostomy is performed to decompress the stomach and prevent gastric reflux through the fistula into the trachea and lungs.

7. Crying increases the amount of air swallowed through the fistula, worsens gastric distention, and increases the risk of gastric reflux.

8. Rationales: _____

Expected outcome 3

The patient will exhibit no complications from aspiration.

Interventions

1. Assess for respiratory complications, noting:
• increased respiratory rate and effort
• increased heart rate
• severe retractions and nasal flaring
• cyanosis
• diminished breath sounds
• arterial or capillary blood gas values showing low oxygen level
• serial X-rays to indicate changes over time (improvement or worsening of aspiration pneumonia)
• culture results indicating infection.

2. Continue ventilatory assistance if present.

3. Prepare and administer antibiotics by the ordered route.

4. Use sterile technique for all care, treatments, and procedures, including sterile solutions for irrigation, dressings, and suctioning equipment.

5. Additional individualized interventions: _____

Rationales

1. These are signs of respiratory distress and complications involving the lungs. Early assessment promotes prompt treatment.

2. Assistance ensures respiratory stability.

3. Prophylactic antibiotics help prevent possible aspiration pneumonitis.

4. Sterile technique reduces the possibility of introducing pathologic organisms.

5. Rationales: _____

COLLABORATIVE PROBLEM

Altered nutrition: less than body requirements related to inability to take oral feedings and withholding of food and fluids

Expected outcome

The patient will maintain optimal nutritional status.

Interventions

1. Calculate calorie needs based on the infant's weight and age.

2. Weigh the infant daily or as needed, and report a loss greater than 50 g in a 24-hour period (depending on the infant's birth weight).

3. Test heelstick blood glucose levels with a reagent strip every 1 to 2 hours or as needed.

4. Administer and monitor peripheral parenteral nutrition with an infusion-control device. The amount depends on the infant's size and condition.

Rationales

1. This ensures optimal calorie intake for weight gain.

2. This is a good gauge of whether nutritional needs are being met.

3. Glucose stores are limited and quickly used up in the infant, causing the potential for hypoglycemia.

4. Peripheral parenteral nutrition is a short-term treatment that provides up to 2,500 kcal/day to maintain the infant's glucose and fluid needs when food and water are withheld. Solutions of less than 12% dextrose are given peripherally. Using an infusion-control device minimizes the risk of infusing too much solution too quickly.

5. Administer and monitor TPN if indicated (see *Comparing types of parenteral nutrition,* page 330). Follow these guidelines:

• Carry out all aspects of procedure with strict aseptic technique. Also, ensure that fluids are prepared in the pharmacy under strict sterile conditions, using a laminar flow hood.
• Position and restrain the infant.
• Prepare an umbilical artery catheter (UAC) or central vein for infusion with intralipids administered through a separate line.

• Prime the I.V. tubing and filter with glucose solution, removing all bubbles. Do not use a filter to administer intralipids.
• Label the solution and mark the time on the tape.

• Assist with passing the catheter through the vein after the area is anesthetized with a local injection.
• Use an infusion-control device with a pressure alarm to regulate the infusion rate.
• Tape all connections to prevent disconnection; clamp lines when connections are open.
• Monitor and maintain TPN administration as follows:
– Change the filter, dressings, and connecting tubing daily.
– Clean the infusion site daily, using an antiseptic solution as ordered.
– Use transparent occlusive dressings, such as Op-Site, for dressings and to secure the I.V. line.
– Culture the filter fluid as policy dictates.
– Check the infusion rate, patency of tubing, and site for infiltration every hour.
– Record all vital information and changes regarding TPN on a flow sheet.

6. To discontinue TPN, gradually wean the infant while increasing oral or enteral feedings.

5. TPN may be administered to meet the infant's nutritional needs for a prolonged period if the infant dose not meet the criteria for surgery; it can provide up to 4,000 kcal/day if necessary. TPN satisfies the infant's caloric, protein, carbohydrate, intralipid, mineral, and vitamin requirements. The total volume of the infusion solution varies; amounts are calculated daily, based on the infant's weight, use of a radiant warmer and phototherapy, and other factors. Fungal or bacterial infection or sepsis is a complication of TPN because the high glucose content of the solution provides a good medium for bacterial growth.
• Sterile technique prevents contamination and the entry of microorganisms into the highly concentrated solution, which provides an excellent medium for bacterial growth.
• This prevents displacement of the catheter.
• Because TPN solutions are hyperosmotic, large central veins are used to rapidly dilute the solutions. A UAC may be used for the infusion of TPN and intralipids. Silicone or Silastic catheters with single or multiple lumens are used.
• This prevents air embolism. Filters are not used with intralipids because intralipid molecules cannot pass through a filter.
• This allows monitoring of the amount infused over a specific period and prevents overinfusion.
• This prevents possible catheter displacement.

• This ensures infusion of the correct amount of fluid at the correct rate, minimizing the risk of fluid overload.
• This prevents hemorrhage or air embolism.

• Monitoring and maintaining TPN administration is vital to preventing such complications as local skin irritation, hyperglycemia or hypoglycemia, metabolic acidosis, hemorrhage, pulmonary embolism, and infection.

6. This intervention maintains glucose levels, prevents rapid shifts in fluid balance, and allows assessment of the infant's ability to tolerate feedings.

Comparing types of parenteral nutrition

Parenteral nutrition is a specialized feeding method used to provide nutrients and maintain fluid and electrolyte balance in the patient who cannot eat normally. The solution is delivered through a peripheral or central vein. An infant whose GI tract cannot be used or who has high metabolic needs that cannot be met by oral or enteral feedings is a candidate for parenteral nutrition.

Types of parenteral nutrition include peripheral and total. The chart below compares these types.

Method	Indications	Nutrient solutions
Peripheral parenteral nutrition Administered through a peripheral vein	• Short-term therapy in patients who require 2,500 kcal/day or less • Adjunct to oral or enteral feedings	• Dextrose 5% in water • Dextrose 10% in water • Amino acid solution • Protein hydrolysates • Fat emulsions
Total parenteral nutrition Administered through a large central vein	• Long-term therapy in patients who require more than 2,500 kcal/day (provides up to 4,000 kcal/day)	• Admixtures of dextrose in water (20% to 50%) and crystalline amino acids • Fat emulsions • Total nutrient admixtures (lipids premixed with dextrose and crystalline amino acids)

7. Administer and monitor gastrostomy tube feedings, when indicated, as follows:
• Secure the tube after placement.
• Aspirate the tube before each feeding and measure residual stomach contents; if you find amounts greater than 2 ml, withhold feedings.
• Start with small amounts of dilute feeding and increase as tolerated (volume and osmolality).
• Assess abdominal girth every 2 hours and observe for diarrhea.
• Allow for feedings by gravity.

• Ensure initial feedings of 4 to 5 ml every 4 hours for neonate.
• Provide a pacifier for the infant to suck on.

8. Provide mouth care every 2 hours.

9. Review daily, or according to hospital policy, results of the following tests: serum glucose, electrolyte, blood urea nitrogen, aspartate aminotransferase (AST), and alanine aminotransferase (ALT) levels; hematocrit; prothrombin time and partial thromboplastin time; urine for glucose, osmolality, and specific gravity; and weekly serum ammonia and triglyceride levels.

10. Additional individualized interventions: _____

7. Feedings through a gastrostomy tube may be ordered until the defect can be surgically corrected.
• This prevents tube dislodgment.
• Residual stomach contents require the withholding of feedings to prevent distention.

• This allows for feedings to be gradually increased as tolerated, preventing fluid imbalances.
• Increased abdominal girth and diarrhea indicate distention from overfeeding and osmolality imbalances.
• Pressure exerted to instill feedings may cause gastric perforation.
• This is the optimal amount for a neonate.

• A pacifier provides oral stimulation for the tube-fed infant.

8. This prevents mucosal drying that occurs with parenteral and enteral feedings.

9. Test results allow monitoring of the effects of nutritional support. Monitoring of lipid infusion and hepatic and renal function is necessary, as is monitoring of other changes that typically occur with TPN.

10. Rationales: _____

NURSING DIAGNOSIS

Risk for fluid volume deficit related to fluid loss through indwelling tube and food and fluid being withheld

Expected outcome

The patient will maintain optimal fluid and electrolyte balance.

Interventions

1. Calculate fluid requirements daily.

2. Weigh the infant every day or as its condition permits.

3. Assess fluid intake and output every hour.

4. Monitor urine output every hour, and report an output of less than 3 ml/kg/hour.

5. Monitor the rate and amount of I.V. fluid infused, and note any infiltration.

6. Monitor urine specific gravity at each voiding.

7. Additional individualized interventions: _____

Rationales

1. Fluid needs vary according to individual infant weight and fluid losses from various routes.

2. Weight gains and losses reflect fluid gains and losses and help determine the infant's fluid needs.

3. Hourly assessment ensures optimal fluid balance by indicating the need for fluid replacement.

4. Adequate urine output should be 3 ml/kg/hour, with a specific gravity of 1.005 to 1.020. Low urine output and increased specific gravity result from low fluid intake.

5. I.V. fluids provide an adequate method to replace fluids. Fluid replacement is calculated and monitored to provide an adequate daily fluid amount based on the infant's body weight and to prevent hypervolemia.

6. These measures provide data related to possible inadequate fluid intake.

7. Rationales: _____

NURSING DIAGNOSIS

Impaired skin integrity related to irritation at stomal site because of secretions

Expected outcome

The patient will maintain skin integrity around the stomal site.

Interventions

1. Assess gastrostomy or esophagostomy stoma for redness, excoriation, and other changes.

2. Use sterile technique when caring for the stoma.

3. Apply a protective covering around the stoma, such as a skin barrier (Op-Site or HolliHesive), or keep the stoma clean and exposed to air.

4. Keep the area clean and dry.

5. Additional individualized interventions: _____

Rationales

1. These changes indicate possible inflammation and skin breakdown, destroying the body's first line of defense and allowing for infection.

2. This prevents contact with contaminants.

3. These preparations protect the skin from irritants.

4. This helps maintain skin integrity and prevents irritation and excoriation.

5. Rationales: _____

Nursing diagnosis

Anxiety (parental) related to impending surgery and threat of child's death

Expected outcome

The parents will express minimal anxiety.

Interventions

1. Allow and encourage parental expression of feelings and fears about the loss of the "perfect child."

2. Reinforce the infant's normal and healthy aspects and the possibility that surgery will correct the defect, leaving no visible effects.

3. Provide accurate information about:
• infant's condition
• defect's cause, occurrence, and type
• special procedures and equipment
• preparation for surgery and care after surgery.

4. Additional individualized interventions: _____

Rationales

1. This promotes a trusting relationship and a secure environment, decreasing parental anxiety.

2. Positive reinforcement helps to reduce parental stress and sadness and to increase positive feelings about the surgical correction.

3. Information reduces anxiety and maximizes understanding. (See the "Preoperative care" plan, page 284, and the "Postoperative care" plan, page 277, for more information.)

4. Rationales: _____

Nursing diagnosis

Ineffective family coping: compromised related to guilt and emotional conflict caused by crisis associated with infant's defect and postponement of surgery

Expected outcome

The parents will develop appropriate coping mechanisms.

Interventions

1. Assess the parents' expressions of anxiety and use of coping mechanisms.

2. Help the parents to express their feelings about the loss of the "perfect child," the need for a prolonged stay in an intensive-care nursery, and changes in the infant's appearance because of gastrostomy tube feedings or other treatments.

3. Provide consistent and accurate information about the infant's condition.

4. Encourage the parents to hold and care for their infant.

5. Additional individualized interventions: _____

Rationales

1. Assessment helps to identify and develop constructive coping strategies.

2. This helps to maintain a trusting, secure environment and shows your acceptance of the parents' concerns and fears.

3. Understanding the infant's progress and condition helps parents cope.

4. Parental involvement promotes bonding.

5. Rationales: _____

Documentation checklist
During the hospital stay, document:
❐ patient status and assessment findings, especially history of polyhydramnios (hydramnios), Apgar scores, gestational age by examination, whether catheter can be passed from nose or mouth to stomach, congenital anomalies, excessive drooling, feeding difficulties, gastric distention, and respiratory effort, including coughing, choking, or cyanosis during feedings
❐ changes in patient status
❐ pertinent laboratory and diagnostic findings, especially serum calcium, phosphorus, total protein, and glucose levels; complete blood count with differential; platelet counts; ABG studies (oxygen, carbon dioxide, bicarbonate, and pH); culture results; and results of chest X-rays, upper GI series, and contrast studies with bronchoscopy
❐ patient's response to treatment
❐ family's reaction to the diagnosis and surgery
❐ parent-infant interaction
❐ family teaching guidelines, especially any respiratory or feeding needs that will continue at home and the need for long-term follow-up
❐ discharge planning guidelines.

Associated plans
❐ Respiratory distress syndrome
❐ Necrotizing enterocolitis
❐ Postoperative care
❐ Preoperative care

Additional nursing diagnoses
❐ Altered family processes related to guilt associated with infant's defect
❐ Dysfunctional grieving (parental) related to loss of the perfect child
❐ Impaired gas exchange related to aspiration
❐ Ineffective breathing pattern related to pulmonary scar tissue, chronic lung damage
❐ Ineffective infant feeding pattern related to TEF
❐ Knowledge deficit (parental) related to lack of information
❐ Risk for altered parenting related to interruption in bonding process
❐ Risk for aspiration related to TEF
❐ Risk for infection related to aspiration of secretions, feedings

Transient tachypnea of the newborn

Definition
Also called retained lung fluid or wet lung, transient tachypnea of the newborn (TTN) develops at birth or shortly afterward and lasts from a few hours to 2 to 4 days. It often affects full-term infants and preterm infants of 34 to 37 weeks' gestation frequently born by cesarean birth. Fluid remaining in the lungs affects breathing because the lymphatics, which are attempting to reabsorb the fluid as fast as possible, become engorged, delaying reabsorption. This results in a splinting of the lung, preventing effective ventilation. It does not occur in infants born vaginally because the thoracic cavity is squeezed during the infant's passage through the vaginal canal, expelling some lung fluid.

The prognosis is good because the condition usually runs its course in about 1 to 4 days without any resultant chronic lung disorder.

This plan focuses on care of the infant who is at risk for retaining or who has retained lung fluid after birth.

Etiology and precipitating factors
• Retention of fetal lung fluid because of delayed or slowed reabsorption
• Aspiration of large amounts of amniotic fluid from perinatal stress or asphyxia, large-for-gestational-age infant of diabetic mother, or difficult transition of breech birth
• Cesarean birth, in which the infant is not subject to the vaginal squeezing during delivery that helps remove pulmonary fluid and does not experience the stress alarm initiated by labor to begin lung fluid reabsorption because birth is imminent

Physical findings
Maternal history
• Perinatal conditions or diseases that necessitate cesarean birth
• Difficulty during delivery
• Diabetes mellitus

Infant status at birth
• Full term or preterm
• Apgar score indicating respiratory difficulty
• Difficult presentation at birth
• Cesarean birth

Integumentary
• Skin duskiness
• Possibly central cyanosis

Pulmonary
• Persistently high respiratory rate
• Possibly chest retractions and nasal flaring
• Possibly expiratory grunt from trying to eject trapped alveolar air
• Possibly cyanosis when breathing room air

Diagnostic studies
• Chest X-ray to reveal hyperinflation, fluid in fissures, costophrenic angles, and flattened diaphragm; patches of collapse may be seen
• Arterial blood gas (ABG) studies may reveal slightly decreased pH with partial pressure of carbon dioxide slightly elevated, but both within normal ranges (see appendix I, Normal laboratory values for the newborn).

COLLABORATIVE PROBLEM
Risk for respiratory deficiency related to obstruction (two expected outcomes)

Expected outcome 1
The patient will maintain optimal respiratory functioning.

Interventions
1. Assess the infant for changes or difficulty in breathing, including:
• increased respiratory rate, depth, and difficulty
• central cyanosis and dusky skin
• grunting, nasal flaring, and retractions
• secretions in airway.

Rationales
1. Identifying changes or difficulty in breathing permits differentiation of TTN from more serious respiratory distress disorders and allows for appropriate treatment. The normal respiratory rate for a full-term infant ranges from 40 to 60 breaths/minute.

2. Monitor ABG studies and (if used) pulse oximetry or transcutaneous monitoring device for oxygen level.

3. Review chest X-rays.

4. Additional individualized interventions: _____
_____

2. Monitoring allows detection of changes. Results should fall within normal limits, with oxygen at the optimal level.

3. X-rays show fluid in the lungs and rule out pneumothorax.

4. Rationales: _____
_____

Expected outcome 2

The patient will maintain a patent airway and optimal respiratory function.

Interventions

1. Elevate the head of the bed slightly, and position the infant with its head supported in the side-lying position or with a shoulder roll in the supine position. Do not hyperextend the infant's neck. The infant may need to be positioned with its head lowered and feet elevated.

2. Change the infant's position from side to side every 2 hours.

3. Maintain a neutral thermal environment.

4. If appropriate, suction secretions from the nasopharynx as needed.

5. Administer warmed, humidified oxygen at 40% or less by hood, mask, or other method, as ordered.

6. If the infant's respiratory status does not improve or if it further deteriorates (possibly from fatigue), provide continuous positive airway pressure (CPAP) or other mechanical ventilation as ordered.

7. If a transcutaneous PO_2 sensor is used, calibrate it according to the manufacturer's directions and rotate the sensor position every 3 to 4 hours. Apply and monitor the pulse oximeter (if used) to measure oxygen levels. Correlate settings with ABG values.

8. If a transcutaneous PO_2 sensor is used, place the high and low alarms in the ON position, and watch for causes of abnormal readings.

9. Additional individualized interventions: _____
_____

Rationales

1. The side-lying and supine positions with the head elevated promote ease of breathing and maximize lung expansion. Lowering the head promotes drainage of secretions. The infant's condition determines the best position.

2. The side-lying position relieves pressure and prevents aspiration.

3. This conserves energy and minimizes oxygen demand.

4. Suctioning clears the airway of secretions and mucus; if the obstruction is too far down for the catheter to reach, it may be more feasible to wait for the lymphatics to absorb the secretions.

5. Oxygen delivery maintains normal partial pressure of oxygen (PO_2) and pink skin color with minimal respiratory effort (see the "Respiratory distress syndrome" plan, page 297, for various methods).

6. CPAP or a brief period of mechanical ventilation may be indicated to maintain airway patency.

7. These steps ensure safe use of the monitoring device and accurate readings. A pulse oximeter is preferred because it gauges oxygen saturation by fiber-optic light without producing heat that might burn the skin.

8. These alarms signal excessively high or low oxygen levels.

9. Rationales: _____
_____

NURSING DIAGNOSIS

Knowledge deficit (parental) related to the infant's condition, treatment, and ability to overcome temporary respiratory distress

Expected outcome

The parents will receive information about the infant's status and care needs and will express understanding of that information.

Interventions

1. Identify what the parents' need and want to learn, and assess their readiness and ability to learn.

2. Inform the parents about:
• cause of the infant's condition
• treatment being given
• special procedures and equipment
• progress and prognosis.

3. Reassure the parents about their ability to care for the infant.

4. Answer the parents' questions and clarify aspects of care as needed.

5. Additional individualized interventions: _____

Rationales

1. This provides the basis for developing a teaching plan that matches the parents' needs and abilities.

2. Information reduces the parents' anxiety and concerns.

3. Encouragement shows your support of the parents' ability to care for the infant after discharge.

4. Addressing the parents' questions and concerns reinforces learning and decreases anxiety about caring for the infant.

5. Rationales: _____

Documentation checklist

During the hospital stay, document:
❐ patient status and assessment findings, especially the type of delivery, maternal history (including history of diabetes mellitus), Apgar scores, gestational age by examination, color, and respiratory effort
❐ changes in patient status, especially respiratory effort
❐ pertinent laboratory and diagnostic findings, especially serum calcium, phosphorus, total protein, and glucose levels; ABG results (oxygen, carbon dioxide, bicarbonate, and pH levels); complete blood count with differential; and chest X-ray results
❐ patient's response to treatment
❐ family's reaction to the diagnosis
❐ parent-infant interaction
❐ family teaching guidelines
❐ discharge planning guidelines.

Associated plans
❐ Cesarean section birth
❐ Respiratory distress syndrome
❐ Pregnancy complicated by diabetes mellitus

Additional nursing diagnoses
❐ Anxiety (parental) related to unknown potential for complications
❐ Ineffective airway clearance related to retained lung fluid
❐ Ineffective family coping: compromised related to fear, guilt over condition of infant, admission to special care unit
❐ Risk for altered parenting related to lack of knowledge, unrealistic expectations for infant
❐ Risk for infection related to retained lung fluid

Appendices, selected references, and index

Appendix A: NANDA taxonomy of nursing diagnoses

The currently accepted classification system for nursing diagnoses is that of the North American Nursing Diagnosis Association (NANDA). It is organized around nine human response patterns: exchanging, communicating, relating, valuing, choosing, moving, perceiving, knowing, and feeling.

The complete taxonomic structure is listed here. The series of numbers before each diagnosis is its classification number, used to determine the placement of the diagnosis within the taxonomy. The number of digits delineates the level of abstraction of the nursing diagnosis (more specific diagnoses are assigned longer numbers).

Pattern 1. Exchanging (Mutual giving and receiving)

1.1.2.1	Altered nutrition: More than body requirements
1.1.2.2	Altered nutrition: Less than body requirements
1.1.2.3	Altered nutrition: Risk for more than body requirements
1.2.1.1	Risk for infection
1.2.2.1	Risk for altered body temperature
1.2.2.2	Hypothermia
1.2.2.3	Hyperthermia
1.2.2.4	Ineffective thermoregulation
1.2.3.1	Dysreflexia
1.2.3.2	Risk for autonomic dysreflexia
1.3.1.1	Constipation
1.3.1.1.1	Perceived constipation
1.3.1.1.2	Colonic constipation
1.3.1.2	Diarrhea
1.3.1.3	Bowel incontinence
1.3.1.4	Risk for constipation
1.3.2	Altered urinary elimination
1.3.2.1.1	Stress incontinence
1.3.2.1.2	Reflex urinary incontinence
1.3.2.1.3	Urge incontinence
1.3.2.1.4	Functional urinary incontinence
1.3.2.1.5	Total incontinence
1.3.2.1.6	Risk of urinary urge incontinence
1.3.2.2	Urinary retention
1.4.1.1	Altered (specify type) tissue perfusion (renal, cerebral, cardiopulmonary, gastrointestinal, peripheral)
1.4.1.2	Risk for fluid volume imbalance
1.4.1.2.1	Fluid volume excess
1.4.1.2.2.1	Fluid volume deficit
1.4.1.2.2.2	Risk for fluid volume deficit
1.4.2.1	Decreased cardiac output
1.5.1.1	Impaired gas exchange
1.5.1.2	Ineffective airway clearance
1.5.1.3	Ineffective breathing pattern
1.5.1.3.1	Inability to sustain spontaneous ventilation
1.5.1.3.2	Dysfunctional ventilatory weaning response (DVWR)
1.6.1	Risk for injury
1.6.1.1	Risk for suffocation
1.6.1.2	Risk for poisoning
1.6.1.3	Risk for trauma
1.6.1.4	Risk for aspiration
1.6.1.5	Risk for disuse syndrome
1.6.1.6	Latex allergy
1.6.1.7	Risk for latex allergy
1.6.2	Altered protection
1.6.2.1	Impaired tissue integrity
1.6.2.1.1	Altered oral mucous membrane
1.6.2.1.2.1	Impaired skin integrity
1.6.2.1.2.2	Risk for impaired skin integrity
1.6.2.1.3	Altered dentition
1.7.1	Decreased adaptive capacity: Intracranial
1.8	Energy field disturbance

Pattern 2. Communicating (Sending messages)

2.1.1.1	Impaired verbal communication

Pattern 3. Relating (Establishing bonds)

3.1.1	Impaired social interaction
3.1.2	Social isolation
3.1.3	Risk for loneliness
3.2.1	Altered role performance
3.2.1.1.1	Altered parenting
3.2.1.1.2	Risk for altered parenting
3.2.1.1.2.1	Risk for altered parent/infant/child attachment
3.2.1.2.1	Sexual dysfunction
3.2.2	Altered family processes
3.2.2.1	Caregiver role strain
3.2.2.2	Risk for caregiver role strain
3.2.2.3.1	Altered family process: Alcoholism
3.2.3.1	Parental role conflict
3.3	Altered sexuality patterns

Pattern 4. Valuing (Assigning relative worth)

4.1.1	Spiritual distress (distress of the human spirit)
4.1.2	Risk for spiritual distress
4.2	Potential for enhanced spiritual well-being

Pattern 5. Choosing (Selecting alternatives)

5.1.1.1	Ineffective individual coping
5.1.1.1.1	Impaired adjustment
5.1.1.1.2	Defensive coping
5.1.1.1.3	Ineffective denial
5.1.2.1.1	Ineffective family coping: Disabling
5.1.2.1.2	Ineffective family coping: Compromised
5.1.2.2	Family coping: Potential for growth
5.1.3.1	Potential for enhanced community coping
5.1.3.2	Ineffective community coping
5.2.1	Ineffective management of therapeutic regimen (individuals)
5.2.1.1	Noncompliance (specify)
5.2.2	Ineffective management of therapeutic regimen: Families
5.2.3	Ineffective management of therapeutic regimen: Community
5.2.4	Effective management of therapeutic regimen: Individual
5.3.1.1	Decisional conflict (specify)
5.4	Health-seeking behaviors (specify)

Pattern 6. Moving (Involving activity)

6.1.1.1	Impaired physical mobility
6.1.1.1.1	Risk for peripheral neurovascular dysfunction
6.1.1.1.2	Risk for perioperative positioning injury
6.1.1.1.3	Impaired walking
6.1.1.1.4	Impaired wheelchair mobility
6.1.1.1.5	Impaired wheelchair transfer ability
6.1.1.1.6	Impaired bed mobility
6.1.1.2	Activity intolerance
6.1.1.2.1	Fatigue
6.1.1.3	Risk for activity intolerance
6.2.1	Sleep pattern disturbance
6.2.1.1	Sleep deprivation
6.3.1.1	Diversional activity deficit
6.4.1.1	Impaired home maintenance management
6.4.2	Altered health maintenance
6.4.2.1	Delayed surgical recovery
6.4.2.2	Adult failure to thrive
6.5.1	Feeding self-care deficit
6.5.1.1	Impaired swallowing
6.5.1.2	Ineffective breast-feeding
6.5.1.2.1	Interrupted breast-feeding
6.5.1.3	Effective breast-feeding
6.5.1.4	Ineffective infant feeding pattern
6.5.2	Bathing or hygiene self-care deficit
6.5.3	Dressing or grooming self-care deficit
6.5.4	Toileting self-care deficit
6.6	Altered growth and development
6.6.1	Risk for altered development
6.6.2	Risk for altered growth
6.7	Relocation stress syndrome
6.8.1	Risk for disorganized infant behavior

6.8.2	Disorganized infant behavior
6.8.3	Potential for enhanced organized infant behavior

Pattern 7. Perceiving (Receiving information)

7.1.1	Body image disturbance
7.1.2	Self-esteem disturbance
7.1.2.1	Chronic low self-esteem
7.1.2.2	Situational low self-esteem
7.1.3	Personal identity disturbance
7.2	Sensory or perceptual alterations (specify visual, auditory, kinesthetic, gustatory, tactile, olfactory)
7.2.1.1	Unilateral neglect
7.3.1	Hopelessness
7.3.2	Powerlessness

Pattern 8. Knowing (Associating meaning with information)

8.1.1	Knowledge deficit (specify)
8.2.1	Impaired environmental interpretation syndrome
8.2.2	Acute confusion
8.2.3	Chronic confusion
8.3	Altered thought processes
8.3.1	Impaired memory

Pattern 9. Feeling (Being subjectively aware of information)

9.1.1	Pain
9.1.1.1	Chronic pain
9.1.2	Nausea
9.2.1.1	Dysfunctional grieving
9.2.1.2	Anticipatory grieving
9.2.1.3	Chronic sorrow
9.2.2	Risk for violence: Self-directed or directed at others
9.2.2.1	Risk for self-mutilation
9.2.3	Post-trauma syndrome
9.2.3.1	Rape-trauma syndrome
9.2.3.1.1	Rape-trauma syndrome: Compound reaction
9.2.3.1.2	Rape-trauma syndrome: Silent reaction
9.2.4	Risk for post-trauma syndrome
9.3.1	Anxiety
9.3.1.1	Death anxiety
9.3.2	Fear

Appendices

Appendix B:
Selected daily dietary allowances — maternal

The following chart shows selected daily dietary allowances for pregnant, lactating, and nonpregnant women.

Nutrient	Pregnant women	Lactating women		Nonpregnant women		
		Months 1 through 6	Months 7 through 12	Ages 15 to 18	Ages 19 to 24	Ages 25 to 50
Calcium	1,200 mg	1,200 mg	1,200 mg	1,200 mg	1,200 mg	800 mg
Folate	400 mcg	280 mcg	260 mcg	180 mcg	180 mcg	180 mcg
Iodine	175 mcg	200 mcg	200 mcg	150 mcg	150 mcg	150 mcg
Iron	30 mg	15 mg	15 mg	15 mg	15 mg	15 mg
Magnesium	320 mg	355 mg	340 mg	300 mg	280 mg	280 mg
Niacin	17 mg NE*	20 mg NE	20 mg NE	15 mg NE	15 mg NE	15 mg NE
Phosphorus	1,200 mg	1,200 mg	1,200 mg	1,200 mg	1,200 mg	800 mg
Protein	60 g	65 g	62 g	44 g	46 g	50 g
Riboflavin	1.6 mg	1.8 mg	1.7 mg	1.3 mg	1.3 mg	1.3 mg
Selenium	65 mcg	75 mcg	75 mcg	50 mcg	55 mcg	55 mcg
Thiamine	1.5 mg	1.6 mg	1.6 mg	1.1 mg	1.1 mg	1.1 mg
Vitamin A	800 mcg RE†	1,300 mcg RE	1,200 mcg RE	800 mcg RE	800 mcg RE	800 mcg RE
Vitamin B_6	2.2 mg	2.1 mg	2.1 mg	1.5 mg	1.6 mg	1.6 mg
Vitamin B_{12}	2.2 mcg	2.6 mcg	2.6 mcg	2.0 mcg	2.0 mcg	2.0 mcg
Vitamin C	70 mg	95 mg	90 mg	60 mg	60 mg	60 mg
Vitamin D	10 mcg	10 mcg	10 mcg	10 mcg	5 mcg	5 mcg
Vitamin E	10 mg TE‡	12 mg TE	11 mg TE	8 mg TE	8 mg TE	8 mg TE
Zinc	15 mg	19 mg	16 mg	12 mg	12 mg	12 mg

*NE: niacin equivalent
†RE: retinol equivalent
‡TE: tocopherol equivalent

Appendix C: Substance use and fetal and neonatal abnormalities

All drugs used by the gravida are potentially teratogenic and drugs crossing the placental barrier may affect the fetus. A correlation does not necessarily exist between maternal reaction to a drug and fetal response to a drug. Any drug use (over-the-counter or prescribed) should be discussed with the doctor and decided by the risk-benefit ratio. The following list includes drugs taken by the gravida and their reported effects on the fetus.

Chemical substance use by the patient may adversely affect the fetus or neonate, either directly or indirectly. Fetal effects depend largely on gestational age, drug potency, and dosage. Maternal drug reaction and fetal response do not necessarily correlate. Neonates exposed to drugs in utero or through breast-feeding may exhibit physical, emotional, and intellectual changes immediately or as the child matures. Food and Drug Administration drug category ratings assist in determining the risk-benefit ratio.

This chart shows the fetal and neonatal effects of selected substances used by pregnant women.

Maternal drug or substance	Reported effects on fetus or neonate
Alcohol	Hypoglycemia; fetal alcohol syndrome; cardiac anomalies; craniofacial anomalies; prenatal and postnatal growth retardation; brain, spinal, and cardiac defects; mental retardation and other neurobehavioral abnormalities
Amphetamines	Thrombocytopenia, transposition of the great vessels, cleft palate
Anesthetics	
Conduction anesthesia	Acidosis, bradycardia, seizures, death, hypotension, myocardial depression
General anesthesia	Chromosomal anomalies, methemoglobinemia, respiratory depression
Local anesthesia (paracervical)	Acidosis, bradycardia, seizures, myocardial and neurologic depression
Antacids	Anomalies, electrolyte imbalances
aspirin	Hemorrhage, premature closing of ductus arteriosus, prolonged gestation
Barbiturates	Withdrawal symptoms, increased anomalies, diminished sucking, diminished serum bilirubin levels, neonatal bleeding
chlorothiazide	Thrombocytopenia, sodium and water depletion
cocaine	Cardiac, central nervous system (CNS), and genitourinary anomalies; dysmorphic features, skeletal defects; atresias; small-for-gestational-age status; neurobehavioral abnormalities
Corticosteroids	Accelerated fetal lung maturation, adrenal suppression, increased incidence of fetal anomalies and death
diazepam	Withdrawal symptoms, anomalies, hypothermia
insulin	Hypoglycemia, skeletal defects, death
lysergic acid diethylamide (LSD)	Chromosomal damage
magnesium sulfate	Hypermagnesemia, CNS depression, peripheral neuromuscular blockage

Maternal drug or substance	Reported effects on fetus or neonate
Marijuana	High-pitched cry, disturbed sleep-wake cycle with short periods of quiet sleep
Nicotine	Low birth weight, stillbirth
morphine, heroin, and methadone	Intrauterine growth restriction, withdrawal symptoms, respiratory depression, death
phenytoin	Patent ductus arteriosus, pulmonary atresia, cleft lip, cleft palate or gum, syndactyly, polydactyly, diaphragmatic hernia, microencephaly, anencephaly
Radioactive iodine	Abnormal thyroid function, hypothyroidism, thyroid destruction
reserpine	Anomalies, bradycardia, hypothermia, lethargy, respiratory difficulties from nasal congestion, increased secretions
Tobacco	Low birth weight, neonatal thyroid enlargement, strabismus, frequent respiratory or ear infections

Appendix D:
Aspects of psychological care — maternal

Pregnancy and parenthood require many maternal psychological as well as physiologic adjustments. The diagnoses, expected outcomes, and nursing interventions and rationales presented here will help to plan health care related to potential problems arising from maternal anxiety, stress, depression, grief, deprivation, undeveloped parenting skills, and self-concept disturbances. These nursing diagnoses and interventions complement the maternal health care plans in this book.

NURSING DIAGNOSIS

Anxiety related to pregnancy and its outcome

Expected outcome

The mother will state that she feels minimal anxiety.

Interventions

1. Determine maternal anxiety level; consider the following:
• mild symptoms (increased alertness, ability to recognize threatening feelings and to learn and comprehend)
• moderate symptoms (periodic inattention, decreased ability to communicate or learn, and need for direction)
• severe symptoms (severely impaired ability to perceive and communicate details and inability to learn)
• panic (distorted perception, inability to communicate or function in everyday living and to learn).

2. Assess behavioral changes associated with anxiety, including irritability and restlessness; rapid speech, repetitive statements and questions, and quivering voice; hand wringing and hand tremors; insomnia, tension, and apprehension; inability to maintain eye contact; inability to concentrate and retain information and a short attention span; inability to communicate and reduced intellectual functioning.

3. Assess physiologic changes associated with anxiety, including increased blood pressure and pulse and respiratory rates; palpitations; perspiration and cold, clammy hands; nausea and vomiting; headache and dizziness; tremors; dry mouth; and dilated pupils.

4. Provide calm, accepting environment for maternal expression of feelings and concerns.

5. Acknowledge the mother's anxiety. Assist her to identify her symptoms and describe how she is experiencing anxiety.

Rationales

1. Anxiety levels may range from mild to panic, with each level accompanied by behavioral and physiologic symptoms. Anxiety is a generalized feeling or tension related to a perceived threat.

2. Behavioral changes become apparent during anxiety states; they increase in severity as anxiety increases.

3. Anxiety stimulates the autonomic nervous system, causing physiologic responses.

4. An accepting, peaceful, nonthreatening environment encourages the mother to externalize her feelings and fears and to identify these emotions and their causes. Accepting the mother's feelings validates them, allowing her to discuss them without fear of ridicule or rejection.

5. Recognizing the behavioral and physiologic manifestations of anxiety defines and validates the anxiety level and, consequently, the steps to reduce it.

Appendices

6. Assist the mother to identify source of stressors during perinatal period.

7. Assist and support the mother to identify and use coping mechanisms that help decrease anxiety (talking, crying, walking, or keeping busy, for example).

8. Inform the mother of all procedures and expectations, presenting accurate information and answering her questions.

9. Allow the mother and significant other, if appropriate, to participate in all decisions.

10. Suggest and teach relaxation techniques if appropriate.

11. Additional individualized interventions: _____

6. Discussion of stressors helps to identify and resolve anxiety.

7. Coping mechanisms temporarily help protect or distance a person from a real or perceived threat.

8. Information reduces the mother's fear of the unknown.

9. Participation in all decisions helps them maintain control over their care and well-being.

10. These techniques may help to relieve anxiety.

11. Rationales: _____

NURSING DIAGNOSIS

Ineffective individual coping related to stress or potential complications of perinatal period and to life changes because of this crisis

Expected outcome

The mother will demonstrate positive coping skills.

Interventions

1. Assess maternal internal and external stressors and use of coping skills, including current stressors and concerns; ability to cope and use coping mechanisms; illness or physical limits to coping ability; ability to accept assistance with coping; and existing support systems.

2. Assist the mother to identify effective coping skills or new behaviors or techniques.

3. Suggest and initiate problem-solving development by:
• role playing
• improving sending and receiving skills by communication
• openly discussing alternative solutions
• developing alternative coping strategies.

4. Support the mother's helpful coping behaviors and existing or possible support systems.

5. Assist the mother to develop goals and define ways and methods to achieve them.

6. Additional individualized interventions: _____

Rationales

1. Effective coping requires the ability to identify and manage stressors by solving problems and adapting to change. Pregnancy is a situational crisis that creates the need for increased coping abilities and adaptation.

2. As the mother uses coping skills effectively, her feelings of autonomy and her ability to cope with stressors will increase.

3. These techniques increase the mother's problem-solving ability, needed to deal more effectively with crises.

4. This supports the mother's continued success in using effective coping behaviors and existing support systems. It may also encourage her to develop a broader support base if familiar supports are ineffective.

5. This encourages independence and positive results in dealing with pregnancy-related stress.

6. Rationales: _____

COLLABORATIVE PROBLEM

Risk for postpartum depression related to physiologic and psychological stresses of pregnancy

Expected outcome

The mother will exhibit no signs of postpartum depression.

Interventions

1. Assess factors predisposing the mother to postpartum mental illness, such as:
• family history of postpartum depression
• previous depression or psychiatric problem during pregnancy
• maternal doubt regarding competence to care for infant
• few or no support systems
• disinterest in infant
• fatigue and overwhelmed feeling
• marital problems, family crisis
• preoccupation with discomfort and physical problems
• low self-esteem.

2. Observe for responses indicating maternity blues, such as:
• mood swings
• tearful and weepy behavior
• "let down" and depressed feelings
• quiet, passive, discouraged feelings
• poor concentration and despondency
• minimal interest in infant
• failure to participate in care.

3. Allow the mother to express her feelings and questions. Maintain a supportive and nonjudgmental attitude.

4. Reassure the mother about her abilities to care for her infant and her coping abilities.

5. Inform the mother that feeling "let down" is normal after delivery. Protect her privacy so she can cry and vent her feelings.

6. Include the mother in all planning and activities related to her infant's care.

7. Suggest referral or follow-up visits if depressed feelings are unresolved.

8. Encourage the patient to identify her social support system.

9. Additional individualized interventions: _____

Rationales

1. Postpartum emotional changes may be transitory; responses can range from maternity blues (30% to 80% of all childbirths) to psychosis (1% to 2%). Role changes and increased responsibilities cause stress for the new mother adapting to physiologic changes that occur post partum.

2. This condition usually occurs and subsides within the 1st week after delivery (although the symptoms may be prolonged). However, in rare instances, maternity blues may develop into depressive psychosis.

3. This provides an atmosphere of trust in which the mother can vent and deal with feelings of inadequacy or other concerns.

4. The mother may be concerned about her ability to care for her infant and her coping abilities.

5. This allows the mother to feel that this response is normal and will pass.

6. This instills self-confidence in the mother as she begins parenting.

7. Counseling may prevent postpartum psychosis.

8. A strong social support network helps the mother with coping skills.

9. Rationales: _____

Appendices

Nursing diagnosis

Dysfunctional grieving related to infant death or malformation

Expected outcome

The mother will openly express her grief.

Interventions

1. Stay with the parents when the physician informs them of the infant's death or malformation. Ensure their privacy.

2. In case of infant's death, call clergy, if requested.

3. Answer questions or give information in simple terms.

4. Remain present and listen; minimize speaking to allow the parents to express their feelings, cry, or show anger, guilt, or other feelings. Use touch to show your support.

5. Prepare the infant for viewing by parents. Stay in the room if they request it.

6. If the infant has a physical malformation, allow the parents to see the infant as soon as possible after being informed.

7. Assess parental responses to loss (death or the "perfect child"), including:
• crying, rage, or silence
• anger at God or themselves
• hostility toward staff
• expression of denial or feelings of guilt
• somatic symptoms, such as shortness of breath, sighing, choking feeling, emptiness in stomach, tightness in throat, and insomnia
• disinterest in activities
• inability to communicate
• ability or inability to vent anger and guilt feelings.

8. Assess for pathologic responses to grieving, such as:
• total denial of the loss
• hostility or cheerfulness with friends and relatives
• psychosomatic disorders or symptoms of illness of the deceased
• deep depression
• loss of social interactions and relationships.

9. Inform the parents about the feelings they can expect throughout the normal grieving process. Emphasize their need to express these feelings. Include that time and understanding assist in resolution of grief.

Rationales

1. The care provider's presence provides support and shows concern and acceptance of parent's feelings. Quiet and privacy allow the parents to express their feelings without fear of judgment or embarrassment.

2. Religious rites and clerical presence support parents' grieving.

3. The parents' grief may preclude them from processing information until the initial shock of loss passes. More information may be given later, as appropriate.

4. Using therapeutic communication techniques demonstrates support, caring, and concern.

5. This offers the parents the opportunity for contact with infant by holding and touching or by taking mementos, such as the crib card or identification band. These actions help the parents eliminate denial and allow them to feel the reality of death.

6. Seeing the infant helps the parents overcome inaccurate images or denial of the infant's abnormality.

7. Grief, a normal process after loss, causes significant emotional pain as well as physical reactions. Initial shock and disbelief give way to denial, which buffers the impact of the loss and allows the parents time to seek ways to respond to the devastating event. Later, when reality cannot be denied, the parents will experience feelings of guilt, anger, and helplessness. Somatic symptoms are common. As the grieving process continues, depression occurs as a response to the loss as well as to the fear and anxiety. The grieving parents eventually reach a state of restitution, which results in gradual acceptance, recovery, and normalcy.

8. Some parents react to grief with pathologic distortions because of their unsuccessful movement through the grieving process.

9. This relieves parents of feeling additional stress about their behavior during the grieving process.

10. Offer information about support groups, booklets that may be helpful as appropriate, and psychiatric counseling with pathologic mourning.

• Offer grief packets, if available (usually consisting of information on support groups and the grieving process)

• Offer memory box, if available (usually including infant picture, crib card, identification bracelet, blanket, and other mementos to serve as a reminder of the infant)

11. Call the parents the day after infant's death and send a card. Send an additional card 2 weeks after the infant's death; call again at 3 and 6 weeks, then again at 6 months if possible.

12. Offer information about the autopsy conference in case the parents want to attend.

13. Suggest meeting with the doctor after discharge in 3 to 4 months.

14. Additional individualized interventions: _____
_____

10. Support groups, self-help materials, and counseling provide additional support, if needed, especially for parents of infants who have congenital anomalies and who may need continual support over a long period.
• Grief packets serve as written guidelines for parents so they know what to expect of themselves.

• Memory boxes help the parents cope with the loss by having tangible reminders of their infant.

11. Consolation and caring are shown to parents. Continued contact with parents helps them to know they have help available if they need it.

12. This helps them understand the infant's illness and cause of death.

13. The doctor can assess the parents' grieving process and special needs.

14. Rationales: _____
_____

NURSING DIAGNOSIS

Altered health maintenance related to lack of material resources and support system

Expected outcome

The mother will keep prenatal appointments.

Interventions

1. Assess factors associated with lack of prenatal care:
• low socioeconomic status
• health beliefs and practices
• personal strengths and reliability
• scarcity of clinics and low-cost or free prenatal care
• use of drugs or alcohol
• lack of supportive family or paternal relationships.

2. Assist the mother to define and clarify prenatal needs.

3. Inform the mother about resources available for prenatal care.

4. Support the decision to contact an agency for care.

5. Monitor ongoing management of prenatal care by mother.

6. Additional individualized interventions: _____
_____

Rationales

1. Ideally, all potential mothers should receive prenatal care starting at 6 to 8 weeks of pregnancy and continuing to the expected date of confinement. Physical examination, measurements, weight gains, nutritional and activity instruction, vital signs, and laboratory tests are monitored to prevent perinatal complications and injury to the fetus or infant. Most preterm births and infants born with complications occur in mothers who have not had prenatal care.

2. Some pregnant women are unaware of the need for prenatal care, especially if they are young or in their teenage years.

3. This information is not always readily available or the mother is not always informed about health care agencies.

4. Supporting the mother's effort to seek adequate, affordable care helps to establish and maintain maternal-infant health.

5. Periodic contact shows interest and support in mother's ability to maintain health.

6. Rationales: _____
_____

Nursing diagnosis

Risk for altered parenting related to knowledge deficit in infant care and inadequate role identity

Expected outcome

The parents will demonstrate appropriate infant care techniques.

Interventions

1. Assess parent teaching needs in infant care; including:
- parity and infant care experience
- stated knowledge deficit
- parental expectations related to self and infant
- perceptions of parenting and behaviors
- role priorities as stated
- learning readiness
- education and communication level.

2. Provide demonstrations and return demonstrations in infant care as follows:
- bathing the infant, sponge and tub baths
- dressing the infant
- caring for cord and circumcision areas
- holding the infant
- feeding the infant
- preparing the infant's feedings
- ensuring infant safety.

3. Provide information about parenting groups.

4. Provide referrals or follow-ups as needed for Visiting Nurse Association, physician, and clinic visits.

5. Provide a positive learning environment, encourage the parents to ask questions, and clarify information for them.

6. Additional individualized interventions: _____

Rationales

1. The teaching plan is based on data collected from parents about their perceptions, experiences, interests, and education levels.

2. Knowledge base is necessary for effective parenting and role identity. Return demonstrations give the parents hands-on experience and increase parental comfort level in providing infant care (see appendix J, Parent teaching guides).

3. These groups help new parents explore their expectations, behaviors, and roles.

4. Medical and nursing attention supports well-baby care after discharge.

5. These approaches and actions facilitate and reinforce parental learning.

6. Rationales: _____

Nursing diagnosis

Body image disturbance related to temporary, pregnancy-induced changes in appearance

Expected outcome

The mother will verbalize a positive self-concept and body image.

Interventions

1. Assess maternal feelings concerning change in appearance, including:
- expression of how mother sees herself
- verbalization of adaptability to changes
- unkempt appearance and inability to maintain self-care
- withdrawal or hostility.

Rationales

1. Society places great importance on appearances. Changes in body shape and size, although gradual, need to be accepted by mother as normal during pregnancy.

2. Assist mother to develop goals and actions to pre-serve self-esteem and self-image; include:
- clothing selection
- becoming and easy-to-care-for hair style
- appropriate weight gain
- attractive accessories
- moderate cosmetic use.

3. Accept mother as an individual with individual needs during her pregnancy.

4. Stress positive features of pregnancy, downplay nega-tive ones.

5. Additional individualized interventions: _____
_____

2. Attractive appearance during pregnancy helps pre-serve a positive self-image and prevents possible nega-tive reactions from others.

3. This attitude promotes a trusting relationship.

4. This helps promote a positive maternal attitude.

5. Rationales: _____
_____

Appendix E:
Preparing for nonemergency surgery

When a pregnant woman has nonemergency, acute but nonemergency, or scheduled surgery—for instance, for ectopic pregnancy, spontaneous abortion, or cesarean section—nursing care proceeds according to general preoperative guidelines, which are reviewed below.

• Obtain a full maternal health history, including data on gynecologic and obstetric histories, gestational age, expected date of confinement, outstanding medical problems, and drug allergies. Perform a physical assessment. Obtain fetal heart sounds, if applicable.

• Review the results of complete blood count, blood typing and screen. Report abnormalities to the primary doctor. Make sure ordered blood is available.

• Determine the extent of the mother's knowledge of the surgical procedure and of anesthesia. Witness an informed consent before administering preoperative medication.

• Withhold food and fluids.

• Inform the mother of what she can expect postoperatively. Discuss:
   – length of time in recovery room
   – availability of pain medication
   – pulmonary hygiene measures, for example, turning, coughing, deep-breathing, spirometry. Demonstrate these exercises for the patient and have her return the demonstration, if her condition permits.
   – circulatory hygiene measures, for example, leg exercise and progressive ambulation
   – I.V. apparatus, abdominal dressing, perineal pad, and indwelling catheter.

• Establish where family members can be contacted and inform them of the patient's progress.

• Contact clergy, if the patient requests.

• Prepare the operative site. Assist with morning care, toilet. Catheterize, and start an I.V. infusion as indicated. Remove the patient's nail polish, jewelry, or prosthetic devices. If the patient wants to wear her wedding band during surgery, tape or tie it to her hand. Attach (and note placement of) religious articles to the patient's hospital gown if she desires. Apply thromboembolic stockings, as indicated.

• Record vital signs, reporting unexpected findings to primary doctor and to the operating room staff.

• Administer preoperative medications, as ordered. Thereafter, the patient should remain in bed. Ensure that both side rails are raised and that the call device is within the patient's reach.

• Document all activities and findings.

Appendix F: Selected methods of family planning

The following chart highlights selected family planning methods that commonly are available and chosen by patients seen in the maternal health care setting.

Method and examples	How the method works	Advantages	Disadvantages
Natural family planning methods: cervical mucus rhythm, basal body temperature rhythm, calendar rhythm, symptothermal, fertility awareness	Couple abstains from sexual intercourse during fertile period	• Require no devices, prescriptions, or use of medication • Morally acceptable to people whose religious beliefs forbid use of mechanical or chemical contraception	• Require high degree of motivation and training • Limit sexual spontaneity • May require protracted periods of sexual abstinence • Require observation and record-keeping associated with menstrual cycle • Rhythm method has highest incidence of failure (pregnancy)
Withdrawal before ejaculation (coitus interruptus)	Prevents deposition of semen in vagina	• Requires no devices, preparations, prescriptions, or use of medication	• Effectiveness depends on correct and consistent use, which is influenced by age, education, degree of motivation, and training and experience in contraceptive use • Requires absolute cooperation of and control by partners; is associated with high level of sexual frustration for both partners • Seminal fluid remaining on vulva may cause fertilization
Barrier methods: male and female condoms; diaphragm; cervical cap; spermicides—spermicidal foams, gels, creams, and suppositories	Mechanical barriers (condom, cap, and diaphragm) prevent sperm penetration; spermicides immobilize or chemically destroy sperm	• Except for diaphragm and cap, barrier methods require no prescriptions or ingestion of systemic medications • May protect against sexually transmitted (ST) infections; male latex condoms are highly effective against transmission of human immunodeficiency virus	• Condom application requires interruption of foreplay; new condom must be applied for each intercourse; some partners report diminished sensations; condoms have limited storage life; some condoms are made of latex and can cause an allergic reaction if either partner is latex sensitive; female condoms have high failure rate • Diaphragms may develop tears or holes; require fitting initially and again after childbirth or abortion; should be used with spermicidal agent; should remain in place at least 8 hours after intercourse; to apply diaphragm, user must be comfortable handling genital area • Cervical cap must be fitted; may remain in place up to 48 hours; should be used with spermicide • Spermicidal agents are messy and may cause local irritation in either partner; multiple coitus necessitates repeated application of spermicidal agent; incorrect or inconsistent use is associated with high failure rate

Method and examples	How the method works	Advantages	Disadvantages
Hormonal contraceptives: estrogen and progestin combination (the pill) or progestinal agent alone (the minipill); subdermal implants of levonorgestrel, Depo-Provera injections	Inhibit ovulation, impair sperm transport, render endometrium inhospitable to implantation of fertilized ovum	• Most effective reversible method of birth control • Separate use from sexual activity • Regulate irregular menstrual cycles • Are associated with reduced incidence of menstrual blood loss, anemia, dysmenorrhea, premenstrual symptoms, functional ovarian cysts, endometrial and ovarian cancers, salpingitis, pelvic inflammatory disease (PID), various benign breast diseases, toxic shock syndrome, and rheumatoid arthritis • Depo-Provera lasts for 3 months	• May be morally unacceptable to people who believe life begins at conception • Necessitate comprehensive physical assessment and annual cervical cytologic examination • Cause metabolic changes that may lead to cardiovascular diseases, especially deep-vein thrombosis and pulmonary embolism • May lead to range of adverse metabolic effects many of which are estrogen-dose related • Not recommended for women over age 40 with systemic or chronic disease • Absolute contraindications for oral contraceptives include known or suspected pregnancy, undiagnosed genital bleeding, thromboembolic disorders, hyperlipidemia, uncontrolled hypertension, diabetes mellitus with vascular changes, coronary artery disease, cerebrovascular accident, estrogen-dependent breast or endometrial carcinoma, and liver dysfunction or tumors • Relative contraindications for oral contraceptives include heavy cigarette smoking and history of migraine or vascular headaches, varicose veins, cardiac or renal disease or dysfunction, gestational diabetes or prediabetes, depression, sickle cell disease, and cholestatic disease during pregnancy • Require ingesting medication 21 or 28 days per month; missed doses may necessitate use of backup barrier contraceptive • May lead to multiple drug interactions • Associated with nutritional deficiencies, cervical mucorrhea, vaginitis, and weight gain • Progestinal agents cause fewer adverse effects but are associated with increased failure rate, ectopic pregnancy, and irregular bleeding • Subdermal implants require subcutaneous insertion of six polysiloxane capsules into upper arm; replacement after maximum 5-year cycle may be difficult because of local fibrosis • Injections are not accepted by everyone and are required every 3 months, possibly leading to noncompliance

Method and examples	How the method works	Advantages	Disadvantages
Intrauterine devices (IUDs): chemically inert devices, copper or progesterone-impregnated devices	Cause intrauterine inflammatory response that is toxic to sperm and fertilized ovum	• Second only to oral contraceptives as most effective reversible birth control method; effectiveness measured in years; copper IUD is effective for 6 to 8 years • Separate use from sexual activity • Affect genital tract only • Require no motivation or learning • Inexpensive	• May be expelled; extrauterine expulsion may result in penetration or perforation of adjacent structures • Pregnancy may occur with device in utero • Contraindicated in known or suspected pregnancy, uterine bleeding, PID, and cervical or uterine cancer • Relative contraindications include nulliparous status, high risk for ST infection, history of ectopic pregnancy or fallopian tube reconstructive surgery, endometriosis, uterine leiomyoma, impaired coagulation, valvular heart disease, and Wilson's disease • May cause cramping, ulceration, pain, and increased bleeding during or between menstrual periods; contribute to pelvic infection; increase risk of spontaneous abortion and ectopic pregnancy • Uterine perforation or interruption of pregnancy may occur during insertion • Progesterone-releasing IUD must be changed yearly
Sterilization; tubal ligation	Terminates fertility by means of surgical transection of oviduct by occlusion, ligation, partial excision, or fulguration	• One-time procedure that may be performed on outpatient basis • Essentially 100% effective and should be considered permanent; virtual infallibility may provide psychological comfort and security	• Possible coagulation burns of adjacent structures during surgery • Mortality (although low) associated with use of general anesthesia • Unacceptable to certain religious, political, and professional groups • Surgical reversal expensive and success rate of 50% to 80%

Appendix G: Fluid and nutritional needs in infancy

Infant fluid-electrolyte and nutritional-caloric needs depend on the infant's weight and gestational age because these determine GI capacity and metabolic rates and capabilities.

Fluid and electrolyte requirements

Fluid and electrolyte requirements vary with each infant. Factors that usually increase the infant's fluid-electrolyte requirements include insensible water loss, phototherapy, radiant warming, abnormal losses preoperatively and postoperatively, vomiting and diarrhea, and labile body or ambient temperatures. In general, the healthy full-term infant (40 weeks' gestation) needs about 100 ml/kg/day of fluid. Sodium, potassium, and chloride needs for the full-term infant are sodium, 2 mEq/kg/day; potassium, 2 mEq/kg/day; and chloride, 2 to 4 mEq/kg/day. Smaller and less mature, the preterm infant has a greater proportion of body weight as water and needs up to 200 ml/kg/day of fluid. Sodium needs range from 3 to 4 mEq/kg/day; potassium and chloride needs vary.

Nutritional and caloric needs

The goal is to supply metabolic needs for growth and for replacement of losses through urine, feces, sweat, and tissue breakdown. The full-term infant needs 100 to 120 kcal/kg/day. Both full- and preterm infants need proteins, carbohydrates, and fats as follows:
• protein: 2.5 to 4 g/kg/day (10% to 15% of caloric intake)
• carbohydrates: 10 to 15 g/kg/day (45% to 55% of caloric intake)
• fats: 5 to 7 g/kg/day (40% to 50% of caloric intake).
Note: To gain 1 g of weight, the infant must store 2 to 3 calories from nutrients composed of about 60% to 80% water, 30% protein, and the rest fat. A low-birth-weight infant must store 20 to 40 calories daily to maintain growth. (See Nutritional and caloric content of milk and formulas and Proposed schedule for feeding a low-birth-weight infant, for more information).

Nutritional and caloric content of milk and formulas

Milk product	kcal/dl	Protein (g/dl)	Carbohydrate (g/dl)	Fat (g/dl)
Breast milk	67	1.2	7	3.8
Cow's milk	67	3.3	4.8	3.7
Enfamil	67	1.5	7	3.7
Gerber with Iron	67	1.5	7.2	3.7
Good Start	67	(100% whey protein)	7.4	3.5
Pregestimil	67	2.2	8.8	2.8
Premature	67 to 100	2.8	9	3.7
Similac with Iron	67	1.5	7.2	3.6

Proposed schedule for feeding a low-birth-weight infant

The following chart shows a recommended schedule for feeding a low-birth-weight infant. If the mother is breast-feeding, the infant does not need to receive a glucose feeding first but may be put straight to the breast.

Infant weight	First feeding	Formula feeding
2 lb, 7 oz to 3 lb, 2 oz (1,250 to 1,500 g)	5% to 10% glucose (3 ml); follow with 5 ml in 2 to 3 hours	5 ml every 2 to 3 hours; increase 1 ml every other feeding up to 10 to 15 ml
3 lb, 2 oz to 4 lb, 3 oz (1,500 to 2,000 g)	5% to 10% glucose (5 ml); follow with 8 ml in 2 to 3 hours	8 ml every 2 to 3 hours; increase 1 ml every other feeding up to 10 to 15 ml
2,000 g or more	5% glucose (15 ml); repeat if tolerated	15 ml every 3 hours; increase 5 ml every other feeding up to 30 ml

Appendix H:
Assessing vital signs in the infant

This guide to assessing the newborn infant's vital signs presents normal ranges for body temperature, heart and respiratory rates, and blood pressure. In a preterm infant, weight and gestational age affect vital signs; therefore, normal ranges vary from one preterm infant to the next.

Measurement	Normal values	Nursing implications
Temperature Fetus: 99.7° to 100° F (37.6° to 37.7° C)	Full-term infant: • 97.7° to 98.6° F (36.5° to 37° C) axillary Preterm infant: • Temperature varies with weight and gestational age	• Measure temperature when infant is admitted to the nursery. • Continue to monitor temperature frequently, and notify the nurse practitioner or doctor if the temperature drops below 97.5° F (36.4° C). • Institute measures to conserve body heat, such as keeping the infant's head covered and keeping the infant dry.
Heart rate	• Fetus: 110 to 160 beats per minute • Full-term infant: 120 to 160 beats per minute (apical) • Preterm infant: 130 to 170 beats per minute (apical)	• Take the infant's heart rate at the apical site and count for 1 full minute using an appropriate stethoscope. • Monitor for bradycardia (less than 120 beats per minute) or tachycardia (more than 160 beats per minute). • Keep in mind that infant crying or activity will increase the heart rate and that sleep may decrease the heart rate to less than 100 beats per minute in some full-term infants.
Respiratory rate	• Full-term infant: 40 to 60 breaths per minute • Preterm infant: respiratory rate varies with gestational age and infant's condition	• Count the breaths for 1 full minute by observing the rise and fall of the abdomen; auscultate with a stethoscope. • Monitor for tachypnea (more than 60 breaths per minute). • Keep in mind that crying or activity will increase the infant's respiratory rate.
Blood pressure	• Full-term: 60 to 80 mm Hg systolic; 40 to 50 mm Hg diastolic • Preterm infant: blood pressure range varies depending on gestational age	• Use a blood pressure cuff that is appropriately sized because the wrong sized cuff can affect the reading. • Consider using the following devices to measure an infant's blood pressure: – *Doppler instrument* (to reflect changes in ultrasound frequency caused by blood movement translated to audible sound by a transducer in the cuff) – *Transducer device* (connected to the umbilical artery catheter to directly measure blood pressure in newborn infants) – *Dinamap blood pressure device* (to electronically measure blood pressure). • Keep in mind that crying, activity, and sleep may cause blood pressure fluctuations.

Appendix I:
Normal laboratory values for the newborn

This chart shows laboratory tests that may be ordered for the newborn, with normal ranges when available. Note that ranges may vary among institutions. Because test results for the preterm infant usually reflect weight and gestational age, preterm infant ranges vary with the infant.

Test	Normal range: Full-term infant	Normal range: Preterm infant
Blood		
Acid phosphatase	7.4 to 19.4 units/L	—
Albumin	3.6 to 5.4 g/dl	3.1 to 4.2 g/dl
Alkaline phosphatase	40 to 300 units/L (1 week)	134 to 308 units/L
Alpha-fetoprotein	up to 10 mg/L, with none detected after 21 days	
Ammonia	90 to 150 mcg/dl	—
Amylase	0 to 1,000 IU/hour	—
Bicarbonate	20 to 26 mmol/L	18 to 26 mmol/L
Bilirubin, direct	less than 0.5 mg/dl	less than 0.5 mg/dl
Bilirubin, total	less than 2.8 mg/dl (cord blood)	less than 2.8 mg/dl (cord blood)
0 to 1 day	2.6 mg/dl (peripheral blood)	1 to 6 mg/dl (peripheral blood)
1 to 2 days	6 to 7 mg/dl (peripheral blood)	6 to 8 mg/dl (peripheral blood)
3 to 5 days	4 to 6 mg/dl (peripheral blood)	10 to 12 mg/dl (peripheral blood)
Bleeding time	2 minutes	—
Arterial blood gases		
ph	7.35 to 7.45	—
$Paco_2$	35 to 45 mm Hg	—
Pao_2	50 to 90 mm Hg	—
Venous blood gases		
pH	7.35 to 7.45	—
Pco_2	41 to 51 mm Hg	—
Po_2	20 to 49 mm Hg	—
Calcium, ionized	2.5 to 5 mg/dl	2.5 to 5 mg/dl
Calcium, total	7 to 12 mg/dl	6 to 10 mg/dl
Chloride	95 to 110 mEq/L	100 to 117 mEq/L
Clotting time (2 tube)	5 to 8 minutes	—

Test	Normal range: Full-term infant	Normal range: Preterm infant
Blood (continued)		
Creatine kinase	10 to 300 IU/L	—
Creatinine	0.3 to 1 mg/dl	1.3 mg/dl
Digoxin level	greater than 2 ng/ml possible; greater than 30 ng/ml probable	—
Fibrinogen	0.18 to 0.38 g/dl	—
Glucose	30 to 125 mg/dl	20 to 125 mg/dl
Glutamyltransferase	14 to 331 units/L	52 to 233 units/L
Hematocrit	52% to 58%	45% to 55%
	53% (cord blood)	—
Hemoglobin	17 to 18.4 g/dl	15 to 17 g/dl
	16.8 g/dl (cord blood)	—
Immunoglobulins, total	660 to 1,439 mg/dl	—
IgG	398 to 1,244 mg/dl	—
IgM	5 to 30 mg/dl	—
IgA	0 to 2.2 mg/dl	—
Iron	100 to 250 mcg/dl	—
Iron-binding capacity	100 to 400 mcg/dl	—
Lactate dehydrogenase	357 to 953 IU/L	—
Magnesium	1.5 to 2.5 mEq/L	—
Osmolality	270 to 294 mOsm/kg H_2O	—
Partial thromboplastin time	40 to 80 seconds	—
Phenobarbital level	15 to 40 mcg/dl	—
Phosphorus	5 to 7.8 mg/dl (birth)	5.6 to 8 mg/dl (birth)
	4.9 to 8.9 mg/dl (7 days)	6.1 to 11.7 mg/dl (7 days)
Platelets	100,000 to 300,000/mm³	120,000 to 180,000/mm³
Potassium	4.5 to 6.8 mEq/L	3.9 to 6 mEq/L
Protein, total	4.6 to 7.4 g/dl	4.3 to 7.6 g/dl
Prothrombin time	12 to 21 seconds	—
Red blood cell count	5.1 to 5.8 (1,000,000/mm³)	4.4 (1,000,000/mm³)
Reticulocytes	3% to 7% (cord blood)	up to 10%
Sodium	136 to 143 mEq/L	—

Test	Normal range: Full-term infant	Normal range: Preterm infant
Blood (continued)		
Theophylline level	5 to 10 µg/ml	—
Thyroid-stimulating hormone	less than 7 microunits/ml	—
Thyroxine (T$_4$)	10.2 to 19 mcg/dl	7.5 to 15.5 mcg/dl
Transaminase		
glutamic-oxaloacetic (aspartate)	24 to 81 units/L	—
glutamic-pyruvic (alanine)	10 to 33 units/L	—
Triglycerides	36 to 233 mg/dl	—
Urea nitrogen (BUN)	5 to 25 mg/dl	3.1 to 25.5 mg/dl
White blood cell (WBC) count	18,000/mm^3	10,000 to 20,000/mm^3
eosinophils-basophils	3%	—
immature WBCs	10%	16%
lymphocytes	30%	33%
monocytes	5%	4%
neutrophils	45%	47%
Urine		
Casts, WBC	present first 2 to 4 days	—
Osmolality	50 to 600 mOsm/kg	—
pH	5 to 7	—
Phenylketonuria (PKU)	no color change	—
Protein	present first 2 to 4 days	—
Specific gravity	1.006 to 1.008	—
Cerebrospinal fluid		
Calcium	4.2 to 5.4 mg/dl	—
Cell count	0 to 15 WBCs/mm^3; 0 to 500 RBCs/mm^3	—
Chloride	110 to 120 mg/L	—
Glucose	32 to 62 mg/dl	—
pH	7.33 to 7.42	—
Pressure	50 to 80 mm Hg	—
Protein	32 to 148 mg/dl	—
Sodium	130 to 165 mg/L	—
Specific gravity	1.007 to 1.009	—

Appendix J: Parent teaching guides

How to bathe your infant

Now that you've brought your infant home, you'll want to keep him clean by giving him sponge or tub baths. How often you bathe him is up to you. If the weather is warm, you may want to bathe him daily and sponge him off every few hours. In cold weather, however, you may reduce the number of baths to one every 2nd or 3rd day. Why? Because the heating system in your home probably keeps the humidity low; by reducing the number of baths, you protect the infant from itchy, dry skin.

No matter which type of bath you give your infant, never leave him unattended in the water, even for a few seconds. If you turn away to reach for soap or powder, always hold your infant firmly with one hand. If the telephone or doorbell rings, wrap him in a towel and take him with you.

Before bathing your infant, review these helpful guidelines:
• Give him a sponge bath the first 3 or 4 weeks after his birth, until his belly button heals. If he has been circumcised, wait until the circumcision heals,

too. Then you can begin tub bathing.
• Set a regular time for his bath, for instance, after his morning feeding and bowel movement.
• Establish a regular place to bathe him. Select a spot that's warm, away from drafts, and at a comfortable height for you.
• Keep bath supplies together in a tray or basket so you won't have to search for them.
• Place the bath supplies within easy reach.
• Test the water temperature by placing a few drops on the crook of your arm; the water should be comfortably warm but not hot.
• Give your infant time to get used to tub baths. If he doesn't like being placed in water, soap him on a towel outside the tub, and put him in the tub only to rinse him. (This home care aid shows you how.) Chances are, he'll soon begin to enjoy the water.
• Use your hands or a soft cloth and mild, unscented soap to bathe your infant. Start with his face, using warm

water only. Using soap, bathe his head from front to back; scrub it well, using your fingertips. Soap and rinse his head at least three times a week, and just rinse it the other days.
• Wash only the outer areas of your infant's ears. When you do, use a soft cloth or cotton ball rather than a cotton-tipped stick. Never insert anything in his ears.
• Wipe eyes from inner to outer direction using a cotton ball and warm water.
• Clean genitals with cotton balls or wash cloth and warm water. For girls, wipe the area from front to back.
• Take special care when holding your infant. Remember, he'll be slippery when he's wet and soapy.
• After completing the bath, don't rub a lot of baby oil on his skin; it may clog his pores. You can prevent chafing by using lotion, cream, or baby powder. If you use powder, apply it lightly.
• Dress the infant in a loose shirt, diaper, and other clothing as weather dictates. A cotton receiving blanket may also be used.

Giving a sponge bath

1. Before you begin, make sure room and bathwater are comfortably warm. Gather unscented soap and two towels (or towel and soft cloth). Place towel or bath blanket on clean, level, sturdy surface. Place infant on the towel. NEVER leave infant unattended. Always keep one hand on the infant. Then, as you support your infant under his shoulders, undress him except for his diaper.

2. Next, take the other towel (or the cloth) and lay it across his legs and stomach to keep him warm. Wet the top end of the towel and gently wipe his face.

3. Then, soap his neck, chest, arms, and hands. Make sure you wash between all his skin folds. Now, dampen the top end of the towel again and rinse his neck, chest, arms, and hands. Make sure you remove any soap trapped in his skin folds, too. Then take a dry area of the towel and lightly pat him dry. Be gentle—remember, his skin is delicate.

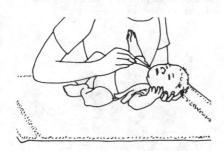
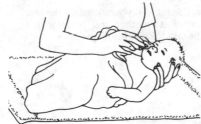
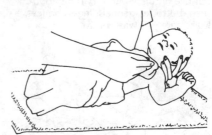

Appendices

4. To bathe your infant's back, gently but firmly support his head with your hand and turn him on his side. Make sure you pat him dry after washing and rinsing him.

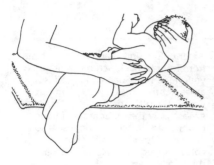

5. Then, remove the diaper. Soap and rinse his abdomen, buttocks, genitals, legs, and feet. Dab gently around his belly button; be especially careful if it hasn't healed yet. Again, pat him dry.

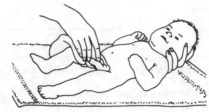

6. After you finish bathing your infant, you may want to apply powder or cornstarch around his genitals and buttocks before putting on a clean diaper. Never shake powder directly on the infant. Put it first on your hands, and then apply it from your hands to the infant. Then dress him immediately, so he doesn't become chilled.

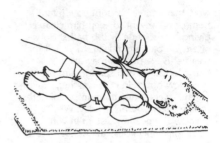

Giving a tub bath and shampoo

To give your infant a tub bath and shampoo, you'll need a tub or basin of warm water, soap, shampoo, a large towel, and a soft cloth.

Remember: You can shampoo the infant's head anytime, but don't place him in a tub of water until his belly button and circumcision have healed.

1. First, lay the towel on a secure surface and place your infant on it. Next, wash and rinse his face with the moistened cloth, and then shampoo his hair.

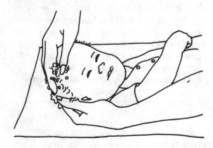

2. To rinse your infant's hair, hold him in a football carry over the tub. Securely support his head with your hand. Wet the cloth and gently wipe the shampoo from his hair. Then, immediately dry his face and hair with an end of the towel.

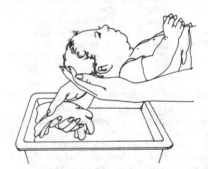

3. Take off your infant's shirt and soap his neck, chest, arms, hands and back, as you would for a sponge bath. Then remove his diaper and soap his abdomen, buttocks, genitals, legs, and feet. Make sure you wash between his toes.

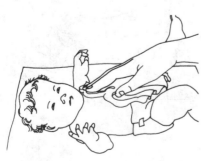

4. Carefully lift your infant by holding his ankles together, and gently soap all the skin folds in his diaper area.

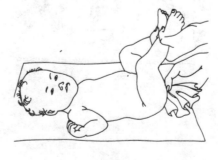

5. Then, with one hand supporting your infant's head and your other hand holding his feet and ankles, place him in the tub to rinse him. Keep him in a sitting position, as shown here.

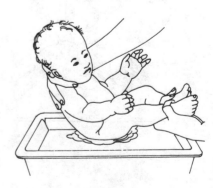

Giving a tub bath and shampoo *(continued)*

6. As you continue to support his head, take the wet cloth and thoroughly rinse his body.

7. When you finish rinsing him, *carefully* lift him out of the tub and immediately wrap him in the towel to keep him warm. Next, pat him dry. Apply powder or cornstarch around his genitals and on his buttocks, if you want. Then, put a clean diaper on him and dress him quickly.

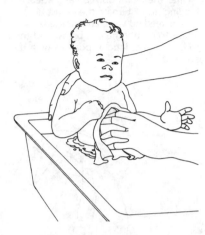

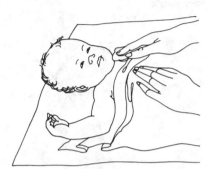

Breast-feeding the infant

As you begin breast-feeding, remember that many substances are eliminated from your body through breast milk. Some common ones include alcohol, barbiturates, bromides, cathartics or laxatives, diuretics, narcotics, oral contraceptives, anticonvulsants, radioactive isotopes (used for tests), steroids, sulfonamides, and tetracycline. Consult your doctor about the effects of any pre-scribed medication or over-the-counter drug.

1. First, thoroughly wash and dry your hands before each feeding. Remember, stress interferes with the let-down reflex, so do your best to relax. Select a position for breast-feeding — either sitting or side-lying. If you choose a side-lying position, make sure your back is comfort-ably supported and the arm closer to the bed is raised. Hold the infant between your arm and side, as shown, so the infant's head is level with your breast. Support the infant with your arm.

2. Hold the infant on your lap at breast level, as shown, so the infant doesn't stretch the breast while feeding. (You can place the infant on a pillow for sup-port and height, if necessary.) If you decide to sit up, select a comfortable chair and support your feet with a stool.

3. If you had a cesarean section — or if you gave birth to twins and want to nurse them simultaneously — use the football carry (see page 364). Place the infant alongside you on a pillow, as shown here.

　Give the infant time to become accus-tomed to the position and to look for the breast. Remember, don't rush. Tension will inhibit both you and your infant.

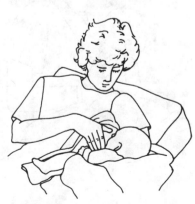

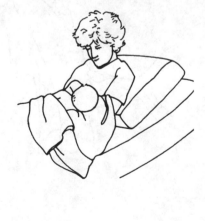

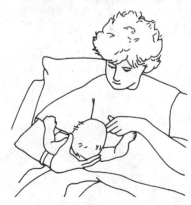

Appendices

4. Now, stimulate the infant's rooting reflex. Place your thumb on the upper breast and, with fingers, form the letter "C"; lift breast towards infant's mouth Keep fingers and thumb back from areola. Some mothers find that they do not need to keep their fingers in place for the entire feeding but only until the infant latches on. Brush the nipple against the infant's cheek. In response, the infant will turn toward your breast. (Don't touch the infant's cheek or head with your supporting arm, because the infant may turn toward the arm and away from the breast.)

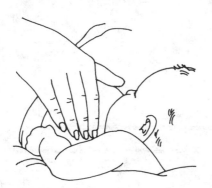

5. Make sure your infant has the entire nipple and most of the areola in his mouth. Otherwise, he won't be able to adequately compress the milk ducts and will have difficulty expressing milk.

When the infant is feeding properly, you'll see his jaws moving up and down rhythmically and he will swallow regularly. If he is having difficulty, make sure the nipple is on top of his tongue—not beneath it.

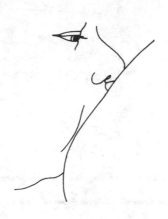

6. Normally, the infant's nose will not sink into the breast, obstructing his breathing. If it does, gently depress the breast with your fingers, as shown here.

Offer the infant both breasts at each feeding and alternate the breast he begins feeding with. Encourage the infant to empty the first breast and then to continue as long as possible with the second.

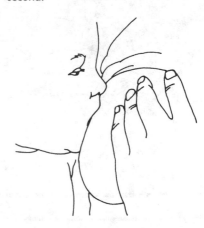

7. To avoid nipple soreness, limit feeding to 7 minutes for each breast initially; then gradually increase the time.

To remove the infant from the first breast, break the suction by gently inserting a fingertip into the infant's mouth, as shown.

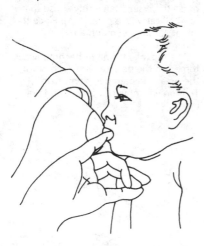

8. You can also break suction by gently pressing down on your breast until the infant's grip is broken or by gently pulling down the infant's chin, as shown here. *Important:* Use one of these techniques when removing the infant from the breast. Otherwise, the nipple may be injured.

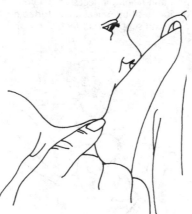

9. Before encouraging the infant to take the other breast, you'll want to burp (bubble) him. Sit the infant upright, and support his head or chin. Place a diaper, blanket, or towel nearby, because the infant may burp up fluid as well as gas. Then, gently pat or stroke the infant's back. Pounding and other forceful motions aren't necessary and may hurt the infant.

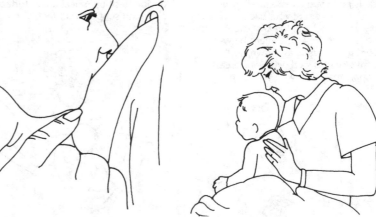

10. Alternately, you may hold the infant upright against your shoulder and rub the infant's back. (Make sure to protect your shoulder with a diaper, blanket or towel). Or, position the infant prone over your knees, as shown here, and gently rub his back.
Note: A breast-fed infant probably won't swallow as much air as a bottle-fed infant. As a result, he probably won't burp as much.

11. Now position the infant at your other breast. When the infant is satisfied, burp him again. (Keep in mind that several feeding patterns exist. You'll want to accommodate the infant's preferences.)
Hint: Put a safety pin on your bra strap to remind you which breast to start with at the next feeding.

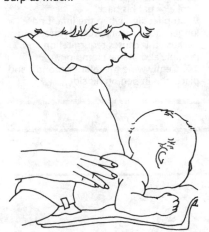

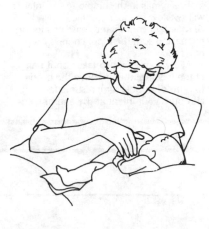

Some do's and don'ts for breast-feeding

As young as he is, a newborn infant has a personality of his own. As a result, breast-feeding may not go smoothly at first. You may become anxious and frustrated—and stress, as you know, can inhibit milk flow and compound the problem.

Remember, breast-feeding is a new experience for you and your infant. You'll need several weeks to become acquainted with your infant's unique problems and preferences. Here are some helpful tips:
• Don't try to nurse the infant when he's drowsy. Instead, spend a few minutes playing with him until he seems alert.
• Arouse the infant's interest in nursing by manually expressing a few drops of milk before encouraging him to take the nipple. Tasting the milk tends to stimulate his sucking reflex.
• If the infant has difficulty grasping the nipple, try rolling your nipple between your fingers first. Or, try applying a breast shield. It'll help draw out the nipple, which may be flattened because of breast engorgement. Don't use this device routinely, because it prevents the infant from completely compressing the milk ducts and emptying the breast.
• If your infant needs supplemental feedings or fluid, breast-feed him before you give him the supplement. This way, he won't lose interest in breast-feeding.

If your breasts are sore, use the breathing and relaxation techniques you learned for delivery. This may reduce pain while you breast-feed.
• If milk flows quickly from your breast, the infant may have difficulty swallowing fast enough. To help prevent him from choking, sit him in a more upright position. Or, if he wishes, let him stop and rest periodically while nursing.
• Once the infant begins to nurse, don't touch his head. You may distract him from nursing.
• If, despite all your efforts, the infant won't feed, don't panic. He will let you know when he's hungry by crying. Plan to feed him as soon as he tells you he's hungry. If you let the infant set his own schedule, you'll have fewer problems feeding him.

Bottle-feeding the infant

1. Thoroughly wash your hands before feeding the infant.
2. Seat yourself comfortably in a chair with arms.
3. Hold the infant in the crook of your arm. Hold the bottle in the hand of your other arm. Hold the infant with his head slightly elevated to decrease the chance of aspiration or choking. The formula should be at room temperature. *Note:* Don't microwave the formula; this can destroy some of the nutrients.
4. Always hold the infant for feedings.

Do not prop the bottle with your infant in a supine position.
5. Insert the nipple in the infant's mouth; hold the bottle at an angle and maintain milk in the nipple so the infant will swallow formula, not air.
6. Maintain your infant's ease of sucking by making sure the nipple hole is properly sized.
7. Allow your infant to take about half of the feeding; then remove the bottle to burp or bubble him; resume feeding and burp your infant at the end of feed-

ing. Burp the infant more often if he swallows a large amount of air or has been crying vigorously.
8. Burp the infant by holding him on your shoulder or placing him on your lap in a sitting position with support. Stroke or pat his back.
9. Stop feeding when the infant no longer sucks. Refrain from overfeeding because this causes regurgitation and possible abdominal cramping.
10. Gently wipe the infant's mouth, and place him in bed on his side.

How to hold the infant

You won't hurt the infant by holding him firmly. His bones are flexible. They won't break when he is carried. But remember, his neck muscles are weak and his head must be supported with a hand or an arm. Here are some ways to hold him.

Vertical hold
First, place a towel on your shoulder to protect your clothing. Remove any sharp objects from shirt pockets before holding the infant. Then, support the infant against your shoulder, placing one hand under his buttocks and supporting his head with your other hand. You may use this hold for walking or talking to your infant because he is positioned close enough to hear your voice.

Horizontal hold
Support the baby's head in the crook of the arm and place the other arm under the buttocks. This hold is excellent for rocking and comforting the baby.

Football carry
Lay the infant along your forearm, supporting the infant's head with your hand and his side with your hip. This frees your other hand, for example, to answer the telephone.
Note: if you had a cesarean section, you may use this hold to breast-feed your infant.

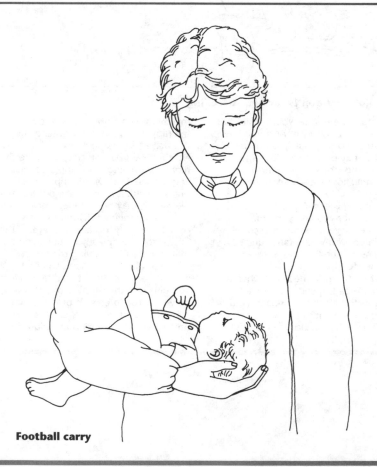

Football carry

Postpartum exercises

After giving birth, you should maintain a regular exercise program to regain your strength, promote healing, and restore your figure. Discuss an appropriate regimen with your doctor before you leave the hospital. Use the exercises shown in this aid as a guide. Begin with the first exercise, and add a new one every day or so, as you become stronger. Perform each exercise five times twice a day, or as directed by your nurse, nurse midwife, or doctor. *Note:* If you've had a cesarean section, you should not perform any of these exercises until you've received your doctor's or nurse-midwife's approval.

Tummy crunch
This exercise is used to tone the abdomen and strengthen abdominal muscles.

1. First, lie flat on your back with your knees slightly bent, as shown. Breathe in deeply so your chest rises. Then, slowly exhale and tightly pull in your abdominal muscles. Hold these muscles tight while counting to five; then relax.

2. While lying in the same position, raise your head. As you do, try to keep the rest of your body still. Bring your head as close as possible to your chest; then, slowly return to starting position.

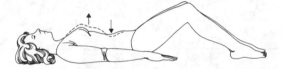
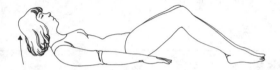

Abdominal stretch
This exercise is used to tone the abdomen and strengthen abdominal muscles.

3. Lie on your back with your legs apart and knees slightly bent. Stretch your arms straight out from your shoulders. Slowly raise them, until your hands meet directly above your chest. Without bending your elbows, lower your arms to the starting position.

4. Next, again lie flat with your legs straight. Raise your head and slightly bend one knee. Using your opposite hand, reach toward this knee, but don't touch it. Return to the starting position and repeat with your other leg and hand.

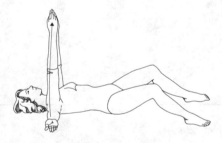
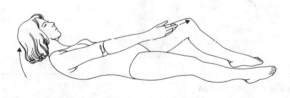

Bent-leg raises
This exercise is used to tone the abdomen.

5. Bend one knee. Bring your knee toward your chin and your heel toward your buttock. Return to starting position and repeat with your other leg.

6. Lie flat, with arms at your sides. Bend one knee toward your chin; then straighten your leg until it's perpendicular to the floor, as shown. Lower this leg and repeat with your other leg.

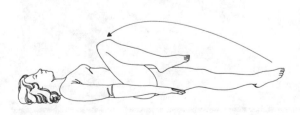
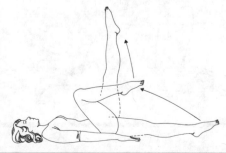

Sit-ups

This exercise is used to tone the abdomen and strengthen abdominal muscles.

7. Sit upright with your knees bent and feet flat on the floor. Clasp your hands behind your head and lean back at about a 45-degree angle to the floor, as shown. Hold this position for several seconds; then sit upright again.

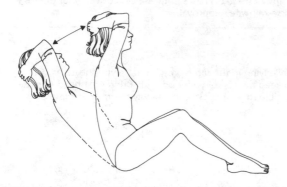

Leg raises

This exercise is used to tone the abdomen.

8. For this exercise, lie flat, as you did for exercise number 6. This time bend *both knees* toward your chin, and then straighten them, until your legs are perpendicular to the floor. Lower your legs.

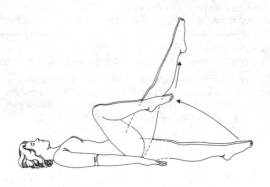

Pelvic tilt

This exercise is used to tone the abdomen and strengthen abdominal and pelvic muscles.

9. Lie with your knees bent and your feet flat on the floor, close to your buttocks. Keep your feet apart. Raise your buttocks slightly off the floor. As you raise your buttocks, tighten them and push your lower back down. Hold this position for several seconds; then return to the starting position.

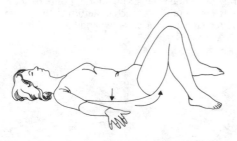

10. Repeat exercise number 9, but this time raise your head and tighten your abdominal muscles as you lift your buttocks.

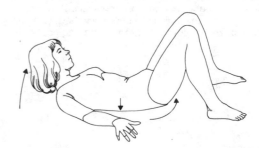

Modified pelvic tilt

This exercise is used to tone the abdomen and strengthen abdominal and pelvic muscles.

11. Rest on your elbows and knees, as shown here, with your arms and legs perpendicular to your body. Hump your back upward (see arrow), tighten your buttocks, and draw in your abdomen. Then relax and take a deep breath.

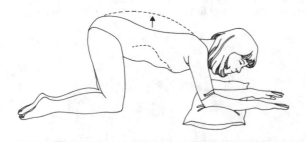

Appendix K: Overview of isolation precautions

Infectious disease precautions are essential in all health care settings. The Centers for Disease Control and Prevention (CDC) recently revised its isolation precaution recommendations for health care facilities, creating two tiers — standard precautions and transmission-based precautions.

Standard precautions

Standard precautions combine the former universal blood and body fluid precautions with body substance isolation. The rationale for standard precautions is that the blood, tissues, and body fluids of all patients must be considered potentially infectious. The specific substances covered by standard precautions include blood and all other body fluids, body secretions, and body excretions, except sweat, even if blood is not visible. Standard precautions should also be followed in the presence of nonintact skin and exposed mucous membranes.

Standard precautions are designed to decrease the risk of transmission of microorganisms from both recognized and unrecognized sources of infection. They should be followed at all times, with every patient. Appropriate protective barriers must be used — such as gloves, gowns, masks, and eye wear — whenever exposure to blood or body fluids is anticipated, such as during any procedure that involves blood or spraying, spattering, or generating droplets of blood or body fluids. Hand washing is absolutely essential to reducing the risk of infection transmission. Wash hands after removing gloves, between patient contacts, after touching contaminated patient care equipment, and after coming in contact with blood or body fluids (whether or not gloves were worn). Preventing injuries from needles, scalpels, and other sharp instruments is also a key step in avoiding infection by bloodborne pathogens. These items should be discarded immediately or as soon as feasible in an approved puncture-resistant container. Avoid recapping needles and bending, shearing, or breaking contaminated needles.

Transmission-based precautions

Transmission-based precautions go beyond standard precautions, aiming to interrupt infection transmission in health care facilities. Transmission-based precautions apply to patients with known or suspected communicable infections and to patients colonized with a resistant microbe. These precautions fall into three general categories: airborne precautions, droplet precautions, and contact precautions. Typically, infection control programs in health care facilities specify the use of one or more of these precaution categories in conjunction with standard precautions.

Airborne precautions

Airborne precautions apply to patients with known or suspected infections caused by airborne pathogens, such as tuberculosis, varicella, and rubeola. These are transmitted when a susceptible person inhales the small droplet nuclei that remain suspended in the air for long periods or when such a person inhales dust particles that contain the infectious microbe. Precautions include placement of the patient in a private room with negative air pressure, respiratory protection for health care workers, and the patient's use of a surgical mask during transport.

Droplet precautions

Droplet precautions are intended to reduce the transmission of infections spread by large-particle droplets. Droplet transmission occurs when such particles come into contact with the eyes or mucous membranes of a susceptible person's nose or mouth, such as when an infected person coughs, sneezes, or undergoes cough inducing procedures such as suctioning. Precautions include use of a private room or placement with a roommate infected with the same microbe. In addition to standard precautions, a surgical mask should be worn when coming within 3' (1 m) of a patient requiring droplet precautions.

Contact precautions

Contact is the most common transmission mode for nosocomial infections. Contact precautions reduce the risk of direct or indirect contact with microbes. These precautions include use of a private room, placement with a roommate infected with the same microbe, proper hand washing, use of gloves and clean, nonsterile gowns, and the cleaning and disinfecting of any shared patient care equipment.

Strict contact precautions are modified for resistant organisms such as vancomycin-resistant *Enterococcus* and methicillin-resistant *Staphylococcus aureus*. Besides the contact precautions already mentioned, strict precautions would include wearing a gown when coming in contact with the patient or his environment and avoidance of public areas by the patient.

Selected references

Barnes, L.P. "Patient Teaching. Critical Pathways: Linking Discharge Planning and Family Teaching," *MCN* 22(2):103, 1997.

Bickley, L., et al. *Bates' Guide to Physical Examination and History Taking,* 7th ed. Philadelphia: Lippincott-Raven Pubs., 1998.

Blackburn, S.T., and VandenBerg, K.A. "Assessment and Management of Neonatal Neurobehavioral Development," in *Comprehensive Neonatal Nursing Care: A Physiologic Perspective,* 2nd ed. Edited by Kenner, C., et al. Philadelphia: W.B. Saunders Co., 1998.

Brazelton, T.B. *Neonatal Behavioral Assessment Scales,* 3rd ed. Cambridge: Cambridge University Press, 1995.

Corbett, J.V. *Laboratory and Diagnostic Procedures with Nursing Diagnoses,* 4th ed. New York: Appleton & Lange, 1996.

"Critical Concepts in Fetal Monitoring" (5 videotapes). Washington, D.C.: Association of Women's Health, Obstetric, and Neonatal Nurses, 1996.

Grodner, M., et al. *Foundations and Clinical Applications of Nutrition: A Nursing Approach.* St. Louis: Mosby–Year Book, Inc., 1996.

Guyton, A.C., and Hall, J.E. *Human Physiology and Mechanisms of Disease,* 6th ed. Philadelphia: W.B. Saunders Co., 1997.

Hauth, J.C., and Merenstein, G.B. *Guidelines for Perinatal Care,* 4th ed. Elk Grove Village, Ill.: American Academy of Pediatrics and American College of Obstetricians and Gynecologists, 1997.

Kenner, C., et al. *Comprehensive Neonatal Care: A Physiologic Perspective,* 2nd ed. Philadelphia: W.B. Saunders Co., 1998.

Kim, M.J., et al. *Pocket Guide to Nursing Diagnoses,* 7th ed. St. Louis: Mosby–Year Book, Inc., 1997.

Loudermilk, D.L., et al. *Maternity and Women's Health Care,* 6th ed. St. Louis: Mosby–Year Book, Inc., 1997.

Malnight, M., and Wahl, J.R.F. "An Alternative Approach for Neonatal Clinical Pathways," *Neonatal Network* 16(4):41-49, 1997.

Merenstein, G.B., and Gardner, S.L. *Handbook of Neonatal Intensive Care,* 4th ed. St. Louis: Mosby–Year Book, Inc., 1998.

Nichols, F.H., and Zwelling, E. *Maternal-Newborn Nursing: Theory and Practice.* Philadelphia: W.B. Saunders Co., 1997.

Tappero, E.P., and Honeyfield, M.E. *Physical Assessment of the Newborn: A Comprehensive Approach to the Art of Physical Examination,* 2nd ed. Petaluma, Calif.: NICU Ink, 1996.

Veccji, C.J., et al. "Neonatal Individualized Predictive Pathway (NIPP): A Discharge Planning Tool for Parents," *Neonatal Network* 15(4):7-13, 1996.

White, R. *Recommended Standards for Newborn ICU Design.* South Bend, Ind.: Memorial Hospital, 1996.

Index

Boldface page numbers refer to major entries; i refers to an illustration; t refers to a table.

Boldface page numbers refer to major entries; i refers to an illustration; t refers to a table.

Index

Index

Boldface page numbers refer to major entries; i refers to an illustration; t refers to a table.

Boldface page numbers refer to major entries; i refers to an illustration; t refers to a table.